ANNUAL REVIEW
OF NURSING RESEARCH

Volume 23, 2005

Annual Review of Nursing Research

Volume 23, 2005

Alcohol Use, Misuse, Abuse, and Dependence

JOYCE J. FITZPATRICK, PhD, RN, FAAN
Series Editor

JOANNE SABOL STEVENSON, PhD, RN, FAAN
MARILYN SAWYER SOMMERS, PhD, RN, FAAN
Volume Editors

Become a subscriber to the ANNUAL REVIEW OF NURSING RESEARCH series and receive a 10% discount. See the last page of this volume for more information.

Springer Publishing Company, Inc.
11 West 42nd Street
New York, NY 10036

06 07 08 09 10 / 5 4 3 2 1

ISBN-0-8261-4135-8
ISSN-0739-6686

ANNUAL REVIEW OF NURSING RESEARCH is indexed in *Cumulative Index to Nursing and Allied Health Literature* and *Index Medicus*.

Typeset by International Graphic Services, Inc., Newtown, PA.

Printed in the United States of America by Maple-Vail Book Manufacturing Group.

Contents

Contributors   vii

Preface   ix
   Joyce J. Fitzpatrick

Part I: Perspectives on Alcohol Use Research and Measurement Issues

1. The Case for Alcohol Research as a Focus of Study   3
    by Nurse Researchers
    JOANNE SABOL STEVENSON AND MARILYN SAWYER SOMMERS

2. Measurement of Alcohol Consumption: Issues and Challenges   27
    MARILYN SAWYER SOMMERS

3. Moderate Drinking and Cardiovascular Disease   65
    JOAN A. MASTERS

**Part II: Research on Alcohol Use, Misuse, Abuse,
and Dependence through the Life Span**

4. Alcohol Consumption During Pregnancy   101
    CARA J. KRULEWITCH

5. Alcohol, Children, and Adolescents   135
    CAROL J. LOVELAND-CHERRY

6. College Students' Alcohol Use: A Critical Review   179
    CAROL J. BOYD, SEAN ESTEBAN MCCABE, AND MICHELE MORALES

7. Alcohol Misuse, Abuse, and Addiction in Young and   213
    Middle Adulthood
    SANDRA M. HANDLEY AND PEGGY WARD-SMITH

8.   Alcohol Use, Misuse, Abuse, and Dependence in Later Adulthood   245
     JOANNE SABOL STEVENSON

Part III: Alcohol Challenges in
Selected Populations and Situations

9.   Alcohol Use and Alcohol-Related Problems Among Lesbians   283
       and Gay Men
     TONDA L. HUGHES

10. Alcohol and Risky Behaviors   327
     COLLEEN M. CORTE AND MARILYN SAWYER SOMMERS

Part IV: Alcohol Intervention Research

11. Alcohol Brief Interventions   363
     DEBORAH FINFGELD-CONNETT

Index   389

Contents of Previous Volumes   405

Contributors

Carol J. Boyd, PhD, RN, FAAN
Director, Substance Abuse Research
  Center
Professor, Nursing and Women's
  Studies
School of Nursing
University of Michigan
Ann Arbor, MI

Colleen M. Corte, PhD, RN
Assistant Professor, Department of
  Public Health, Mental Health, and
  Administrative Nursing
College of Nursing
University of Illinois at Chicago
Chicago, IL

**Deborah Finfgeld-Connett, PhD,
  APRN, BC**
Associate Professor
Coordinator, Mental Health Nurse
  Practitioner Program
Sinclair School of Nursing
University of Missouri at Columbia
Columbia, MO

**Sandra M. Handley, PhD, RN,
  CARN, CS-FNP**
Administrator, Nurse Practitioner
Student Health and Wellness
University of Missouri at Kansas City
Kansas City, MO

**Tonda L. Hughes, PhD, RN,
  FAAN**
Research Director, Center of
  Excellence in Women's Health
Associate Professor, Public Health,
  Mental Health, and
  Administrative Nursing
College of Nursing
University of Illinois at Chicago
Chicago, IL

**Cara J. Krulewitch, PhD, RN,
  CNM**
Assistant Professor, Department of
  Family and Community Health
School of Nursing
University of Maryland
Baltimore, MD

**Carol J. Loveland-Cherry, PhD,
  RN, FAAN**
Professor and Executive Associate
  Dean for Academic Affairs
School of Nursing
University of Michigan
Ann Arbor, MI

Joan A. Masters, PhD, APRN, BC
Assistant Professor
School of Nursing
Duquesne University
Pittsburgh, PA

Sean Esteban McCabe, PhD, MSW, MA
Assistant Research Scientist
Substance Abuse Research Center
Ann Arbor, MI

Michele Morales, PhC, MSW
Research Assistant
Substance Abuse Research Center
Ann Arbor, MI

Marilyn Sawyer Sommers, PhD, RN, FAAN
Professor and Associate Dean for
    Research
College of Nursing
University of Cincinnati
Cincinnati, OH

Joanne Sabol Stevenson, PhD, RN, FAAN
Professor, Graduate Program
Mount Carmel College of Nursing
Columbus, OH

Peggy Ward-Smith, PhD, RN
Assistant Professor
School of Nursing
University of Missouri at Kansas City
Kansas City, MO

Preface

This 23rd volume in the *Annual Review of Nursing Research (ARNR)* series is focused on alcohol use, misuse, abuse, and dependence. This topic is timely and important as there is much that is known and much that requires further research. Drs. Joanne Stevenson and Marilyn Sommers, well known scholars in this area, have served as the volume editors. They selected the content areas for the chapters and edited these into a comprehensive volume. Throughout the chapters distinctions are made among positive aspects of alcohol use, misuse (e.g., during pregnancy), abuse (e.g., binge drinking among college-age students), and dependence.

In the first chapter, Drs. Stevenson and Sommers make the case for alcohol research as a focus of study by nurse researchers. In chapter 2, Marilyn Sommers discusses the issues and challenges in the measurement of alcohol consumption for purposes of research. Joan Masters tracks the research on moderate drinking and cardiovascular disease in chapter 3. Chapters 4 through 8 follow a developmental progression from alcohol-related research in pregnancy through old age. Cara Krulewitch delineates research on alcohol consumption during pregnancy in chapter 4; Carol Loveland-Cherry discusses alcohol, children and adolescents in chapter 5; Carol Boyd, Sean Esteban McCabe, and Michele Morales provide a critical review of college students' alcohol use in chapter 6; Sandra Handley and Peggy Ward-Smith review research on alcohol misuse, abuse and addiction in young and middle adulthood in chapter 7; and Joanne Sabol Stevenson discusses alcohol use, misuse, abuse and dependence in later adulthood in chapter 8. In chapter 9, Tonya Hughes describes alcohol use and alcohol-related problems among lesbians and gay men. Colleen Corte and Marilyn Sommers review research on alcohol and risky behaviors in chapter 10. The final chapter, chapter 11, includes a delineation of alcohol intervention research.

As with previous ARNR volumes, it is important to acknowledge the contributions of the nurse scholars who wrote chapters for this volume. In addition, we would like to acknowledge the ARNR Advisory Board members who have supported this effort over the past several years. And, most importantly, recognition is due to the volume editors for their special efforts in bringing this important area of research to the attention of nurses and other health professionals.

Joyce J. Fitzpatrick, PhD, RN, FAAN
Series Editor

PART I

Perspectives on Alcohol Use Research and Measurement Issues

Chapter 1

The Case for Alcohol Research as a Focus of Study by Nurse Researchers

Joanne Sabol Stevenson and Marilyn Sawyer Sommers

ABSTRACT

Sixty percent of the U.S. population drinks alcohol. Although numerous investigators have shown that low-volume alcohol intake has positive influences on cardiovascular health, bone density, and cognition, there is a fine line between positive, neutral, and negative ramifications of alcohol consumption on health. Alcohol accounts for 7% of the global burden of disease and injury from all causes and for 10% to 11% of all illnesses and death each year worldwide. So alcohol use is a two-edged sword.

Psychiatric nurses have a long history of involvement with alcoholic patients, and alcohol users, misusers, and abusers comprise a significant percentage of the patient load in every specialty and subspecialty of nursing. Yet nursing education has neglected this important area of content in general nursing curricula, staff development has not trained mainstream nurses to routinely assess for alcohol problems among hospital patients, and primary care providers have failed to do case finding.

During the past 25 years, the federal government has funded curricular and faculty development programs to bring alcohol information into the core of health provider training. The process has been halting and minimally successful at best. One ramification of the inattention to alcohol-related education is the dearth of nurse-scientists engaged in programs of research in the field of alcohol abuse. A federally funded faculty development program in the 1990s focused attention on this issue, and a small cadre of nurses were trained to do related research. Several of the authors in this volume are members of that group.

A brief overview of the focus of each of the remaining chapters in this volume is presented. A rationale is provided for the importance of this area of research for nursing knowledge and quality patient care in essentially all areas of nursing practice. Finally, several burning research questions are posed that would most appropriately be answered through nursing research.

Keywords: nursing history, alcohol education, project MAINSTREAM, nursing faculty development, nursing curricula, alcohol-related research

Approximately 60% of Americans consume alcohol (ethanol). In the primary care population, 38% are low-risk drinkers (see chapter 2, Table 2.1 for definitions of alcohol consumption and the following patterns of drinking), 9% are at-risk drinkers, 8% are problem drinkers, and 5% are dependent drinkers (Manwell, Fleming, Johnson, & Barry, 1998). Alcohol misuse and abuse are significantly related to over 100,000 preventable deaths in the United States each year (Dawson, 2000, 2001). Alcohol misuse is a global as well as a national health care problem. The World Health Organization (WHO) estimated that substance abuse (alcohol and other drugs of abuse) accounts for 7% of the entire global burden of disease and injury from all causes, measured by an indicator that combines both morbidity and premature mortality. In more developed countries, alcohol accounted for a much higher proportion of disease and injury burden than in the poorer developing countries; in developed countries, WHO estimated that alcohol accounts for 10% to 11% of illness and death each year (WHO, 2000). The Global Status Report on Alcohol (WHO, 1999) noted that morbidity from alcohol has a greater impact on health worldwide than malnutrition or poor sanitation. Hence, alcohol plays a critical role in the health and illness of the world's population

Alcohol misuse and abuse are associated with several high-profile health problems—heart dysrhythmias and failure, numerous cancers, hypertension, type II diabetes, violence, fires and falls, motor vehicle crashes, depression, and suicide. Persistent alcohol abuse is linked to diseases of the gastrointestinal tract, central nervous system, cognition and memory, and peripheral vascular system, as well as liver and kidney failure. Alcohol abuse costs the U.S. economy about $185 billion annually (National Institute on Alcohol Abuse and Alcoholism [NIAAA], 2000), primarily due to lost productivity from alcoholic illness, injury, and crime (Harwood, 2000). This figure does not include future monies lost due to premature deaths from alcoholism. These data strongly support the position that alcohol abuse is an important health and social issue in the United States.

Notwithstanding the myriad facts and figures indicating their importance in health care and every specialty of nursing, alcohol-related problems generally have been invisible to all but psychiatric nurses, and even they have been concerned primarily with inpatient and outpatient treatment of alcohol dependents. Assessment for alcohol abuse has merited little or no attention in most nursing textbooks and clinical courses. Although it is an issue for all body systems, all age groups, and all sites of care, it has been given short shrift in nursing curricula and usually relegated to a minimal number of clock hours of lecture in the psychiatric nursing course.

The unfortunate ramification of neglecting to teach nursing students the important role that alcohol plays in health and illness and failing to teach and reinforce the necessity of alcohol-related assessments of all patients beginning with school-age children is a glaring absence of alcohol use and abuse assessment across all health systems and all patient populations by nurses in professional and advanced practice.

Acute hospital patients in particular are overrepresented among subpopulations that misuse or abuse alcohol. In-hospital prevalence figures range from 25% to 30% for men and 8% to 10% for women (Hearne, Connolly, & Sheehan, 2002; Schneekloth et al., 2001; Watson, 2000). Unfortunately, less than 50% of in-patients are assessed for alcohol use (Kouimtsidis et al., 2003). The prevalence figures are slightly less in primary care, but they still are about 20% for men and 8% for women (Fiellin, Reid, & O'Connor, 2000; Fleming, Manwell, Barry, & Johnson, 1998; Reid, Fiellin, & O'Connor, 1999; Roeloffs, Fink, Unutzer, Tang, & Wells, 2001). These findings have not changed for either the prevalence or the rate of assessment by health personnel over the past 20+ years (Schneekloth et al., 2001). The finding that assessment efforts by nurses and physicians have not improved over the past two decades is alarming.

In addition, there are few nurse-scientists with programs of research in the field of alcohol-related knowledge development. Although alcohol abuse is a leading cause of morbidity and mortality and heavily implicated in damage to all organs of the body that lead to hospitalizations, long-term disabilities, and death (McGinnis & Foege, 1993; McIinnis & Powell, 1994), it is virtually invisible within mainstream nursing care and nursing science. Even the National Institute of Nursing Research does not fund alcohol-related studies and has been exceedingly slow to partner with the NIAAA for joint calls for proposals.

One goal for this 23rd volume of the *Annual Review of Nursing Research* is to bring alcohol-related research out of the closet and clarify its relevance for mainstream nursing care and research. Alcohol misuse is not just a psychiatric problem; it is a mainstream, main street and suburb, total population problem that has major significance in primary care, trauma and emergency care, acute medical and surgical care, obstetrics, pediatrics, and geriatrics, as well as community health, home care and long-term care. No nursing care provider is untouched by it.

HEALTH EFFECTS OF ALCOHOL USE, MISUSE, ABUSE, AND DEPENDENCE

The influence of alcohol use permeates all of the nursing practice specialties and serves as a confounder, albeit usually ignored, in many nursing studies, whether descriptive or experimental in design and covering all age groups. It is important to emphasize the distinction between alcohol consumption and alcohol dependence because their influence on nursing specialties differs greatly, although there is some overlap. Psychiatric nurses and addiction nurses deal, in the main, with the psychological and social problems and cognitive decrements associated with alcohol dependence. Home care and long-term care nurses provide service during the terminal illnesses of chronic alcohol dependents. The disease conditions that are wholly attributable to alcohol use include alcoholic dementia, psychoses, polyneuropathy, cardiomyopathy, gastritis, fatty liver, hepatitis, liver cirrhosis, fetal alcohol syndrome (FAS), fetal alcohol effect (FAE), and ethanol or methanol poisoning (Rehm, Room, Graham, et al., 2003). These few, relatively small subpopulations of alcohol-affected patients, unfortunately, have been viewed as the main population of alcohol users who come in contact with nurses. The facts, however, present quite a different story.

About 44% of adults 18 years and older in the United States are current drinkers, another 22% are former drinkers, and only 34% are lifetime abstainers (Dawson, Grant, Chou, & Pickering, 1995). Former drinkers include those who stopped drinking for non-health-related causes, addicts or abusers who stopped to ameliorate their alcohol problems, and those who are commonly referred to as "sick quitters," meaning they stopped due to a medical illness (including taking prescription drugs that are incompatible with alcohol). Alcohol consumption per se is associated with both positive and negative biomedical consequences, quite separate from the myriad problems of alcohol addiction (Whitfield et al., 2004).

The quantity, frequency, and patterns of alcohol consumption are very important factors in health protection, morbidity, and mortality worldwide. On the matter of health protection, 20 to 72 g of alcohol per day (13.6 g = 1 standard drink [NIAAA, 2004]) was found to be protective for coronary artery disease and ischemic stroke in meta-analyses (Correo, Bagnardi, Zambon, & La Vecchia, 2004; Rehm, Room, Monteiro, et al., 2003). For self-perception of health, 100 to 199 g per week odds ratio (OR) 0.58, 95% confidence interval (CI) 0.38–0.89) was deemed optimal alcohol intake for nonsmokers compared with abstainer-nonsmokers (Poikolainen, Vartiainen, & Korhonen, 1996). However, the net effect of alcohol use in coronary artery disease is still negative; the global death rate from cardiovascular disease (CVD) is 600,000, and the prevented deaths is 332,000, so the net excess deaths from alcohol use is 268,000 (Rehm, Room, Monteiro, et al., 2003). Overall, alcohol consumption accounts for 3.2% of global deaths among the eight WHO regions and 4.0% of the global disability-adjusted life years lost to premature disability (Rehm, Room, Monteiro, et al., 2003). The conditions and diseases wherein alcohol is a major contributor (higher level of intake than 80 g per day), according to several meta-analyses, include lip and oropharyngeal cancer, esophageal cancer, laryngeal cancer, liver cancer, female breast cancer, epilepsy, hypertension, coronary (ischemic) heart disease, cardiac arrhythmias, hemorrhagic stroke, esophageal varices, gastro-esophageal hemorrhage, liver cirrhosis (all causes), acute and chronic pancreatitis, spontaneous abortion, low birth weight, and psoriasis (Rehm, Room, Graham, et al., 2003). Many of these diseases in their prodromal stages fall within the practice realm of primary and acute care nurses on a daily basis; yet queries about quantity/frequency of alcohol use, misuse, and abuse rarely are part of the routine intake information gathered by either nurses or physicians (Schneekloth et al., 2001). Furthermore, patient education about the negative effects of alcohol misuse and abuse do not come close to paralleling the prevalence of routine patient teaching about the negative effects of tobacco products. Those integrative literature reviews conducted for the remaining chapters of this volume that encompass the kinds of health problems noted above uncovered a dearth of studies or contributions to the science by nurse-investigators. This area of knowledge development to inform evidence-based nursing practice is ripe for new programs of research involving myriad nurse scientists and their graduate students.

There is general agreement among investigators about the high level of alcohol involvement in all types of unintentional injuries (Li, Kevl, Smith, & Baker, 1997; Waller, Hill, Maio, & Blow, 2003). A meta-analysis by Smith, Branda, and Miller (1999) estimated that alcohol was involved in 38.5% of all non-traffic-related injury deaths (fires/burns, hypothermia, drownings, falls, gunshot wounds, and poisonings) and 39.7 % of all traffic fatalities (including pedestrians) in the United States in 1999. Smith et al.'s findings also showed that alcohol was involved in 30% to 57% of violent deaths, and Greenfield (1998) found that 37% of violent crimes were committed under the influence of alcohol (homicide, sexual assault, robbery, and assault).

Unfortunately, the relationship between alcohol and interpersonal violence or violent crimes is difficult to capture, although a meta-analysis of 129 studies showed associations between alcohol and violence (Lipsey, Wilson, Cohen, & Derzon, 1997). However, intimate partner violence reportedly involves alcohol more often than other crimes (Leonard & Roberts, 1999), and women are most vulnerable to partner attack when they (alone or in addition to the partner) are under the influence of alcohol (Chase, O'Farrell, Fals-Stewart, & Murphy, 2003; Chermack, Walton, Fuller, & Blow, 2001; Greenfield, 1998; Kaufman-Kantor & Asdigian, 1997; Testa & Parks, 1996). These data indicate that trauma nurses have routine encounters with alcohol-related injuries and patients who should be carefully assessed for alcohol misuse or abuse. Also when conditions permit, brief interventions would be appropriate nursing actions. Research reported by one team of nurse-researchers has demonstrated that hospitalization for an alcohol-related injury alone, coupled with screening for alcohol use, can be a powerful intervention to decrease drinking in the year following injury (Sommers, Dyehouse, & Howe, 2001). Many more nurse-investigators need to become involved to answer numerous other questions about alcohol, unintentional injuries, and effective health-promoting nursing actions.

Pregnancy, labor and delivery, and postpartum nursing are all areas where nurses routinely encounter women who use or abuse alcohol (and other substances). Thankfully, maternal-child nurses are probably the most sensitive and up-to-date about the issues, because alcohol intake during pregnancy is correlated with fetal alcohol effects (see chapter 4 in this volume for a review of this area of research). Because any amount of alcohol consumption at any time during pregnancy or breast-feeding is risky, the message to be given to patients is clear and unambiguous. In addition, voluntary organizations and governmental bureaus have produced brochures, posters, and other media about these risks. That makes it easier for nurses, physicians, and other health care providers to all be on the same page and present a united front to pregnant women. Nevertheless, the area merits more research by nurses, most notably to develop and test effective protocols for teaching prevention to future and current parents, change substance use behaviors among recalcitrant pregnant women, and construct evidence-based best practices to care for children with FAS or FAE.

The role of pediatric nurses in prevention and intervention in alcohol-related health problems is complex. It includes teaching and helping children with FAS and FAE to avoid personal use of alcohol as they grow up. A more common condition involving alcohol and children is child abuse and injury, which was estimated to be directly attributable to adult alcohol use in 16% of cases (English, Holman, Milne, Hulse, & Winter, 1995; Ridolfo & Stevenson, 2001). Nurses in this case have a responsibility to report to proper authorities suspicions about the abuse, but they are not otherwise involved in resolving the situation because it is a legal matter. The much more common situation for pediatric nurses is the realization that parents of their young patients are misusing or abusing alcohol and that it is having a negative effect on the health of the children. Examples include parental noncompliance in the management of asthma, type I diabetes, and cystic fibrosis. Descriptive studies of incidence and prevalence, theory development, and interventions development and testing in this area are virtually nonexistent. It is an open book waiting for discovery by pediatric nurse-investigators.

In summary, opportunities for nursing programs of research abound in alcohol use, misuse, and abuse-related investigations, as well as the more traditional area of alcohol dependence. It is hoped that some nurses-scientists and graduate students will be stimulated by one or another of the review chapters in this volume and will initiate a program of research on alcohol or other substance abuse.

HISTORICAL OVERVIEW OF NURSING RESEARCH AND EDUCATION IN SUBSTANCE ABUSE

Early Research by Nurse-Scientists

Some nurses have been interested in alcohol-related research since at least the mid-1970s. One small but important group of nurse-researchers began their careers at the University of Illinois–Chicago. Elizabeth Burns and colleagues conducted important research on the effects of various amounts of alcohol consumed by pregnant rats on the developing brains of their progeny over the full course of pregnancy and beyond. Burns et al. refuted previously held assumptions that dangers from heavy alcohol use were limited to the first trimester of pregnancy and that low or moderate levels of alcohol had no deleterious effects on fetal brain development, especially during later pregnancy (Burns, Kruckeberg, Kanak, & Stibler, 1986; Burns, Kruckeberg, Stibler, Cerven, & Borg, 1984; Kruckeberg et al., 1984; Stibler, Burns, Kruckeberg, Cerven, & Borg, 1985; Stibler et al., 1983). This group of studies influenced the later recommendations to pregnant women about the dangers of alcohol intake at any time during pregnancy.

One of Burns's doctoral students, Karleen Kerfoot, showed that social drinking during lactation also is problematic. The concentration of alcohol in human milk was measurable 30 minutes after ingesting one standard drink and continued to be measurable for several more hours (Kerfoot, Kruckeberg, & Burns, 1985). Burns wrote a review of the then existing body of research on effects of alcohol and other stressors during the brain growth spurt that was published in volume 8 of the *Annual Review of Nursing Research (ARNR)* (Burns, 1990).

Another of Burns's doctoral students, Mary Haack, became interested in the drinking behavior of nurses and nursing students. Haack conducted three studies that informed the nursing service and education communities about alcohol use and abuse among nurses. She found that nursing students drank more than other professional college students (Haack & Harford, 1984), that family history of drinking was associated with heavier drinking among nursing students (Haack, Harford, & Parker, 1988), and that stress-related drinking among nursing students appeared to be increasing (Haack, 1988).

Sullivan studied nurses who were recovering from alcohol and other chemical dependence (1987a) and compared their personal, family, and professional lives (1987b) with nurses who were not dependent. She and her colleagues also described nurses' sexual problems (Sullivan, 1988) and the disciplinary actions applied by the state boards (Sullivan, Bissell, & Leffler, 1990). At about the same time, Gerace (1988) reported on the alcohol use of 160 nurse educators in the Midwest and compared the findings with national data on American women. She found that nurse-educators drank more often but in lower quantities. After about 1990, this trend toward focusing alcohol and drug abuse research on nursing students and nurses abated. Sullivan and Handley reviewed this corpus of studies on alcohol use and abuse by nurses, including a number of qualitative studies, in volume 10 of the ARNR (1992).

The next year, Sullivan and Handley published a comprehensive review of the alcohol and drug abuse research on various client groups that had been conducted by nurses and was cited in the CINAHL database (1993). This review, of course, left out any studies by nurses that were published in journals not included in Cumulative Index to Nursing and Allied Health Literature (CINAHL). Interestingly, there were five publications attributed to one investigator, three to another, and five nurse investigators had two citations each; hence it would appear that a small cadre of nurses were interested enough in the field to publish more than once. This review chapter appeared in volume 11 of the ARNR (Sullivan & Handley, 1993). Included in the 1993 chapter were several studies about the attitudes of nurses and nursing students toward alcohol and drug-abusing and -dependent patients, as well as, outcomes of educational interventions to counteract the generally negative attitudes.

The next era of nurse involvement in the field of alcohol abuse research occurred during the late 1980s, and its primary focus was on educating nursing faculty about alcohol problems and treatment so they could teach nursing students and graduate nurses about the myriad health-related challenges that evolve from alcohol misuse and abuse. The secondary focus was research training for the purpose of developing programs of research in alcohol and other substance abuse.

Nursing, Substance Abuse, and the National Institutes of Health

Although the care of persons with substance abuse disorders has long been within the domain of nursing, federal agencies responsible for funding research and other programs in substance abuse were not knowledgeable about nursing education or nursing science. Beginning in the 1970s, the American Nurses Association Cabinet (originally called the Commission) on Nursing Research actively lobbied the U.S. Congress to create an Institute of Nursing Research within the National Institutes of Health (NIH). In light of this goal, cabinet members met at least annually with the director of the NIH and selected institute directors. These meetings had the dual purpose of explaining and promoting nursing research as a legitimate scientific discipline with legitimate claims to institute status and promoting immediate funding opportunities for individual nurse-scientists within relevant institutes.

It was within this context that, in 1985, newly elected research cabinet member Eleanor Sullivan met for the first time with Enoch Gordis, director of the National Institute on Alcohol Abuse and Alcoholism. Sullivan explained the reason for her visit and bluntly asked, "Are you funding any research by nurses?" Gordis responded in the negative and noted, "We have never really thought about that" (personal communication, Eleanor Sullivan, 2004). Dr. Sullivan then went on to explain the essence of nursing science and what it could contribute to the developing science of substance abuse.

In 1986, during Sullivan's second visit with Gordis, he indicated that the NIAAA and the National Institute on Drug Abuse (NIDA) were about to issue a call for contract applications to develop curricula to educate health professionals and that, for the first time, nursing programs would be eligible to submit proposals (personal communication, Eleanor Sullivan, 2004). Three nurse educators won contracts in this competition: Elizabeth Burns (Ohio State University), Olga Church (University of Connecticut–Storrs), and Madeline Naegle (New York University). The curricula from the three universities were disseminated widely and have been available to guide the education of nursing students and nurses for several years (Burns, Ciccone, & Thompson, 1991; Church, Fisk, & Neafsey, 1990; Naegle, 1989, 1991, 1992, 1993). The curriculum developed by the Ohio State University team for undergraduate students, graduate students, and continuing education learners was published as a book by Springer Publishing Company (Burns, Thompson, & Ciccone, 1994).

In 1990, Sullivan, then dean of the School of Nursing, University of Kansas, was appointed by Gordis to serve on the NIAAA National Advisory Council on Alcohol Abuse and Alcoholism. This council advised the secretary of health and human services, the director of NIH, and the director of the NIAAA on program and policy initiatives in the field of alcohol abuse and alcoholism research. It also prioritized research applications for funding. This appointment was a watershed event for nursing within the NIH in that a nurse was appointed to a nonnursing institute advisory council.

EFFECTS OF THE FACULTY DEVELOPMENT PROGRAM ON SUBSTANCE ABUSE IN NURSING

In 1989, the NIAAA, NIDA, and Office of Substance Abuse Prevention (OSAP) announced the Faculty Development Program (FDP) to prepare health professional faculty for education and research in the area of alcohol and substance abuse. The request for applications was open to medicine, nursing, pharmacy, and social work. The program objectives targeted development of faculty fellows in substance abuse prevention, screening, education, research, case management, rehabilitation, and referral.

FDP Funding and Purposes

Over several funding cycles, 11 university nursing programs were supported (see Table 1.1). Nurse leaders in substance abuse also were appointed to the Special Review Committee assembled by the NIAAA to review the applications. These nurses were E. Gerald Bennett (Medical College of Georgia), Laina Gerace (University of Illinois), Edith Heinemann (University of Washington), Stella Shiber (Johns Hopkins), and Eleanor Sullivan (University of Kansas).

The specific objectives of the funded projects were to (1) expand the level of faculty knowledge and clinical expertise in alcohol and other drug abuse; (2) expand and strengthen curricular offerings on substance abuse at graduate and undergraduate levels; (3) enlarge and strengthen community networks of interdisciplinary professionals, including nurses, to serve as resources in addressing community service and training needs in the area of substance abuse; and (4) evaluate programmatic effects on faculty, curricula, and students. The FDP projects fostered change at the individual level (faculty fellows and students) and at the school or college level (curriculum) (Gerace, Sullivan, Murphy, & Cotter, 1992). Each funded project was required to make permanent changes in the curricular plan and required courses of the academic unit's nursing programs.

Each grant provided salary support, travel funds, and educational resources for the three to five faculty fellows. In addition, funds were made available to promote collaboration across programs. For example, Burns at Ohio State hosted a meeting of nursing and interdisciplinary fellows from the University of Michigan, Case Western Reserve, University of Kentucky, and University of Cincinnati to develop networks and collaborative projects. In addition, fellows presented papers and networked each year at the Association of Medical Education and Research in Substance Abuse (AMERSA). The NIAAA, NIDA, and OSAP administrators were particularly interested in encouraging and facilitating programs of research among faculty who were new to research or new to the field of substance abuse research.

FDP's Contributions to Knowledge Development

The FDP made several important contributions to advancing nursing science and training nurse scientists. Substance abuse had long been the purview of psychiatric nursing, but through the FDP, nurses with expertise in acute care,

TABLE 1.1 Nursing Participation in the NIAAA/NIDA/OSAP Faculty Fellow
Program

Date of Award	College/ university	Program director	Faculty fellows	ATOD federal funding by faculty fellows, 1990–1996
1989	University of Illinois– Chicago	Laina Gerace	Tonda Hughes, Fran Cotter, Susan Dudas, Marie Talashek*	Hughes: F32DA005466 (1992–1994) Patterns of drug use and abuse among women
1989	University of Washington	Shirley Murphy	Susan Flagler, Sharon Fought, Rebecca Kang, Marcia Killien	Murphy: T32DA007257-01 (1991–1996) Nursing research training: Substance abuse
1989	University of Kansas	Eleanor Sullivan	Julia Hagemaster, Sandra Handley, Ardyce Plummer, Sarah Stanley	None located on CRISP
1990	Herbert H. Lehman College	Kem Louie	Barbara Backer, Sarah Beaton, Alicia Georges (partial listing)	None located on CRISP
1990	New York University	Madeline Naegle	No data available	No data available
1990	Ohio State University	Elizabeth Burns	Joanne Stevenson, Mary Ellen Wewers, Jeanne Clemment	Stevenson: R15AA010031 (1994–1997) Alcohol abuse in older women in acute care hospitals Wewers: M01RR000034 (1990–1997) Nicotine, neuroregulators, and dysphoric states among smokers Wewers: R29NR003213 (1992–1997) Cigarette smoking, opioid peptides, and mood states

(continued)

TABLE 1.1   *(continued)*

Date of Award	College/ university	Program director	Faculty fellows	ATOD federal funding by faculty fellows, 1990–1996
1990	University of Cincinnati	Janice Dyehouse	Joan Tiessen, Dianne Felblinger, Carole Kenner, Nancy Savage, Marilyn Sommers*	Dyehouse: R01AA010355 (1995–1999) Brief strategies—alcohol-related nontraffic injuries Kenner: U84/ CCU508718 (1994–1998) Perinatal alcohol users: Identification and intervention Sommers: R49/ CCR510153 (1994–1997) Preventing alcohol-related vehicular injury—brief strategy
1990	University of Connecticut	Olga Church	No data available	No data available
1990	University of South Florida	Ona Riggin	Barbara Redding, Cynthia Selleck (partial listing)	None located on CRISP
1990	University of Texas Health Sciences Center–Houston	Marianne Marcus	Dorothy Otto (partial listing)	None located on CRISP
1992	Case Western University	Karen Budd	SusanAuvil-Novak, Rhonda Draper, Mollena Martinez, Diana Morris, Caroline Pritchard	None located on CRISP

*Co-project directors
Note. ATOD = alcohol, tobacco, and other drugs; CRISP = Computer Retrieval of Information on Scientific Projects (http://crisp.cit.nih.gov/crisp/crisp_query.generate_screen); NIAAA = National Institute on Alcohol Abuse and Alcoholism; NIDA = National Institute on Drug Abuse; OSAP = Office of Substance Abuse Prevention

community health, parent–child health, child and adolescent health, and adult and older adult health explored problems of substance abuse in their target populations, and several received federal funding for their research (see Table 1.1). For example, Carole Kenner (parent–child nursing expert, University of Cincinnati) received funding from the Centers for Disease Control and Prevention (CDC) to test an intervention to reduce fetal alcohol syndrome, Joanne Stevenson (older-adult health nursing expert, Ohio State University) received funding from the NIAAA to study alcohol abuse in older women, and Marilyn Sommers (trauma nursing expert, University of Cincinnati) received funding from the CDC's National Injury Center to study the effectiveness of brief interventions following alcohol-related vehicular crashes. In addition to the federal grants shown in Table 1.1, several fellows received research or demonstration program funding from state grant mechanisms, foundations, and other nongovernmental sources.

Alcohol and Substance Abuse Content in Nursing Curricula

Prior to FDP funding, several studies by nurses explored substance abuse education and nurse competencies in substance abuse screening and treatment. Bartek, Lindeman, Newton, Fitzgerald, and Hawks (1988) found that the majority of medical surgical nurses in their sample ($N = 83$) had limited classroom and clinical experience with alcoholism. Sullivan and Hale (1987) studied registered nurses' ($N = 1026$) beliefs about alcoholism and found that those who had received their nursing education in hospital diploma programs and those with master's degrees had more positive attitudes about alcoholism than either baccalaureate-prepared nurses or nurses with doctoral degrees. Hoffman and Heinemann (1987) implemented a national survey with schools of nursing as the unit of analysis ($N = 336$) to determine the current curricular offerings in substance abuse. They found that the majority of nursing schools in their sample (72%) required only 1 to 5 clock hours of instruction on alcohol and drug abuse content during their entire undergraduate curricula. These data supported the need for the FDP in nursing education (Heinemann & Hoffman, 1989; Murphy, 1989) and served as a justification for the substance abuse teacher-training focus of the faculty fellows.

A variety of curricular products emerged from the FDP grants to fill the gap in nursing programs. Murphy (1991) proposed an empirically based substance abuse course for graduate students in nursing with a theoretical model using Prochaska and DiClemente's (1984) stages of change. Three project directors (Gerace, Sullivan, and Murphy), along with Fran Cotter, the chief of the Health Professions Educational Program at the NIAAA, laid out a definitive road map for both future faculty development and curricular change in substance abuse (Gerace et al., 1992). The University of Kansas faculty, in conjunction with the American Nurses Foundation and the Speas Memorial Trust, developed an alcohol and other drug abuse (AODA) curriculum for practicing nurses that they delivered through 2-day workshops (Hagemaster, Handley, Plumlee, Sullivan, & Stanley, 1993).

Outcome studies followed. Gerace and her colleagues at the University of Illinois–Chicago implemented a clinical evaluation program to improve the recognition of and responses to substance-misusing patients by advanced practice nurses and graduate students (Gerace, Hughes, & Spunt, 1995; Talashek, Gerace, Miller, & Lindsey, 1995). Marcus, Rickman, and Sobhan (1999) developed a collaborative effort between university faculty and acute care nurses and found that these nurses acquired essential knowledge and skills about substance abuse over an 18-month training period.

Unfortunately, no longitudinal studies were conducted to evaluate the long-term outcomes of the FDP projects. A final report of the funding program was assembled by the COSMOS Corporation of Bethesda, MD, but it merely assembled the results from each funding site rather than an integrated evaluation of overall outcomes, and the report is no longer in print. Fortunately, three nursing program directors reported on the progress made toward improving nursing competencies in substance abuse and offered recommendations for reality-based learning strategies to enhance student competencies (Marcus, Gerace, & Sullivan, 1996).

Project MAINSTREAM

In 2000, after a hiatus of several years without federal funding for substance abuse education, the Health Resources and Services Administration (HRSA) and the Center for Substance Abuse Treatment (CSAT) of the Substance Abuse and Mental Health Services Administration (SAMHSA) funded a 5-year cooperative agreement to improve health professional education in substance abuse. The Association for Medical Education & Research in Substance Abuse (AMERSA) was chosen to implement the agreement and was charged with three goals (Haack & Adger, 2002):

1. Produce a strategic plan to advise the federal government and others about how to improve health professional education on substance abuse
2. Conduct an interdisciplinary faculty development program (Project MAINSTREAM) for faculty fellows of multiple professions
3. Build regional training networks and a national electronic communications resource that will support an expansion in faculty development

Mary Haack was appointed as the cochair of the strategic planning effort (goal 1) and was the lead author of the strategic plan (Haack et al., 2002). In response to goal 3, a Web site entitled Project MAINSTREAM (Multi-Agency Initiative on Substance Abuse TRaining and Education for America) was developed that can be accessed at www.projectmainstream.net. The purpose of the Web site is to serve as a resource for all health care professional educators who wish to improve their teaching on substance use disorders. It provides materials and links and serves in some ways as a real-time FDP for health professionals who recognize that they need additional training. For goal 2, Project MAINSTREAM announced a 2-year, part-time fellowship for faculty from 16 health professions who were not currently engaged in substance abuse education. The fellows were to develop knowledge and competencies in alcohol and drug screening, assessment, intervention, and referral; identifying and assisting children and adolescents with substance-abusing parents; and serving as resources for their communities in implementing prevention programs. AMERSA currently is training 39 fellows, including some nurses. Mary Haack (University of Maryland), Linda Degutis (Yale University), and Janice Dyehouse (University of Cincinnati) have or are serving as mentors in this program (www.projectmain stream.net, 2004), but are not necessarily mentoring nurse-fellows. This implies that they are recognized as generalist experts in substance abuse.

NONGOVERNMENTAL NETWORKING BY NURSES IN SUBSTANCE ABUSE

In the mid-1980s, Elizabeth Burns initiated the Nursing Interest Group within the International Council on Alcohol and Addictions (ICAA) based in Geneva, Switzerland; subsequently, nurse-investigators presented their blind-reviewed research and other papers in the large multidisciplinary sessions or in the nursing sessions of ICAA conferences. The U.S. nurse-scientists networked actively with nurses and other substance abuse scholars from several countries and continents. Over the next decade, FDP nurse fellows and former fellows presented at ICAA conferences in Brazil, Germany, Italy, Switzerland, the United States, and other countries. Beginning in 1995, Mary Haack assumed leadership of the Nursing Interest Group of the ICAA.

Haack was largely responsible during the mid-1990s for the formation of the American Academy of Nursing Expert Panel on Mental Health, Mental Illness, and Substance Abuse. She served as the first chair of the panel. The panel members participated in the aforementioned Project MAINSTREAM strategic planning process and were involved in writing some sections of the report in keeping with the mission of the academy to participate in health planning and policy development.

The International Network of Nurses in Alcohol, Tobacco, and Drug Misuse and Addiction met for the first time during the International Council of Nurses

(ICN) Centennial Congress in London in June 1999, again in Copenhagen in June 2001, and they plan to continue meeting during each ICN congress. The international network is open to practitioners, educators, researchers, and leaders/ policy makers with the goals of improving education of nurses, improving peer assistance to nurses, improving quality of assessment and treatment of substance-abusing patients, collaboration with other professions, community education, and policy implementation in the member countries. The coordinating organization was the London-based Association of Nurses in Substance Abuse that was formed in 1983 to provide a networking forum for British nurses who were few in number and isolated in their practices. The U.S. partner in the meeting was the National Nurses Society on Addictions that was formed in 1975, but which recently changed its name to the International Nurses Society on Addictions (http://intnsa.org). The latter organization sponsors annual conferences, has an official journal (*Journal of Addictions Nursing*), offers specialty certification at the basic (CARN) and advanced practice levels (CARN-AP), and has an annual research grant program to stimulate research that directly or indirectly impacts addictions nursing.

In 1991, former FDP fellow Marilyn Sommers and Karen Allen of the Midwest Nursing Research Society (MNRS) received approval for their plan to create the Addictions and Substance Abuse Research Section (ASAR) within MNRS. This action formalized substance abuse as a phenomenon meriting knowledge development by nurse scientists in the Midwest. Importantly, several former FDP fellows joined the interest group and became core participants in its activities over time. Indeed, several of the chapter authors in this volume of the *Annual Review of Nursing Research* were FDP fellows and are current members of the MNRS ASAR.

Alcohol-focused nurse educators and nurse researchers have had a patch-work history of successes and lulls over the past 25 years. It is hoped that this 23rd volume of the *ARNR* will serve to interest a new generation of budding nurse-scientists in this important and interesting field of research.

THE FRAMEWORK, GOALS, AND CONTENT AREAS COVERED IN VOLUME 23

In 2002 this volume was commissioned, with Stevenson and Sommers as the coeditors. It was quite a challenge to find a cadre of alcohol-intensive nurse researchers who had the expertise and experience to undertake the complex tasks of reviewing the research literature on the topics that had been chosen. Unfortunately, some chapter topics of interest are missing from this volume, including dual diagnosis (i.e., alcohol and mental health problems combined), alcohol issues among minority populations, and alcohol and women's health.

We are exceedingly proud, however, of the authors and the chapters that are included. They represent a substantial contribution toward gathering the best evidence available through July 2004 on topics intended to generate research questions of importance to nurses and nursing. The framework for the layout of the remaining chapters covers five domains of knowledge development in alcohol research: First, there are two chapters that complete the Part I focus on research and measurement issues: a chapter by Marilyn Sawyer Sommers on the complex issues of measurement in the alcohol research field, followed by a review by Joan A. Masters of the possible protective health effects of low-volume and moderate alcohol consumption. Part II focuses on alcohol-related issues through the life span. Part III covers the special population of lesbians and gay men and the issue of alcohol and high-risk behaviors. Finally, Part IV offers brief interventions featuring the best evidence to date about their efficacy and effectiveness.

Chapter 2 by Marilyn Sawyer Sommers reviews the formidable literature and informs us about the complex issues and challenges of self-reported measures of alcohol consumption. This chapter covers several issues important to measurement, beginning with definitions of terms that are often used too loosely or interchangeably, through various measures to determine use (quantity–frequency), and an evaluation of myriad extant tools developed for epidemiological studies, screening, and individual-level assessment of problem drinking. Sommers presents a comparison and evaluation of the biological markers currently used to measure recent, longer term, and chronic alcohol consumption and from moderate to intoxicating quantities.

Chapter 3 by Joan Masters provides a balanced analysis of the still-controversial notion that low-volume alcohol consumption is protective against certain cardiovascular conditions, most notably myocardial infarction. The controversy arises for some in questioning the validity and reliability of the data underpinning the protection hypothesis. Others accept the fact of the protective quality, but argue that the dangers of overconsumption outweigh the benefits and that it is impractical to expect the public to maintain the low doses that are deemed protective. Also, the effects of low doses over the course of several decades remain understudied.

Chapters 4 through 8 cover alcohol use, abuse, and dependence over the life span. In Chapter 4, Cara Krulewitch reviews the considerable literature on the older concept of fetal alcohol syndrome and brings us up to the present with the more useful term *fetal alcohol effect*. She pays particular attention to the role of alcohol as a tetratogen but also postulates that more attention is needed in heavy, episodic drinking in young women before they become pregnant or prior to pregnancy recognition. Carol Loveland-Cherry evaluates, in Chapter 5, the individual, family, group, and community-focused interventions that have been developed and tested to prevent and treat alcohol challenges among children and adolescents. Next, Carol Boyd and her colleagues review the body of research on young adults during the college years and the special problem of binge drinking in this group. The chapter also addresses the dearth of research on individual- and aggregate-level interventions to decrease college-student binge drinking. In Chapter 7, Sandra Handley and Peggy Ward-Smith review the evidence on alcohol use, misuse, and abuse among young and middle-aged adults. This is the segment of society that has family and job responsibilities, which can be affected negatively by abuse of alcohol. In particular, they note the lack of alcohol- related studies that deal with the developmental differences in young and middle adulthood. Chapter 8, the final chapter in this section, presents a critical review of studies on older adults and their unique biobehavioral and socioemotional issues and challenges in the face of alcohol use, abuse, and dependence. In this chapter, Joanne Sabol Stevenson reviews the evidence about early- and late- onset abuse and the possible connections to genetics, the special case of older women and abuse, and the problem of mixing alcohol with prescription and over-the-counter drugs.

Two important cutting-edge topics in alcohol research are addressed in Chapters 9 and 10. Tonda Hughes provides a substantive elucidation and critique of the research—mostly epidemiological to date—of gay and lesbian alcohol use, abuse, and addiction. She notes the important issues and challenges for future research, including the need for theory-based intervention development and testing. Colleen Corte and Marilyn Sawyer Sommers review their respective areas of expertise to bring together the divergent literatures and theoretical perspectives on alcohol and risk taking. They postulate that risky drinking, in combination with other behaviors, such as risky driving behavior, sexual behav- ior, and violent behavior, escalates the potential for adverse events.

Finally, in Chapter 11 Deborah Finfgeld-Connett offers readers a critique of the body of research on alcohol-related brief interventions. She covers the science work produced to date in the two main areas of practice where the technique has undergone clinical trials: primary care and trauma/emergency care. She also makes the case that brief intervention may be the most appropriate strategy for general practitioners to use to reduce drinking in problem and risky drinkers (nondependents) at least in the short term (over 12 months).

DIRECTIONS FOR FUTURE ALCOHOL AND OTHER SUBSTANCE ABUSE RESEARCH PROGRAMS IN NURSING

Genetics-related research opens myriad possibilities for prevention, early case finding, and precise treatment of alcohol-related addictive conditions. The op- portunities for nurse researchers are rich and varied—any age group, family or community level, biological (bench) or behavioral research or a combination, and any place on the continuum from primary or secondary prevention to chronic disease management or end-of-life care. Alcohol and other substance abuse affects people in every sector of life, and they have an impact on nursing practice across all specialties. The unanswered questions in the alcohol field present an important opportunity for nurse-scientists to add to a body of knowledge that will make substantial difference to the quality of peoples' lives.

Nurse-researchers with a special interest in vulnerable populations have much work in store. Too little is known about the mechanisms of use, misuse, abuse, addiction, and effective treatment of women contrasted to men, ethnic and racial minorities, gays and lesbians, and special groups such as the developmentally disadvantaged and those with dual diagnoses of mental illness and substance abuse. Numerous and diverse programs of research are available for the choosing.

Instrumentation and methodological challenges abound in substance abuse in general, and alcohol abuse in particular. Even something as simplistic as an alcohol biomarker is so complex that no gold standard has been developed. Likewise, scales to capture abuse are numerous, but nothing satisfactory is yet available for mass community screening, primary care assessment, acute care screening, occupational or educational sector testing, and the elderly. There is even need for more sensitive and specific measures to detect drunk driving and to document relapse.

Methodological issues such as sampling and sample accrual need more thoughtful science work. For too long the samples have consisted of captured audiences such as members of the military, patients in veterans' hospitals and clinics, patients in treatment for dependence, and patients in terminal stages of alcohol-related diseases. How do researchers accrue appropriate samples to study binge drinking in non-college-age young adults? What is a valid approach to sampling and measurement of drinking behavior among various socioeconomic groups of older women? If the traditional self-help groups, such as Alcoholics Anonymous, do not work for gays and lesbians, what would work and why? How do physiology, spirituality, and genetics interact in the drinking behavior and addiction tendencies of certain ethnic groups? These are but a few of many research questions waiting to be addressed by well-trained scientists, including nurses.

So much work needs to be done, it will take many motivated scientists considerable time and funding to develop the breakthrough studies to build the knowledge base that will lead to a decrease in the suffering caused by alcohol and other substance abuse. Nurses are in an excellent position to address many of the untapped research questions that exist today.

REFERENCES

Bartek. J. K., Lindeman, M., Newton, M., Fitzgerald, A. P., & Hawks, J. H. (1988). Nurse-identified problems in the management of alcoholic patients. *Journal of Studies on Alcohol, 49*, 62–70.

Burns, E. M. (1990). The effects of stress during the brain growth spurt. In J. J. Fitzpatrick, R. L. Taunton, & J. Q. Benoliel (Eds.), *Annual Review of Nursing Research* (Vol. 8, pp. 57–82). New York: Springer Publishing Co.

Burns, E. M., Ciccone, J. K., & Thompson, A. (Eds). (1991). *An addictions curriculum for nurses and other helping professionals: Undergraduate, graduate and continuing education levels.* Columbus: Ohio State University.

Burns, E. M., Kruckeberg, T. W., Kanak, M. F., & Stibler, H. (1986). Ethanol exposure during brain ontogeny: Some long-term effects. *Neurobehavioral Toxicology and Tertolgy,* 8, 383–389.

Burns, E. M., Kruckeberg, T. W., Stibler, H., Cerven, E., & Borg, S. (1984). Ethanol exposure during brain growth spurt. *Teratology,* 29, 251–258.

Burns, E. M., Thompson, A., & Ciccone, J. K. (Eds.). (1994). *An addictions curriculum for nurses and other helping professionals.* New York: Springer.

Chase, K. A., O'Farrell, T. J., Murphy, C. M., Fals-Stewart, W., & Murphy, M. (2003). Factors associated with partner violence among female alcoholic patients and their male partners. *Journal of Studies on Alcohol,* 64, 137–149.

Chermack, S. T., Walton, M. A., Fuller, B. E., & Blow, F. C. (2001). Correlates of expressed and received violence across relationship types among men and women substance abusers. *Psychology of Addictive Behaviors,* 15(2), 140–151.

Church, O., Fisk, N. B., & Neafsey, P. J. (1990). *Curriculum for nursing education in alcohol and drug abuse: Project NEADA.* Storrs: University of Connecticut School of Nursing.

Correo, G., Bagnardi, V., Zambon, A., & La Vecchia, C. (2004). A meta-analysis of alcohol consumption and the risk of 15 diseases. *Preventive Medicine,* 38, 613–619.

Dawson, D. A. (1994). Heavy drinking and the risk of occupational injury. *Accident Analysis and Prevention,* 26, 655–665.

Dawson, D. A. (2000). Alcohol consumption, alcohol dependence, and all-cause mortality. *Alcoholism: Clinical and Experimental Research,* 24, 72–81.

Dawson, D. A. (2001). Alcohol and mortality from external causes. *Journal of Studies in Alcohol,* 62, 790–797.

Dawson, D. A., Grant, B. F., Chou, S. P., & Pickering, R. P. (1995). Subgroup variation in US drinking patterns: Results of the 1992 national longitudinal alcohol epidemiologic study. *Journal of Substance Abuse,* 7, 331–344.

English, D. R., Holman, C. D. J., & Milne, E. (1992). *The quantification of drug-caused morbidity and mortality in Australia: 1992.* Canberra, Australia: Commonwealth Department of Human Services and Health.

English, D. R., Holman, C. D. J., Milne, E., Hulse, G., & Winter, M. G. (1995). Quantification of morbidity and mortality caused by substance abuse. Second International Symposium on the Social and Economic Costs of Substance Abuse, Montebella, CA, Oct. 2–5, 1995, 21 p.

Fiellin, D. A., Reid, M. C., & O'Connor, P. G. (2000). Screening for alcohol problems in primary care: A systematic review. *Archives of Internal Medicine,* 160, 1977–1989.

Fleming, M. F., Manwell, L. B., Barry, K. L., & Johnson, K. (1998). At-risk drinking in an HMO primary care sample: Prevalence and health policy implications. *American Journal of Public Health,* 88, 90–93.

Gerace, L. M. (1988). Patterns of alcohol use among nurse educators. *Issues in Mental Health Nursing,* 9, 189–200.

Gerace, L. M., Hughes, T., & Spunt, J. (1995). Improving nurses' responses toward substance-misusing patients: A clinical evaluation project. *Archives of Psychiatric Nursing, 9*, 286–294.

Gerace, L. M., Sullivan, E. J., Murphy, S. A., & Cotter, F. (1992). Faculty development and curriculum change in substance abuse. *Nurse Educator, 17*, 24–27.

Greenfield, L. A. (1998). *Alcohol and crime: An analysis of national data on the prevalence of alcohol involvement in crime.* Report prepared for the Assistant Attorney General's National Symposium on Alcohol Abuse and Crime. Washington, DC: U.S. Department of Justice.

Haack, M. R. (1988). Stress and impairment among nursing students. *Research in Nursing and Health, 9*, 125–134.

Haack, M. R., & Adger, H. (Eds.). (2002). *Strategic plan for interdisciplinary faculty development: Arming the nation's health professional workforce for a new approach for substance abuse disorders.* Providence, RI: AMERSA. Retrieved July 16, 2004, from http://www.projectmainstream.net/mainstream/supportdata/SPACdocfinal.pdf

Haack, M. R., & Harford, T. C. (1984). Drinking patterns among student nurses. *International Journal of the Addictions, 19*, 577–583.

Haack, M. R., Harford, T. C., & Parker, D. A. (1988). Alcohol use and depression symptoms among female nursing students. *Alcoholism: Clinical and Experimental Research, 12*, 365–367.

Hagemaster, J., Handley, S., Plumlee, A., Sullivan, E., & Stanley, S. (1993). Developing educational programmes for nurses that meet today's addiction challenges. *Nurse Education Today, 13*, 421–425.

Harwood, H. (2000). *Updating estimates of the economic costs of alcohol abuse in the United States.* Rockville, MD: National Institute on Alcohol Abuse and Alcoholism.

Hearne, R., Connolly, A., & Sheehan, J. (2002). Alcohol abuse: Prevalence and detection in a general hospital. *Journal of the Royal Society of Medicine, 95*, 84–87.

Heinemann, M. E., & Hoffman, A. L. (1989). Nurse educators look at alcohol education for the profession. *Alcohol Health and Research World, 13*, 48–51.

Hoffman, A. L., & Heinemann, M. E. (1987). Substance abuse education in schools of nursing: A national survey. *Journal of Nursing Education, 26*, 282–287.

Kaufman-Kantor, G., & Asdigian, N. (1997). When women are under the influence: Does drinking or drug use by women provoke beatings by men? In M. Galanter (Ed.), *Alcohol and violence—Epidemiology, neurobiology, psychology, family issues: Recent developments in alcoholism* (Vol. 13, pp. 315–336). New York: Plenum.

Kerfoot, K. M., Kruckeberg, T. W., & Burns, E. M. (1985). Maternal ethanol consumption and levels of ethanol in breast milk. *Proceedings of the 34th International, Congress on Alcoholism and Drug Dependence, 34*, 124.

Kouimtsidis, C., Reynolds, M., Hunt, M., Lind, J., Beckett, Drummond, C., et al. (2003). Substance use in the general hospital. *Addictive Behaviors, 28*, 483–499.

Kruckeberg, T. W., Gaetano, P. K., Burns, E. M., Stibler, H. J., Cerven, E., & Borg, S. (1984). Ethanol in pre-weanling rats with dams: Body temperature unaffected. *Neurobehavioral Toxicology and Teratology, 6*, 307–312.

Leonard, K. E., & Roberts, L. J. (1999). The effects of alcohol on the marital interactions of aggressive and non-aggressive husbands and their wives. *Journal of Abnormal Psychology, 107*, 602–615.

Li, G., Kevl, P. M., Smith, G. S., & Baker, S. P. (1997). Alcohol and injury severity: Reappraisal of the continuing controversy. *Journal of Trauma, 42,* 562–569.

Lipsey, M. W., Wilson, D. B., Cohen, M. A., & Derzon, J. H. (1997). Is there a causal relationship between alcohol use and violence? A synthesis of evidence. In M. Galanter (Ed.), *Alcohol and violence—Epidemiology, neurobiology, psychology, family issues: Recent developments in alcoholism* (Vol. 13, pp. 245–282). New York: Plenum Press.

Manwell, L. B., Fleming, M. F., Johnson, K., & Barry, K. (1998). Tobacco, alcohol, and drug use in a primary care sample: 90-day prevalence and associated factors. *Journal of Addictive Diseases, 17,* 67–81.

Marcus, M. T. (2000). An interdisciplinary team model for substance abuse prevention in communities. *Journal of Professional Nursing, 16,* 158–168.

Marcus, M. T., Gerace, L. M., & Sullivan, E. J. (1996). Enhancing nursing competence with substance abusing clients. *Journal of Nursing Education, 35,* 361–366.

Marcus, M. T., Rickman, K. A., & Sobhan, T. (1999). Substance abuse education liaisons: A collaborative continuing education program for nurses in acute care settings. *Journal of Continuing Education in Nursing, 30,* 229–234.

McGinnis, J. M., & Foege, W. H. (1993). Actual causes of death in the United States. *Journal of the American Medical Association, 270,* 2207–2212.

McInnis, E., & Powell, J. (1994). Drug and alcohol referrals: Are elderly substance abuse diagnoses and referrals being missed? *British Medical Journal, 308,* 444–446.

Murphy, S. A. (1989). The urgency of substance abuse education in schools of nursing. *Journal of Nursing Education, 28,* 247–251.

Murphy, S. A. (1991). An empirically based substance abuse course for graduate students in nursing. *Journal of Nursing Education, 30,* 274–277.

Naegle. M. A. (1989). Targets for change in alcohol and drug education for nursing roles. *Alcohol Health and Research World, 13,* 52–55.

Naegle, M. A. (Ed.). (1991). *Substance abuse education in nursing* (Vol. 1) (Publication No. 15-2407). New York: National League for Nursing.

Naegle, M. A. (Ed.). (1992). *Substance abuse education in nursing* (Vol. 2) (Publication No. 15-2463). New York: National League for Nursing.

Naegle, M. A. (Ed.). (1993). *Substance abuse education in nursing* (Vol. 2) (Publication No. 15-2463). New York: National League for Nursing.

National Institute on Alcohol Abuse and Alcoholism (NIAAA). (2000). *Tenth Special Report on Alcohol and Health.* Bethesda, MD: Author.

National Institute on Alcohol Abuse and Alcoholism (NIAAA). (2004). Definition of a standard drink. Retrieved October 1, 2004, from http://www.niaaa.nih.gov/public ations/niaaa-guide/StandardDrinksC hart.htm

Poikolainen, K., Vartianen, E., & Korhonen, H. J. (1996). Alcohol intake and subjective health. *American Journal of Epidemiology, 144,* 346–350.

Prochaska, J. O., & DiClemente, C. C. (1984). The stages of change. In J. O. Prochaska & C. C. DiClemente (Eds.), *The transtheoretical approach: Crossing traditional boundaries of therapy* (pp. 21–32). Homewood, IL: Dow Jones-Irwin.

Rehm, J., Room, R., Graham, K, Monteiro, M., Gmel, G., & Sempos, C. T. (2003). The relationship of average volume of alcohol consumption and patterns of drinking to burden of disease: An overview. *Society for the Study of Addiction to Alcohol and Other Drugs, 98,* 1209–1228.

Rehm, J., Room, R., Monteiro, M., Gmel, G., Graham, K, Rehn, N., et al. (2003). Alcohol as a risk factor for global burden of disease. *European Addiction Research*, 9, 157–164.

Reid, M. C., Fiellin, D. A., & O'Connor, P. G.(1999). Hazardous and harmful alcohol consumption in primary care. *Archives of Internal Medicine*, 159, 1682–1689.

Ridolfo, B., & Stevenson, C. (2001). *The quantification of drug-caused mortality and morbidity in Australia: 1998.* Canberra: Australian Institute of Health and Welfare.

Roeloffs, C. A., Fink, A., Unutzer, J., Tang, L., & Wells, K. B. (2001). Problematic substance use, depressive symptoms, and gender in primary care. *Psychiatric Services*, 52, 1251–1253.

Schneekloth, T. D., Morse, R. M., Herrick, L. M., Suman, V. J., Offord, K. P., & Davis, L. J. (2001). Point prevalence of alcoholism in hospitalized patients: Continuing challenges of detection, assessment, and diagnosis. *Mayo Clinic Proceedings*, 76, 460–466.

Smith, G. S., Branda, C. C., & Miller, T. R. (1999). Fatal non-traffic injuries involving alcohol: Meta-analysis. *Annals of Emergency Medicine*, 33, 659–668.

Sommers, M. S., Dyehouse, J. M., & Howe, S. R. (2001). Binge drinking, sensible drinking, and abstinence after alcohol related-vehicular crashes: The role of intervention versus screening. *Association for the Advancement of Automotive Medicine*, 45, 317–328.

Stibler, H., Burns, E. M., Kruckeberg, T. W., Cerven, E., & Borg, S. (1985). Changes of synaptosomal surface carbohydrates after ethanol exposure during synaptogenesis. In H. Parvez, E. Burns, Y. Burov, & S. Parvez (Eds.), *Progress in alcohol research* (pp. 37–49). Utrecht, Netherlands: VNU Science Press.

Stibler, H., Burns, E. M., Kruckeberg, T. W., Gaetano, P., Cerven, E., Borg, S., et al. (1983). Effect of ethanol on synaptosomal sialic acid metabolism in the developing rat brain. *Journal of the Neurological Sciences*, 59, 21–35.

Sullivan, E. J. (1987a). A descriptive study of nurses recovering from chemical dependency. *Archives of Psychiatric Nursing*, 1, 194–200.

Sullivan, E. J. (1987b). Comparison of chemically dependent and nondependent nurses on familial, personal, and professional characteristics. *Journal of Studies on Alcohol*, 48, 563–568.

Sullivan, E. J. (1988). Association between chemical dependency and sexual problems in nurses. *Journal of Interpersonal Violence*, 3, 326–329.

Sullivan, E. J., Bissell, L., & Leffler, D. (1990). Drug use and disciplinary actions among 300 nurses. *International Journal of Addictions*, 25, 375–391.

Sullivan, E. J., & Hale, R. E. (1987). Nurses' beliefs about the etiology and treatment of alcohol abuse. *Journal of Studies on Alcohol*, 48, 456–460.

Sullivan, E. J., & Handley, S. M. (1992). Alcohol and drug abuse in nurses. In J. J. Fitzpatrick, R. L. Taunton, & A. K. Jacox (Eds.), *Annual Review of Nursing Research* (Vol. 10, pp. 113–125). New York: Springer.

Sullivan, E. J., & Handley, S. M. (1993). Alcohol and drug abuse. In J. J. Fitzpatrick & J. S. Stevenson (Eds.), *Annual Review of Nursing Research* (Vol. 11, pp. 281–297). New York: Springer.

Talashek, M. L., Gerace, L. M., Miller, A. G., & Lindsey, M. (1995). Family nurse practitioner clinical competencies in alcohol and substance use. *Journal of the American Academy of Nurse Practitioners*, 7, 57–63.

Testa, M., & Parks, K. A. (1996). The role of women's alcohol consumption in sexual victimization. *Aggression and Violent Behavior, 1*, 217–234.

Waller, P. F., Hill, E. M., Maio, R. F., & Blow, F. (2003). Alcohol effects on motor vehicle crash injury. *Alcoholism: Clinical and Experimental Research, 27*, 695–703.

Watson, H. (2000). Problem drinkers among acute care inpatients. *Nursing Standards, 14*(40), 32–35.

Webb, G. R., Redman, S., & Hennrikus, D. J. (1994). The relationships between high-risk and problem drinking and the occurrence of work injuries and related absences. *Journal of Studies on Alcohol, 55*, 434–446.

Whitfield, J. B., Gu, Z., Madden, P. A., Neale, M. C., Heath, A. C., & Martin, N. G. (2004). The genetics of alcohol intake and of alcohol dependence. *Alcoholism: Clinical and Experimental Research, 28*, 1153–1160.

World Health Organization (WHO). (1999). Global status report on alcohol. Retrieved September 27, 2004, from http://www.who.int/substance_abuse/PDFfiles/global_alcohol_status_report

World Health Organization (WHO). (2000). Substance abuse: The mission. Retrieved September 27, 2004, from http://www.who.int/substance_abuse

Chapter 2

Measurement of Alcohol Consumption: Issues and Challenges

Marilyn Sawyer Sommers

ABSTRACT

In both the clinical and research settings, nurses assess patterns of alcohol consumption to screen for risk of adverse events or to determine the health consequences of drinking. The purposes of this critical review are to explore issues and controversies surrounding the measurement of alcohol consumption and to critique the existing literature relevant to the research and clinical arenas. An electronic literature search was completed to identify research articles addressing human studies from 1995 through 2004 related to alcohol consumption. Key words included alcohol drinking (subheadings blood, metabolism, psychology, and urine), standard drink, problem drinking, heavy drinking, and ethanol analysis (subheadings blood, urine, and chemistry). The results were in two primary content areas: self-reported alcohol consumption and assessment of consumption by using biological markers.

Self-reported alcohol consumption can be quantified in a variety of ways, such as ounces of ethanol per day, standard drinks per day, drinking occurrences per month, heavy drinking occasions per month, and frequency of perceived drunkenness. The choice of measure depends on setting (clinical vs. research), the role of the variable under study, the capabilities and demographics of the study population, the study design, and the resources available to collect alcohol consumption data.

A variety of biologic instruments are used to assess alcohol consumption, each with sensitivities and specificities that vary by age, gender, and possibly by ethnicity/race. Previous work has focused on the white, male, alcohol-dependent population and non-alcohol-dependent male controls. Some urgency exists to expand the biometrics of alcohol use to minority and older populations as well as to women across the life span.

Keywords: alcohol consumption, ethanol consumption, self-reported alcohol use, alcohol use, alcohol measurement, alcohol biometrics

What constitutes an alcoholic drink, and how do people describe their own alcohol consumption? An alcohol researcher would likely answer in terms of a standard drink (see Table 2.1), whereas patients in an emergency department may have definitions of a single drink that vary from a 1.5 ounce shot to a fifth (of a gallon) of distilled spirits. The general public is remarkably naive about alcohol consumption. Reflecting the age of "super-sized" portions, when college-age drinkers free-pour (pour the amount they believe to be correct) a 12 oz beer or a shot of liquor for a mixed drink, they overpour by as much as 80% (White, Kraus, McCracken, & Swartwelder, 2003). Beverage types are confusing to the public as well. Some wine coolers, while having the look and appeal of wine products, may actually be malt beverages that contain no wine, are brewed like beer, as opposed to fermented like wine, and have the alcohol content of beer. These products can mislead the average consumer, who may equate wine coolers with wine products (Taylor, Drew, Waiters, & Bluthenthal, 2003). Added to this complex picture are the common misconceptions that, whereas "hard" liquor causes alcoholism, beer does not and that alcohol dependence leads to inaccurate self-reporting of drinking no matter what the context. These misperceptions make it clear that collecting data about alcohol consumption is indeed a challenge to scientists and clinicians.

The study of alcohol-related health consequences presents nurse-scientists with a multitude of decisions about alcohol consumption. An extensive body of literature guides the quantification of alcohol intake. Understanding of complex issues, such as what constitutes meaningful variation in drinking (Dawson, 1998b), the most appropriate technique for eliciting quantity/frequency data (Cunningham, Ansara, Wild, Toneatto, & Koski-Jannes, 1999), and the role of underreporting in alcohol measurement (Ivis, Bondy, & Adlaf, 1997), makes the quantification of alcohol consumption a challenge. In addition, there is a growing clinical movement across health care disciplines to implement routine screening and brief intervention (SBI) to manage problem drinking (Chang, Goetz, Wilkins-Haug, & Berman, 2000; Fleming, Barry, Manwell, Johnson, & London, 1997). Clinical programs for SBI must be evidence-based with measurable outcomes if they are to be effective.

TABLE 2.1   Definitions: Alcohol Consumption and Patterns of Drinking

Term	Definition	Source
A Drink; Standard drink	A standard drink contains about 14 g of pure alcohol (% below is ethanol content by volume). Standard drink equivalents include: • one 12 oz bottle of beer (4%–5% alcohol) • one 12 oz bottle of light beer (2.5% alcohol) • one 8.5 oz bottle of malt liquor (6%–10% alcohol) • one 5 oz glass of table wine (12%–14% alcohol) • one 3.5 oz of fortified or desert wine, port (19%–22% alcohol) • one 12 oz wine cooler (4%–5%) • one 2.5 oz of cordial, liqueur, or aperitif (17%–30% alcohol) • one 1.5 oz of 80-proof distilled spirits (e.g., gin, vodka, whiskey) (40% alcohol) • one 1 oz of brandy (60% alcohol)	• Dufour (1999) • National Institute on Alcohol Abuse and Alcoholism (NIAAA 2004). Retrieved October 1, 2004, from http://www.niaaa.nih.gov/ publications/niaaa-guide/ standardDrinksChart.htm • Taproom (2004). Retrieved October 1, 2004, fromhttp:// www.taproom.com/beer/ beerprf.htm • Wikipedia (2004). Retrieved October 1, 2004, from http://www.wikipedia.org/ wiki/Alcoholic_beverage
Abstinence	Consumption of fewer than four standard drinks per year	• NIAAA (1999). Retrieved October 1, 2004, from http://www.niaaa.nih.gov/ databases/dkpat17.htm

(continued)

TABLE 2.1   *(continued)*

Term	Definition	Source
Alcohol abuse	Maladaptive pattern of drinking leading to clinically significant impairment or distress as manifested by at least one of the following within a 12-month period: recurrent use of alcohol, resulting in failure to fulfill major role obligations, recurrent alcohol use in situations in which it is physically hazardous, recurrent alcohol-related legal problems, continued alcohol use despite having persistent or recurrent social or interpersonal problems caused or exacerbated by the effects of alcohol	• Hasin (2003). Classification of alcohol use disorders. National Institute on Alcohol Abuse and Alcoholism. Retrieved October 1, 2004, from http://www.niaaa.nih.gov/publications/arh27-1/5-17.htm
Alcohol consumption	Number of standard drinks ingested by an individual (quantity) per unit time (frequency)	• Sommers et al. (2003)
Alcohol dependence syndrome	Formerly called alcoholism; a psychobiological condition characterized by an inner drive to consume alcohol, continuing to drink in the presence of harm, and experiencing a withdrawal state when drinking is interrupted for some time period (usually within 12 hours but may occur up to 7–10 days after drinking cessation). A maladaptive pattern of drinking, leading to clinically significant impairment or distress as manifested by three or more of the following occurring at any time in the same period: tolerance, withdrawal, impaired control, neglect of activities, time spent in alcohol-related activity, continued use despite problems	• Saunders & Lee (2000) • Hasin (2003). Classification of alcohol use disorders. National Institute on Alcohol Abuse and Alcoholism. Retrieved October 1, 2004, from http://www.niaaa.nih.gov/publications/arh27-1/5-17.htm

TABLE 2.1   *(continued)*

Term	Definition	Source
Alcohol misuse	Consumption of alcohol at a level that can cause damage to the individual's health and well-being; can cause the individual to act in a manner that endangers the lives and safety of other people in the community or prevents the wider community from enjoying a peaceful environment	• Scottish Executive Online (2004). Retrieved October 1, 2004, from http://www.scotland.gov.uk/cru/kd01/red/tpamwr-04.asp
Alcoholism	Primary, chronic disease with genetic, psychosocial, and environmental factors influencing its development and manifestations. The disease is often progressive and fatal. It is characterized by continuous or periodic impaired control over drinking, preoccupation with alcohol, use of alcohol despite adverse consequences, and distortions in thinking, most notably denial	• American Society of Addiction Medicine (ASAM, 2001). Retrieved October 1, 2004, from http://www.asam.org/ppol/Definition%20of%20Alcoholism.htm
Current alcohol use	Consumption of at least one standard drink in the past 30 days (includes binge and heavy use)	• Substance Abuse and Mental Health Services Administration (SAMHSA, 2004). Alcohol use. 2002 National Survey on Drug Use and Health (NSDUH). Retrieved October 1, 2004, from http://www.oas.samhsa.gov/NHSDA/2k2NSDUH/Results/2k2results.htm#chap3
Harmful drinking	Pattern of alcohol use that is currently resulting in problems	• Allen et al. (1997) • Reinert & Allen (2002)
Hazardous drinking	Pattern of alcohol use that poses high risk of future damage to physical/mental health	• Allen et al. (1997) • Reinert & Allen (2002)

(continued)

TABLE 2.1 *(continued)*

Term	Definition	Source
Heavy drinking	Consumption of five or more drinks on the same occasion on at least 5 different days in the 30 days prior to survey for men; four or more drinks on the same occasion on at least 5 different days in the 30 days prior to survey for women. Note: Heavy drinking is sometimes defined as 1 oz or more of ethanol per day (14 or more drinks per week or 2 or more drinks per day; NIAAA, 1999). Retrieved October 1, 2004, from http://www.niaaa.nih.gov/databases/dkpat17.htm)	• SAMHSA (2004). Retrieved October 1, 2004, from http://www.oas.samhsa.gov/NHSDA/2k2NSDUH/Results/2k2results.htm#chap3. Note: Reference does not differentiate between men and women. • Shalala (1995)
Heavy, episodic drinking (also known as 5+ drinking and binge drinking)	Consumption of five or more drinks on the same occasion at least once in the 30 days prior to survey for men; four or more drinks on the same occasion at least once in the 30 days prior to survey for women	• SAMHSA (2004). Retrieved October 1, 2004, from http://www.oas.samhsa.gov/NHSDA/2k2NSDUH/Results/2k2results.htm#chap3. Note: Reference does not differentiate between men and women. • Naimi et al. (2003); Shalala (1995)
Low-level drinking	Consumption at levels lower than those defined by moderate drinking: Women: 1–6 drinks per week Men: 1–13 drinks per week Often used to describe the lower levels of moderate drinking (see below), such as no more than 1–2 drinks, 4 days per week for men or 1 drink, 4 days per week for women.	• Moller (2004) • Gunzerath, Faden, Zakhari, & Warren (2004)

TABLE 2.1   *(continued)*

Term	Definition	Source
Moderate drinking	Consumption of no more than two drinks per day by men and no more than one drink per day by women	• Dufour (1999) • NIAAA (2000a, 2002b). Retrieved October 1, 2004, from http://www.niaaa.nih.gov/publications/harm-al.htm
Problem drinking	Pattern of alcohol use by people who engage in heavy drinking and possibly alcohol abuse but exhibit no symptoms of physical dependence on alcohol	• Walitzer & Connors (1999)
Recommended drinking limits	Women: one standard drink per day and no more than seven standard drinks per week; on any single day no more than three standard drinks. Men: two or fewer standard drinks per day and no more than fourteen standard drinks per week; on any single day no more than four standard per drinks. Note: Recommendations do not apply to special populations such as pregnant women or recovering dependent drinkers.	• NIAAA (2003). Retrieved October 1, 2004, from http://www.niaaa.nih.gov/publications/Practitioner/Note14
Risky (at-risk) drinking	Pattern of alcohol use that may place individuals at increased risk for developing adverse health effects or alcohol dependence	• Allen et al. (1997)

The purposes of this review are to explore issues and controversies surrounding the measurement of alcohol consumption and to critique the existing literature in the area. After an explanation of the concept of a "standard drink," the following self-reported measures will be discussed: the volume, frequency, and variation of consumption; the role of heavy drinking occasions; and the importance of the perception of drunkenness. In addition, the properties and usefulness of laboratory tests will be discussed and critiqued. One psychometric instrument, the Alcohol Use Disorders Identification Test (AUDIT), will also be discussed because of its utility in quantifying alcohol consumption.

The review of literature was accomplished by the following procedure. An electronic search was completed using the Medline, Cumulative Index of Nursing and Allied Health Literature (CINAHL), and psychology and behavioral sciences databases from January 1, 1995, to December 31, 2003, for human studies using the term *alcohol consumption*. The search engine recommended the use of the term *alcohol drinking* (subheadings, including blood, metabolism, psychology, and urine, were used). In addition, searches were completed on the terms *standard drink, problem drinking, heavy drinking, alcohol measurement,* and *ethanol analysis* (subheadings blood, urine, and chemistry). Because a large volume of literature has evolved recently in the area of biological markers for alcohol use, a Medline search was also completed for the years 2000–2004 for the following terms: *biological markers alcohol, CDT [carbohydrate deficient transferrin] alcohol, GGT [γ (gamma) glutamyl transferase] alcohol,* and *MCV [mean corpuscular volume] alcohol.* Relevant articles were culled from the database. In addition, the author used her own compilation of relevant articles collected since 1990 and reviewed the reference lists of relevant articles to locate other articles of interest. During final revisions of the manuscript in 2004, journals relevant to alcohol research were reviewed monthly for articles that would make substantive additions to this review.

MEASUREMENT OF ALCOHOL CONSUMPTION

Since the 1920s, measurement of alcohol consumption has been a focus of research (as summarized in Alanko, 1984, and Room, 1990). Although an extensive body of literature has been written since then to guide the quantification of alcohol intake, there is no general consensus that supports a single measurement strategy. The best measurement technique is the one that is an appropriate match for the research questions/hypotheses; the type, timing, and variability of the drinking pattern to be quantified; and the target population. For example, a short reference period for drinking may minimize recall loss, but longer periods are more likely to demonstrate an atypical pattern of drinking. A 1-week, daily recall method may be an accurate reflection of drinking patterns for a steady drinker, but it may altogether miss the consumption of an infrequent, heavy episodic drinker (Dawson, 1998a; Duffy, 1985). Consensus has emerged around certain universal indicators of alcohol consumption, such as the standard drink and specific frequency and intensity measures (Kadden & Litt, 2004).

Definitions of a Standard Drink

The concept of a "standard drink" was developed as a mechanism to compare the alcohol content across different types of beverages. From a public health perspective, the standard drink was introduced as a means of advising the general public whether or not they were drinking within a reasonable threshold for avoiding harm (International Center for Alcohol Policies, 1999). A standard drink is defined as a suitable, internationally accepted measure for alcohol consumption in grams of alcohol per drink or per day (Turner, 1990). Although international standards at one time ranged from 6.0 g per drink in Australia and New Zealand to 28.0 g per drink in Japan (Turner, 1990), the international consensus is that one standard drink includes 13.6 grams of absolute alcohol (National Institute on Alcohol Abuse and Alcoholism, 1995; Turner, 1990).

Several studies illustrate the need for the concept of the standard drink. Banwell (1999) found that the range of wine provided across 31 licensed premises in Australia ranged from 110 to 230 ml. Kaskutas and Graves (2001) found that self-selected drink size by subjects was 49% above the standard size for beer and 307% above the standard size for spirits. The concept of the standard drink, therefore, has become a necessary measurement tool for all investigators needing to quantify alcohol consumption. To explain the concept of a standard drink to subjects or patients, a card that illustrates standard drink size across the range of drinks (commonly beer, wine, and distilled spirits) is useful (see Table 2.1).

Research assistants should examine the labels of alcoholic beverages where the research is taking place, because local variations, such as increased alcohol content in certain malt liquors as compared with other liquors, occur. An eye to the target population is also warranted. If the investigators are enrolling collage-age women, an analysis of drinking patterns among young women, with attention to "trendy" drinks, such as wine coolers and mixed drinks, is required. International variations also occur. In the United States, 1 fluid ounce (fl oz) is 29.58 ml, whereas in Great Britain 1 fl oz is 28.41 ml (Dufour, 1999). These discrepancies can have important methodological consequences for multisite international studies. They are also important for clinicians who work with alcohol misusers and abusers across communities and cultures.

U.S. Recommendations for Alcohol Consumption

The concept of a standard drink is also used by clinicians to guide counseling and determine the effectiveness of interventions. Current drinking recommendations for healthy adults are to limit alcohol consumption to 1 standard drink per day and no more than 7 standard drinks per week for women, and 2 or fewer standard drinks per day and no more than 14 standard drinks per week for men (NIAAA, 2003). The recommendations do not apply to special populations who may need to reduce drinking further or even abstain, such as women who are pregnant or recovering dependent drinkers. Quantity, frequency, and variation in drinking patterns can be accomplished in a number of ways.

Alcohol Consumption: Quantity and Frequency Measures.

In the quantity/frequency method, an interviewer asks the participant how often he or she consumes alcoholic beverages and how many standard drinks are consumed on each occasion (Serdula, Mokdad, Byers, & Siegel, 1999). The types of survey questions most commonly used to measure quantity/frequency fall into five categories: frequency measures, quantity/frequency (Q/F) measures, graduated frequency measures, short-term recall methods, and diary methods. Using frequency measures, the interviewer queries the respondent on typical drinking frequency in a given time frame (never, daily, weekly, monthly). A subject might be asked, "How many days do you usually drink per year?" A simple frequency question is efficient and limits subject burden. The drawback of using frequency measures alone is that they do not allow researchers to calculate a person's average or total volume of alcohol over time.

Using Q/F measures, the interviewer determines both drinking occurrences and the volume of alcohol consumed per occasion (Dufour, 1999). Volume of drinking alone (quantity) is highly correlated with serious health effects and is a useful predictor of social and physical consequences of drinking (Dawson, 1998b; Dawson, Grant, & Harford, 1995). Frequency measures provide information about the patterns of drinking. Estimates are then calculated by an estimation formula. Together, Q/F measures represent average alcohol intake per unit of time. Q/F measures can be either global (general alcohol intake over time regardless of beverage) or beverage-specific. Global measures might include a formula to calculate average daily alcohol (ethanol) intake, such as

$$\frac{[\text{usual quantity of standard drinks per drinking day}] \times [\text{usual number of drinking days per year}] \times 0.55}{365 \text{ days per year}}$$

when 0.55 is the average ethanol content per drink in ounces (Dawson, 1998b). This formula is based on no specified reference period and requires two questions (How many standard drinks do you usually drink each day that you drink? and How many days do you usually drink per year? [Dawson, 1998b; Dufour, 1999]). To account for individuals' beverage choices, the ethanol content of 0.55 can be replaced by 0.54 for beer, 0.48 for wine, and 0.61 for spirits (Dawson, 1998b).

The type of beverage, as compared to the total ethanol intake, may be relevant for some studies. Two teams of investigators found conflicting results when testing the hypothesis that wine or beer consumption placed individuals at a lower risk for liver cirrhosis than spirit consumption (Kerr, Fillmore, & Marvy, 2000; Pelletier et al., 2002). In an extensive review of the literature, Smart (1996) found that behavioral consequences varied with different beverage types. He noted the following: blood alcohol levels rose most quickly with spirits; at the same dosage levels, beer created less impairment than brandy; those who drank beer or beer and spirits had more alcohol-related problems than those who drank wine; and beer drinkers were more likely than others to drink and drive. Although some investigators measure a specific type of beverage, most use the Q/F method to calculate global ethanol intake per unit of time.

Despite the advantages of Q/F measures, they do not detect irregular or seasonal drinking patterns because they require respondents to average alcohol consumption mentally (Dufour, 1999). Cho, Johnson, and Fendrich (2001) found seasonal consumption patterns in a large U.S. sample ($N = 57,758$). Both male and female subjects were more likely to report past 30-day alcohol consumption in January than in March and were more likely to report heavy episodic drinking in July compared with other months. If the investigator wants to measure variations in drinking patterns, other questions are more appropriate (see Alcohol Consumption: Heavy Drinking Occasions and Variable Drinking Patterns).

Interviewers using graduated frequency measures begin with a question eliciting the largest number of drinks consumed by the person on any one drinking occasion during the past year, followed by subsequent questions with progressively lower alcohol quantities (What is the maximum number of standard drinks you have had on any given occasion during the past year? [Cherpitel, 1997]). The advantage to this survey method is that it does not require as much mental calculation as regular Q/F measures. Self-reports obtained from this method may be more accurate than global measures (Dufour, 1999). Along this line, Dawson (1998b) studied total ethanol intake with type of beverage and also volume of ethanol (days of drinking 5 or more standard drinks [5+ drinks] and days of drinking 9 or more standard drinks [9+ drinks]). She found that global measures led to reports of lower levels of consumption (0.47 oz of ethanol per day [oz ETOH/day]) as compared with beverage-specific measures (0.52 oz ETOH/day). She also found the highest amount of ethanol consumption when she included 5+ and 9+ drinking days (0.72 oz ETOH/day). The benefit of graduated frequency measures is that they are more likely than Q/F measures to capture variations in drinking as well as heavy drinking, although they have a higher subject burden and cost than other methods. However, just because beverage-specific measures and 5+/9+ drinking yield higher levels of consumption than global measures, they do not necessarily yield more accurate data.

When using short-term recall methods, interviewers request information about actual alcohol consumption for a short period of time, often the past week. This approach is based on the assumption that respondents have a better short-term memory for exact amounts of drinking over a short period of time as compared to a longer one. The most common approach is to ask respondents to cite the number of standard drinks consumed on each of the 7 days preceding the interview. Although the method is efficient and cost effective, it may overestimate abstinence and underestimate irregular, heavy, episodic drinking (5 or more standard drinks on one occasion for men and 4 or more standard drinks on one occasion for women [5+/4+ drinking]) (Dufour, 1999; Substance Abuse and Mental Health Services Administration (SAMHSA), 2001). In addition, it does not account for seasonal variation.

In diary methods, participants record each drink consumed over a given time frame either retrospectively or shortly after consumption. Perhaps the most detailed diary method is the Timeline Followback (TLFB) method introduced by Sobell and Sobell in the 1970s (Sobell, Maisto, Sobell, & Cooper, 1979; Sobell, Sobell, Leo, & Cancilla, 1988; Sobell, Toneatto, & Sobell, 1994). The TLFB is a retrospective diary method in which participants are asked to record an estimate of the amount of alcohol they consumed on each day for a prescribed period of time (Cunningham et al., 1999). The time frame can vary up to 12 months from the interview date. A calendar serves as a memory aid to enhance recall (Sobell, Brown, Leo, & Sobell, 1996). The TLFB method produces the following variables: drinks per drinking day, drinking days, days of abstinence, heavy drinking occasions (5+ drinking), weeks within the recommended drinking limits, and total ethanol consumption (total grams of ethanol based on standard drinks).

The psychometric properties of the TLFB method have been assessed in several studies. Correlation of self-reported drinking from both participants and collaterals (significant others who provide independent data on participants' drinking) ranged from 0.60 to 0.90 (Sobell & Sobell, 1992). Test–retest reliabilities on the TLFB method have been generally high (0.70 to 1.00) (Sobell et al., 1988). The obvious advantage of the TLFB method is that it provides detailed information on a variety of drinking patterns. A drawback to the retrospective diary method is that it prolongs the interview and increases subject burden. Cunningham et al. (1999) found that when surveys are mailed to respondents, 29% fewer respondents who received the TLFB returned their survey materials as compared with those respondents who received just a graduated frequency measure. Subject participation and retention may be negatively affected by the use of the TLFB procedure.

Alcohol Consumption:
Heavy Drinking Occasions and Variable Drinking Patterns

Measuring the quantity and frequency of ethanol intake is one approach to measuring alcohol consumption. Most scientists also include measures to distinguish meaningful variations in drinking patterns, such as the frequency of heavy, episodic drinking (Dawson, 1998a). Heavy, episodic drinking is defined as five or more drinks on one occasion, or "5+ drinking." Some scientist have been moving away from the term *binge* to refer to 5+ drinking because binge may imply very heavy drinking over a prolonged period of several days (Gill, 2002). Although "heavy, episodic drinking" is a common way to express 5+ drinking on a single occasion (Carey, 2001; Dawson, 1998b; NIAAA, 2002a), Murgraff,

Parrott, and Bennett (1999) recommended the use of the term *risky single-occasion drinking* (RSOD), and Measham (1996) referred to "heavy sessional drinking."

Lange and Voas (2001) raised further questions about the term *binge*. They noted: "It is, we feel, a mistake to use the term *binge* drinking on the basis of its value in predicting problems. Inherent in the concept of binge drinking is recognition that such drinking produces high blood alcohol concentrations (BACs)" (p. 331). They went on to report the results of their study, in which they found that young pedestrians heading into Tijuana, Mexico, from the United States to drink on the weekends had a mean number of 6.2 drinks for men and 4.1 drinks for women. Corresponding blood alcohol concentrations (BACs), respectively, were 0.09% and 0.08%. They concluded that currently used definitions of binge drinking predict relatively low BACs and may not capture the excessive drunkenness quality of the term. Perkins, Linkenback, and DeJong (2001) found a similar range of BACs in binge drinkers and concurred with Lange and Voas on the use of the term *binge*.

For the purpose of this review, the term *heavy, episodic drinking* will be used unless investigators used 5+ drinking as the outcome variable. The benefit of using the more generic term (heavy, episodic drinking) as compared to 5+ drinking is that it reflects gender differences. Heavy, episodic drinking is defined as drinking five or more drinks for men (5+) and four or more drinks for women (4+) on the same occasion on at least 1 day in the past 30 days. Although Midanik (1999) used the same definition (5+ drinking) for both men and women, NIAAA (SAMHSA, 2001) recommended that women be considered heavy, episodic drinkers when they exceed 4+ drinks on one occasion.

Heavy, episodic drinking in college students is assessed differently from other populations. College students are usually asked how often they have engaged in the behavior in the past 2 weeks rather than past month (Alcohol Policies Project, Center for Science in the Public Interest, 2000; NIAAA, 2002a). The reason for a shortened time frame in the college-age population is that heavy, episodic drinking is epidemic on college campuses. Scientists from NIAAA (2002b) reported that 40% to 50% of college students engaged in heavy, episodic drinking in the 2 weeks prior to being surveyed. Given the frequency of heavy, episodic drinking, most experts recommend asking college students about drinking patterns in the previous 2 weeks rather than the previous month.

Several other subtle points merit emphasis when discussing heavy, episodic drinking. Data resulting from questions about 4+/5+ drinking do not take into account the size and weight of the person or the duration of drinking, nor is it synonymous with intoxication (Carey, 2001).

What additional data do measures of variability in drinking provide for the investigator? Several investigators have found that when the dimension of 5+ drinking was combined with average alcohol intake, 5+ drinking identified drinkers at greater risk for alcohol-related problems and/or alcohol-related harm than average alcohol intake alone (Midanik, 1999; Midanik, Tam, Greenfield, & Caetano, 1996; Room, Bondy, & Ferris, 1995). The 4+/5+ definition identifies high-risk samples in different age groups and across gender (Bradley et al., 2001; Luczak, Wall, Shea, Byun, & Carr, 2001) and is particularly useful in survey studies and at a population level (Carey, 2001). These studies support the notion that quantity, frequency, and variability of drinking are crucial in determining risk. At this point, there is some consensus recommending the 4+/5+ definition (Perkins et al., 2001; Wechsler, Dowdall, Davenport, & Castillo, 1995) and the use of the term *heavy, episodic drinking* (Carey, 2001; Lange & Voas, 2001; NIAAA, 2002b) rather than *binge drinking*. Dawson (1998b) used both 5+ and 9+ drinking to further categorize heavy, episodic drinking; this differentiation should be further investigated to determine how well 9+ drinking predicts risk as compared to 4+/5+ drinking.

How does one quantify 5+ drinking episodes? One method is to use the graduate frequency approach. Interviewers ask participants to estimate how often in the past 30 days on one occasion (within 6 hours) they drank at each of the following levels: 12 or more drinks, 8–11 drinks, 5–7 drinks, 3–4 drinks, and 1–2 drinks. The frequency of 5+ drinking is derived by using only the 5–7, 8–11, and 12 or more intervals from the graduated frequency measure (Midanik, 1999). It is important to note that the intervals need to be modified for women to capture 4+ drinking. Of course, one occasion is not equivalent to 1 day. Lapham, Gregory, and McMillan (2003) provided the following example: If an individual has two 12 oz beers with lunch and three 5 oz glasses of wine with dinner, that situation would be considered two drinks on one occasion and three drinks on another. Therefore, it is helpful to define "one occasion" for subjects.

Another aspect of variability is to determine usual versus unusual drinking patterns. Dawson (1998b) recommended differentiating between usual and unusual patterns of drinking as well as type of beverage. She suggested 21 questions, with 7 questions each for beer, wine, or spirits. The questions include the following content for beer: (1) Do you ever drink beer? (2) How often do you drink beer each week? (3) How many beers do you drink on a usual drinking day? (4) What size of beer do you usually drink? (5) What is the most beer you have drunk in one day (heaviest day)? (6) What size beer did you drink on the heaviest drinking day? and (7) How many times in the past year did you drink in the same way that you drank on the heaviest day? Although these questions provide beverage-specific ethanol volumes and also capture variability, they add subject burden and cost to any study.

Alcohol Consumption: Perception of Drunkenness

As noted earlier, Lange and Voas (2001) found that 5+ drinking is not necessarily associated with excessive drinking and alcohol intoxication. Five+ drinking, therefore, cannot be equated to drinking to drunkenness or frequency of intoxication. This variable (frequency of intoxication) has been used as a subjective measure of excessive drinking since the 1960s (Midanik, 1999). Although the amount of alcohol needed to become drunk varies dramatically by consumption patterns, biological factors, and demographics, the mean number of drinks to achieve drunkenness reported by individuals who have been drunk at least once in the last year was 9.8 for males and 5.7 for females (Clark, 1982).

Drunkenness is defined as the amount of alcohol needed to cause intoxication. This measure is assessed by a questions such as, "How many drinks do you think you would have to have before you would feel drunk?" (Clark, 1982; Midanik, 1999) and "In your opinion, the last time you drank alcohol, were you (1) completely sober, (2) slightly drunk, (3) really drunk, or (4) so drunk that you passed out?" This question is followed by "Think back on your last drinking occasion and describe in your own words as accurately as you can what you drank and how much" (Lintonen & Rimpela, 2001).

Perception of drunkenness is a concept that helps investigators understand the consequences of drinking. Midanik (1999) compared three measures of heavy drinking (drunkenness, 5+ drinking, and feeling the effects of alcohol) to determine which was the best predictor of adverse events. She found that the frequency of drunkenness compared to the other measures was the best predictor of adverse social consequences of drinking, alcohol dependence, and alcohol-related harm. Interestingly, Nielsen (1999) found clear ethnic differences in the number of times drunk among 18- to 29-year-olds: the average times drunk in Whites was significantly higher than that of African Americans and Hispanics. Age of first drunkenness is also important. Hingson, Heeren, Winter, and Wechsler (2003) found that college students who reported being drunk before the age of 13 had 1.5 times greater odds of unplanned sex and 1.7 times greater odds of unprotected sex reportedly because of drinking. Thomas, Reifman, Barnes, and Farrell (2000) found that by delaying the onset of drunkenness, adolescents could diminish future levels of alcohol misuse and risk taking. Therefore, the measurement of the perception of drunkenness has particular utility for nurse-scientists investigating the role of alcohol in adolescent risk taking and alcohol-related adverse events.

Recommendations for Measurement of Quantity, Frequency, and Variability

Alcohol consumption can be quantified in a variety of ways, such as average grams or ounces of ethanol per day, standard drinks per day (or week or month), number of drinking occurrences per month, heavy drinking occasions per month, or frequency of perceived drunkenness. The choice of measure depends on the role of the variable in the study, the capabilities and demographics of the study or clinical population, the design of the study, the time available for assessment, and the resources available to collect alcohol consumption data.

Most alcohol research uses the multiplicative function of a quantity measure with a frequency measure (Rehm, 1998) that yields a calculated volume of ounces of ethanol per unit of time or number of standard drinks per unit of time. Measures of variability provide additional information about unusual drinking patterns and heavy, episodic drinking. The most refined procedures include quantity, frequency, and variability. One method to obtain more extensive data is Dawson's (1998b) approach of asking 21 questions, with 7 questions each for beer, wine, and spirits. The TLFB method (Sobell et al., 1996) also provides data on monthly alcohol consumption, both for usual and unusual months.

Capturing heavy, episodic drinking adds to the richness of the data. A disadvantage of using 5+/4+ drinking episodes rather than volume of ethanol or standard drinks is that a 5+/4+ episode is a categorical measure. Continuous data on alcohol consumption are reduced to a dichotomous measure (either 5+/4+ drinking or no 5+/4+ drinking), which is insensitive to differences between 1–2 drinks and 3–4 drinks, or 5 drinks as compared to 12 drinks. If measuring 5+/4+ drinking is critical to the research question, 5+/4+ drinking frequency (number of heavy, episodic drinking occasions per unit of time) is a better measure than 5+/4+ status (ever vs. never) (Carey, 2001).

If a limited time is available to obtain drinking data, two simple quantity/frequency questions are appropriate. Cherpitel (1997, p. 348) recommends: On average, how many days per week do you drink alcohol? and On a typical day when you drink, how may drinks do you have? The investigative team needs to make decisions about the measurement of alcohol consumption based on the methodological losses and gains of each technique. Along those lines, investigators need to consider the truthfulness of self-reported drinking by their subjects.

Critique of the Use of Self-Reported Measures: Quantity-Frequency, Heavy Drinking Occasions, and Variable Drinking Patterns

The measures of alcohol consumption discussed thus far have been derived from self-reported measures of drinking. Research on alcohol consumption has generally supported the use of self-reported data as a valid basis for measuring alcohol intake. Some disadvantages exist, however, and ongoing work is needed to support the validity of self-reported alcohol data.

Review articles (Babor, Brown, & Del Boca, 1990; Babor, Stephens, & Marlatt, 1987; Midanik, 1982b; Sobell & Sobell, 1990) have supported the validity of self-report as long as investigators implement certain methodological strategies during data collection. Sobell and Sobell (1990) noted that self-reports in those who misuse or abuse alcohol are generally truthful as long as the interviews are conducted in a clinical research setting, the respondent is alcohol-free at the time of the interview, and there is an assurance of confidentiality. Embree and Whitehead (1993) recommended four features in the self-reported survey instrument that can increase validity and reliability, including use of (1) detailed but separate questions about quantity, frequency, and variability of drinking; (2) questions of an incremental nature so that answers to each portion of the questions are summed to arrive at a final calculation; (3) a day (24-hour) period of reference; and (4) the concept of a standard drink. Most investigators implementing intervention trials using self-reported measures of alcohol consumption do not include a report of these features in their methods sections. It is difficult, therefore, to determine if investigators are maximizing the accuracy of their outcome measures.

Self-reported measures present several difficulties to investigators. They are usually retrospective rather than prospective in nature, thereby relying on subjects' perceptions of past drinking. They may be affected by factors such as the method of data collection, the setting, and the type of information sought (Kadden & Litt, 2004). The possible consequences of reporting alcohol misuse or abuse is also a consideration. Subjects participating in intervention studies to reduce alcohol-related vehicular crashes (in spite of assurances of confidentiality) may fear legal action if they report drinking to intoxication prior to driving. Pregnant women fear that self-reported alcohol use during pregnancy could have adverse effects on maintaining custody of the infant should a case be brought against them. Treatment status may also affect self-report. Midanik (1982a) found significant overreporting in people entering alcoholism treatment. The concerns about self-reported consumption have some basis in the literature. Although there is a general level of confidence in self-reports, investigators have often found a small proportion of inaccurate respondents (Sobell, Toneatto, Sobell, Leo, & Johnson, 1992; Sommers et al., 2000).

As noted earlier, review articles support the validity of self-report (Babor et al., 1987, 1990; Midanik, 1982b; Sobell & Sobell, 1990). Some investigators, however, illustrated that even when they report statistically significant findings, self-report is by no means an exact reflection of actual drinking patterns. Smith, McCarthy, and Goldman (1995) found a correlation between adolescents' self-reports and collaterals' reports of $r = 0.62$ for the total amount of alcohol consumed and $r = 0.64$ for the most alcohol consumed during any 1 day. Therefore, either the subjects themselves or their collateral informants were somewhat inaccurate. Paradoxically, in many studies when a collateral reports higher amounts of alcohol consumed than respondents, the respondent is considered to be a "denier," and the collateral maintains status as the more valid reporter. When a collateral reports less consumption, the collateral loses status as providing the more valid measure (Midanik, 1982b). The question for investigators becomes, therefore, who is the accurate reporter of alcohol consumption: the respondent or the collateral?

Other investigators compared self-reported alcohol use to biological measures. Sommers et al. (2000) found that the correlation between BAC and estimated blood alcohol concentration (EBAC) calculated from self-report was $r = 0.461$ ($p < .001$) in adults hospitalized after an alcohol-related injury. Although there is a statistically significant correlation, the mean difference between the BAC and EBAC was 91.87 mg/dl in men and 34.29 mg/dl in women. In short, both men and women underestimated their drinking, although self-reports reflected their general patterns of drinking. Fuller, Lee, and Gordis (1988) found that approximately 59% of patients in a treatment program relapsed when self-reported alcohol consumption was used as the primary variable, whereas when laboratory tests of blood and urine were performed as well, 72% of the subjects showed evidence of relapse. When compared with laboratory measures, therefore, self-reported measures of drinking in most settings seem to reflect lower levels of drinking than do laboratory measures.

Self-report has also been found to have monthly variations. Cho et al. (2001) found that self-reported alcohol consumption was significantly more accurate in January than in March. They recommended that investigators consider seasonal variations to minimize seasonal bias.

Finally, no standard self-reported variables are chosen for use across all intervention trials. Inconsistencies among outcome variables and the lack of standardization of assessment methods make cross-trial comparisons difficult. Kadden and Litt (2004) recommended that two measures of self-reported consumption be used for alcohol treatment studies: drinking frequency with the number of days abstinent and drinking intensity with the number of days of heavy drinking (6 or more standard drinks in 24 hours for men and 4 or more standard drinks in 24 hours for women). They also recommended that consequences of drinking be measured by psychometric instruments. To remedy the lack of standardization in intervention trials, a consensus conference at the National Institutes of Health might resolve the situation so that trial results could be compared across intervention trials.

With the qualifications discussed above, scientists generally support the use of self-reported data for research purposes as long as methodological strategies are used to increase their accuracy. Clinicians are uneven in their trust of self-reported alcohol data (Sommers, Dyehouse, Howe, Wekselman, & Fleming, 2002). Future research will refine methods to collect accurate self-reported data. Teasing out the strategies to enhance the accuracy of self-report depending on gender, age, and ethnicity is critical to future research. Choosing the self-reported variables that are most likely to change over time and most likely to lead to improved health in response to interventions is essential to further knowledge development. Assessing the validity and reliability of collateral reports is also an important issue if scientists continue to use collaterals as a source of consumption data. Finally, identifying which biological variables are best used to shore up self-reported variables warrants further investigation. With this issue in mind, the discussion in this chapter moves to a review and critique of laboratory measures of alcohol consumption.

LABORATORY MEASURES OF ALCOHOL (ETHANOL) CONSUMPTION

A variety of laboratory tests is used to determine recent, short-term, and long-term alcohol consumption. Although the terms *alcohol* and *ethanol* (ethyl alcohol) are often used interchangeably, ethanol is one of several types of alcohol and is present in fermented and distilled liquors. To identify levels of immediate alcohol use (within 72 hours of drinking), scientists use blood, breath, saliva, and urine analyses of ethanol levels. These tests determine the ethanol levels or the immediate products from ethanol metabolism in body fluids. To assess drinking that has occurred during the short to mid-range time period (1–6 weeks after heavy drinking), scientists use markers that reflect ethanol effects on body organs or cellular processes. These tests include carbohydrate-deficient transferrin (CDT) and γ glutamyl transferase (GGT). Mean corpuscular volume (MCV) and alanine aminotransferase (ALT) reflect the long-range metabolic and organic changes that occur with more than 6 weeks of heavy drinking.

Tests Used to Assess Drinking during the Immediate Period

Ethyl alcohol is completely miscible (capable of being mixed) in water and is distributed throughout the total body water by simple diffusion (Sommers, Savage, Wray, & Dyehouse, 2003; Venes 2001). Measures of ethanol in body fluids (particularly blood) or exhaled air remain the laboratory standard for quantifying immediate alcohol use.

The concentration of ethanol in all body fluids (as measured in blood, saliva, and urine) can be measured by either gas chromatography or the enzymatic method. Gas chromatography is the reference method (as close to the gold standard as possible) for ethanol levels (Bishop, Duben-Engelkirk, & Fody, 2000; Musshoff, 2002; Nine, Moraca, Virji, & Rao, 1995) and can also be used to quantify other volatile alcohols, such as methanol and isopropanol. An important differentiation exists between gas chromatography and the enzymatic method. Whereas gas chromatography allows the scientist to identify the concentration of each alcohol present, the enzymatic method is not specific to ethanol. The presence of isopropanol and (with some test kits) methanol to prepare the skin prior to venapuncture may interfere with the accuracy of the enzymatic method (Bishop et al., 2000; Ravel, 1995; Sommers, Savage, et al., 2003). In addition, if a subject in a research study or patient has ingested a mixture of alcohols, the enzymatic method will not differentiate among them. Whenever possible, gas chromatography should be used for ethanol analysis of body fluids in clinical and research protocols.

Blood Analysis

Blood alcohol concentration is the level of ethanol in whole blood or serum. After recent drinking, ethanol is rapidly absorbed into the bloodstream from the stomach and small intestine and is distributed into the total body water (Pincus & Abraham, 2001). The BAC is calculated using the weight of ethanol (milligrams [mg]) and the volume of blood (deciliter [dl]). This calculation yields a BAC that can be expressed as a proportion (mg/dl) or as a percentage (% ethanol by volume). It is important to determine whether samples are derived from serum or whole blood. Serum contains more alcohol than whole blood by a factor of 1.18:1. For example, a whole blood specimen with an ethanol level of 100 mg/dl would have a serum ethanol value of 118 mg/dl. Whether serum or whole blood is used, the BAC is the most appropriate measure to quantify immediate alcohol consumption and has a sensitivity and specificity of at least 99% when appropriate controls are in place with gas chromatography (Musshoff, 2002; Sommers et al., 2001). The normal range for BAC is listed in Table 2.2.

Blood alcohol concentration is influenced by both ethanol absorption and metabolism. Factors that affect BAC include rates of ethanol absorption from the gastrointestinal tract, whether or not food was ingested with the ethanol, the amount and type of food ingested, the rate of gastric emptying, the length of the drinking episode, the type of beverage(s) ingested, and the demographics of the individual subject. For individuals with normal liver function, ethanol is metabolized at a rate of one standard drink every 60 to 90 minutes; in general, when a nondependent individual is intoxicated, BAC will be reduced by 15 mg/dl (0.015%) per hour following a drinking episode (Fleming, Mihic, & Harris, 2001).

Critique of the Current Research on BAC

Although the BAC is the metric of choice to determine immediate alcohol use, several issues exist with its interpretation. Women demonstrate a 35% to 45% higher blood ethanol level for a given amount of ethanol than men because the female's body contains proportionately less body water than males (Davies & Bowen, 1999). At a given BAC, an investigator cannot assume that men and women have ingested the same number of standard drinks. Gender differences in alcohol absorption and metabolism remain an important area for investigation. Women who use birth control pills experience a higher, more sustained level of blood ethanol than those who do not. In addition, during the premenstrual

TABLE 2.2   Laboratory Tests to Detect Presence of Alcohol or Physiologic Effects of Alcohol

Laboratory test	Timing*	Normal range**	Sensitivity**	Specificity**
BAC	Immediate	Negative (0–10 mg/dl)	> 99%	> 99%
Saliva alcohol	Immediate	Negative (< 10 mg/dl)	> 99%	> 99%
Breath alcohol	Immediate	Negative (< 10 mg/dl)	> 99%	> 99%
Urine alcohol	Immediate	Negative (< 10 mg/dl)	> 99%	> 99%
Serum and urine methanol	Immediate	Methanol < 1.0 mg/L in blood or urine	Not reported	Not reported
5HTOL/ 5HIAA	Immediate	< 15 pmol/ nmol	Not reported	Not reported
WBAA	Short to mid-range	< 9 micro-moles/liter	67%	77%
CDT	Short-range	0–26 u/L for women; 0–20 u/L for men	82% (range: 12–91%)	97% (range: 87–97%)
GGT	Short-range	Females: 6–45 u/L Males: 5–30 u/L	70% (range: 34–85%)	59–95%
MCV	Long-range	80–100 femtoliters	60% (range: 29–90%)	76–90%
AST	Long-range	6–25 u/L	70% (range: 27–77%)	68%
ALT	Long-range	3–30 u/L	58%	57%

ALT = alanine aminotransferase; AST = aspartate aminotransferase; BAC = blood alcohol concentration; CDT = carbohydrate deficient transferrin; 5HIAA = 5-hydroxyindoleacetic acid; 5HTOL = urine 5-hydroxytryptophol; GGT = γ (gamma) glutamyl transferase; MCV = mean corpuscular volume; u/L = units per liter; WBAA = whole blood associated acetaldehyde.

*Timing of positive test: Immediate range = 0–72 hours after alcohol consumption; short-range = 7–28 days after heavy drinking; mid-range = 4–6 weeks after heavy drinking; long-range > 6 weeks or more of heavy drinking or alcohol dependence.

**Normal ranges and sensitivity/specificity information are from Kaplan et al. (1995); Meerkerk et al. (1999); Ravel (1995); Rukstalis et al. (2002); Sharpe (2001); Sillanaukee et al. (1999); Wallach (2000).

period, peak ethanol levels occur more rapidly and reach a higher level than during ovulation. These differences may occur because fluid shifts during ovulation increase total body water and lead to ethanol dilution (Lucey, Hill, Young, Demo-Dananberg, & Beresford, 1999; Wallach, 2000). Even in light of these gender differences, no recommendations exist to help investigators control for these variations when studying alcohol levels in young women.

Age differences create an equally problematic issue for investigators. Elderly persons become intoxicated and reach higher peak ethanol levels more quickly than younger persons (Wallach, 2000). This effect occurs because of the decrease in body water consequent to aging (Davies & Bowen, 1999; Lucey et al., 1999). Elderly persons of either gender have higher blood ethanol levels than younger persons when ethanol is taken without food. Age differences, however, can be eliminated when ethanol is ingested with a carbohydrate meal (Lucey et al., 1999). As with gender differences, more research is needed to guide future investigations. For study populations across the life span, definitive work is needed so that drinking outcomes as measured with BAC can be compared across age, gender, and eating patterns.

Ethanol elimination rates also remain an area for further study. Estimation of the ethanol elimination rate has been based on either normal volunteers or dependent drinkers (Brennan, Betzelos, Reed, & Falk, 1995); studies of elimination rates have not occurred in the general hospital population, or in the primary care population. Brennan et al. (1995) found that the rate of ethanol elimination was 19.6 mg/dl per hour in a small sample ($N = 24$) of emergency department patients, but further work in this area is necessary with larger samples before ethanol elimination rates can be predicted with accuracy in hospitalized patients.

Breath, Saliva, and Urine Analyses

Although BAC analyzed with gas chromatography is generally considered the gold standard to reflect immediate alcohol use (Musshoff, 2002), ethanol levels can be measured from breath, saliva, and urine. An exhaled breath can be analyzed to determine alcohol consumption in the immediate past. Breath contains ethanol after ingestion because the lung capillaries are permeable to ethanol; there is a fairly consistent equilibrium of ethanol to alveolar air (2,100:1) as compared to blood. Breath ethanol levels can be extrapolated to whole blood ethanol levels by multiplying measured breath ethanol by the factor 2,100 (range 1,837–2,863) (Gibb, Yee, Johnson, Martin, & Nowack, 1984; McClatchy, 1994; Sommers, Savage, et al., 2003).

A drawback to breath ethanol analysis is that several substances such as ketone bodies may interfere with ethanol measurement (Ravel, 1995). Acetylaldehyde, 2-butanol, gasoline, isoprene, isopropanol, and methanol are also measured in small amounts, but the response is so small that it does not interfere with ethanol measurement (Intoximeters, 2002; Sommers et al., 2003). Measurements are also determined by the subject's effort to exhale. If the subject has a chronic lung condition or respiratory muscle weakness, or is unable to follow instructions, the investigator might not be able to obtain an accurate measurement or any measurement at all. Finally, data collection requires subject preparation (see discussion below on saliva analysis).

Analysis of saliva can also be used to determine drinking in the immediate past. By simple diffusion, ethanol is distributed in the total body water and then excreted in saliva. The saliva ethanol/blood ethanol ratio is variable but in the range of 1.04 to 1.14. Scientists have found correlations of 0.96 to 0.99 between saliva ethanol levels and BAC (Bates & Martin, 1997; Wallach, 2000). Data collection for saliva analysis presents some challenges to the investigator. Specimen collection is difficult in individuals with a very dry mouth, and, like breath analysis subjects need adequate preparation for saliva analysis. For 15 minutes prior to testing, subjects cannot ingest ethanol, food, or drink, nor should they rinse with mouthwash. In addition, saliva ethanol testing does not identify an ethanol concentration below 20 mg/dl (Wallach, 2000).

Ethanol is excreted in the urine, which reflects drinking in the immediate period even after blood alcohol levels have fallen to zero. A positive urine ethanol analysis indicates ethanol ingestion within the past 8 hours and is used to confirm recent drinking. Because blood/urine ratios are highly dependent on bladder stasis, the individual's level of hydration, and glomerular filtration rates, urine ethanol levels are generally not used as legal evidence for intoxication. Urine/blood ratios, therefore, are highly variable but usually approximate 1:3 (Jacobs et al., 1994; McClatchy, 1994). False-positive urine ethanol levels may occur in diabetic patients and those with urinary tract infections due to an organism that can ferment ethanol, such as *Candida albicans* (Medical Algorithms Project, 2004; Sommers, Savage, et al., 2003).

Another urine analysis that will reflect drinking that has occurred within the past 12 hours is the urine 5-hydroxytryptophol (5HTOL)/5-hydroxyindoleacetic acid (5HIAA) ratio. 5HTOL and 5HIAA are the products of serotonin metabolism, and without ethanol intake, the urinary ratio of 5HTOL to 5HIAA is very low (< 0.01). When acetaldehyde derived from ethanol competes with the aldehyde formed from serotonin, a switch in the metabolic pathway occurs, and the 5HTOL/5HIAA ratio increases and remains elevated (50 to 100 times normal) for more than 5 to 10 hours after ethanol is cleared from the blood (Helander & Eriksson, 2002; Jones & Helander, 1999). The urine 5HTOL/5HIAA ratio thus becomes a marker for recent ethanol ingestion even after blood, urine, and saliva analyses are negative for ethanol. In particular, it is used as a "morning after" test of abstinence as part of some treatment programs. A person might consume moderate amounts of ethanol the previous evening and provide an early morning urine sample negative for ethanol but with an elevated 5HTOL/5HIAA ratio (Jones & Helander, 1999).

In summary, BAC as measured by gas chromatography is the method of choice to determine drinking in the immediate period. This technique, however, requires a venapuncture and the quality controls inherent with any laboratory analysis. Breath analysis is used widely among investigators because it is a relatively inexpensive and noninvasive technique, but subjects need to be cooperative in order to obtain the measurement. Saliva and urine analyses also provide data on immediate drinking patterns, but just as with the BAC, all measures of immediate drinking can be affected by age and gender, as well as by error introduced during laboratory instrumentation.

To refine our understanding of all of these measurement strategies, more research is needed. Large-scale investigations exploring the effects of gender and age as well as variables such as ingestion of food and the role of organ dysfunction are needed to clarify our understanding of the laboratory measurement of immediate alcohol consumption. Studies that compare BAC to analyses of breath, saliva, and urine in a variety of populations are also needed to explore the differences in the accuracy and precision of measurements across populations.

Tests Used to Assess Drinking during the Short-Term and Mid-Range Period

Several laboratory tests can be used to assess drinking patterns over the short term (several weeks). Short-term drinking results in products from alcohol metabolism. During ethanol metabolism, acetaldehyde molecules are released in a free state and change the structure and function of a wide variety of proteins. In addition, acetaldehyde is a liver toxin (Bishop et al., 2000). In particular, acetaldehyde binds to many proteins, including albumin, hemoglobin, and transferrin. One laboratory test in particular is appropriate to assess a recent period of drinking: the measurement of carbohydrate-deficient transferrin.

CDT is a transferrin isoform (a protein having the same function as another protein and similar composition but is the product of a different gene). Transferrin is a globulin that binds and transports iron; CDT contains fewer sialic acid molecules than normal transferrin and therefore is called carbohydrate-*deficient* transferrin, indicating its abnormal form (Ravel, 1995; Stibler, 1991). CDT elevation with ethanol misuse and abuse is thought to occur from a multistep process not clearly understood at this time (Anton, Stout, Roberts, & Allen, 1998; Sillanaukee, Strid, Allen, & Litten, 2001). It is known that the transferrin abnormality allows the investigator to measure the accumulated effect of alcohol consumption; elevations appear after regular intake of 50 to 80 g of ethanol per day for at least 1 week with a half-life of 15 days during periods of abstinence (Stibler, 1991). CDT is also used to detect chronic use (Figlie, Benedito-Silva, Monteiro, & Souza-Formigoni, 2002).

A variety of gender and life span considerations exist with the use of CDT. It appears to be the most accurate test to predict heavy drinking in men but not in women. Using the criterion for number of drinks per day, sensitivity of CDT for women is 33% and for men 56%. Using the criteria for heavy drinking days, sensitivity of CDT for women is 40% and for men is 72% (Oslin et al., 1998). At similar levels of drinking, ethanol-dependent women present a lower prevalence of abnormal CDT than ethanol-dependent men (Figlie et al., 2002). The reasons for these differences are complex but can be partly explained because women produce CDT under natural conditions such as during pregnancy, estrogen replacement, and anemia; in addition, they may produce less CDT than men in response to heavy drinking (Anton, 2001). CDT also appears to be a more sensitive measure than other laboratory tests to reflect patterns of drinking in men than women. Burke et al. (1998) found that CDT was sensitive to changes in drinking in men with even relatively low alcohol intake (20 to 60 g per day). CDT may be the best single ethanol biological marker available in the primary care male population (Conigrave et al., 2002). Age-related changes also affect the CDT's usefulness. Young men ages 20 to 40 years have higher sensitivities and specificities for CDT (83% and 87%, respectively) as compared with older men and women (Yersin et al., 1995).

In the 20 years that CDT has been available, a series of approximately 100 manuscripts have been published describing the effectiveness of the test as a marker for alcohol consumption. In their comprehensive review, Koch et al. (2004) noted that previous studies do not include adequate samples of women, nor do enough of the investigations include homogenous samples from which sound conclusions can be drawn regarding specificity and sensitivity. The authors also stated that study populations consisting of subjects with a broad spectrum of diseases merit investigation rather than comparing dependent drinkers with controls (abstainers). Much work remains to be done in understanding the usefulness of CDT across relevant subpopulations.

Tests Used to Assess Drinking during the Long-Range Period

For many years, a standard battery of laboratory tests was used to identify problem or dependent drinkers. These tests include γ-glutamyl transferase, mean corpuscular volume, and serum aspartate aminotransferase and alanine aminotransferase.

GGT is an enzyme involved in the transfer of γ-glutamyl residue from peptides to amino acids, water, and other small peptides (Bishop et al., 2000). Because GGT is bound to the surface of the plasma membrane of liver cells, this location makes the release of the enzyme a very sensitive indicator of all hepatobiliary disorders (Kaplan, Jack, Opheim, Toivola, & Lyon, 1995). During periods of heavy drinking, hepatic cellular toxicity occurs with leakage of GGT across the cell membrane into the blood. Because GGT increases can often be noted before the onset of pathological consequences of drinking, serum GGT levels may be used as a screening tool to identify problem drinkers who have no overt physical symptoms (Anton et al., 1998; Ravel, 1995; Sacher & McPherson, 1991).

As with other laboratory markers, age and gender play a role in the specificity and sensitivity of the tests. Normal values are thought to be lower for premenopausal women because of suppression of enzyme activity due to estrogen and progesterone (Bishop et al., 2000). In both men and women, GGT is more affected by drinking intensity (drinks per drinking day) than by frequency (number of days drinking); GGT is helpful in determining intermittent, high-level heavy episodic drinking in men and women (Anton et al., 1998). CDT seems to be a better screen for heavy ethanol use in males, whereas GGT is more accurate in females (Allen, Sillanaukee, & Anton, 1999). GGT also has higher sensitivities and specificities (74% and 70%, respectively) in older as compared to younger men (Yersin et al., 1995).

The mean corpuscular volume is the volume of an average red blood cell. The MCV is calculated by dividing the hematocrit value by the erythrocyte count (Ravel, 1995). Increased MCV occurs with heavy drinking and dependence because of the effects of ethanol on the erythrocyte membrane and perhaps by folic acid deficiency in dependent drinkers (Ravel, 1995). Parmahamsa, Reedy, and Varadacharyulu (2004) speculated that the change in the erythrocyte membrane was due to an increase in microviscosity, consequent decrease in membrane fluidity, and an increased lipid peroxidation leading to structural damage in dependent drinkers. MCV is not helpful for monitoring acute episodes of heavy drinking because of its prolonged half-life (Sommers, Savage, et al., 2003). The highest sensitivities and specificities occur in older men (Yersin et al., 1995).

Serum aspartate aminotransferase and alanine aminotransferase are found in almost every tissue and fluid of the body, with particularly high concentrations in the cells of the heart and liver. They belong to the class of enzymes called transferases and are important in the transfer of amino groups during synthesis and degradation of amino acids. Heavy or chronic drinking leads to increased cell permeability to transferases, cell lysis and necrosis, and release of transferases into the blood. Generally, the sensitivity of AST to detect chronic drinking is somewhat higher than that of the ALT level (Wallach, 2000). Age, gender, and race play a role in the accuracy of tests to predict chronic alcohol use. Childhood, adolescence, and pregnancy elevate ALT levels and render it a less sensitive test for those populations. The ALT is normally 1.5 times higher in African American males and 1.8 times higher in Hispanic males than in European males. In addition, European male values are 40% higher, African American females are 20% higher, and Hispanic females are 40% higher than those of European females (Ravel, 1995). These factors are important in large studies with diverse populations and, if not considered during analysis, may add "noise" to data that masks the effects of drinking.

Summary and Critique: Analysis of Laboratory Measures of Alcohol Consumption

The use of biological markers to assess alcohol consumption is complex and requires considerable analysis of the literature. In particular, the sensitivity and specificity of biological markers vary based on the subjects' ages, gender, drinking patterns, behavior (obesity, smoking) and genetic makeup (Anton, 2001; Meerkerk, Njoo, Bongers, Trienekens, & van Oers, 1999; Sommers, Savage, et al., 2003). Some recommendations can be made based on the current literature. In a population-based study of 4,310 adult men and women across the life span, the association of alcohol consumption to laboratory markers was strongest for the GGT followed by the CDT and MCV (Alte et al., 2003). For studies that enroll men only, Conigrave et al. (2002) recommended the CDT as the best single ethanol marker available in the primary care male population.

Using biological markers in females is much more complex than in males because of the hormonal changes that occur during the childbearing years and pregnancy. The MCV and GGT appear to be the most efficient laboratory markers for detecting heavy drinking during pregnancy (Sarkola, Eriksson, Neimela, Sillanaukee, & Halmesmaki, 2000). In a systematic review of studies including CDT as a marker of dependent drinking, Salaspuro (1999) found that the GGT was a more sensitive marker for heavy drinking in women than was CDT. Sillanaukee, Ponnio, and Seppa (1999) found that the sensitivity of the MCV to predict heavy drinking is higher in women than in men, but not as high as the GGT (60% sensitivity for the GGT in women and 52% sensitivity for the MCV). Therefore, the GGT appears at this time to be the most appropriate single biological marker to assess mid- and long-term drinking in women.

The choice of marker is also dependent on age. Both older men and women become intoxicated and reach higher peak ethanol levels more quickly than do younger persons, probably because of a decrease in total body water that occurs with aging (Wallach, 2000). The sensitivity of both the GGT and MCV increases with age in males (Yersin et al., 1995); both are useful in studies of elderly men. GGT and MCV are more sensitive throughout adulthood in women and may continue to be so in late adulthood, although further work is needed in this area.

Finally, combining several tests is most likely a solution for investigators (Allen et al., 1999; Sillanaukee et al, 1999; van Pelt, Leusink, van Nierop, & Keyzer, 2000). Harasymiw and Bean (2001) found that by using a combination of 25 chemistry and hematology analyses at a cost of $15 per subject, they were able to identify 88% of heavy drinkers and 92% of light drinkers. Sillanaukee et al. (2000) found that, in a sample of approximately 7,000 men and women ages 25 to 74 years, a combined marker (CDT and GGT) called the γCDT performed better than the GGT or the CDT alone, and correlated strongly with alcohol-related factors. The highest sensitivity (95.5%) was found in women.

Many of the studies reported in the literature have small sample sizes and lack reports of power analysis calculations. White males, alcohol dependents, and abstainers are overrepresented in published studies, whereas women, minorities, moderate drinkers, problem drinkers, and healthy populations are underrepresented. Except for alcohol dependents, few studies consider populations with other diseases and disorders. Studies are often clinical in nature, and laboratory measures and equipment lack rigorous quality control specifications. Certainly more work is merited to determine the best laboratory marker or combinations of markers to predict drinking in the immediate, mid-term, and long-term period. Life span and gender issues in particular complicate the sensitivity and specificity of laboratory analyses, but until a gold standard emerges to assess mid- and long-term drinking patterns, a combination of markers appears the best strategy for investigators. In reality, different gold standards are likely warranted for cohorts such as young and middle-aged men, young and middle-aged women, older men, and older women.

ALCOHOL USE DISORDERS IDENTIFICATION TEST (AUDIT)

The AUDIT is a particularly useful psychometric instrument that is used to measure hazardous and harmful drinking and can also be used to quantify consumption. A complete review of psychometric instruments used to assess alcohol consumption is available in Cherpitel (1997) and Sommers, Wray, Savage, and Dyehouse (2003). Through the efforts of a World Health Organization collaborative, the AUDIT was constructed by means of psychometric testing in six countries ($N = 1,905$) (Allen et al., 1997; NIAAA, 2000b; Saunders et al., 1993). The intent of the developers was to construct a brief screening scale to identify individuals with alcohol problems, including those in the early as compared to the dependent phases of alcohol misuse (Reinhart & Allen, 2002). The instrument contains 10 questions that cover three conceptual domains: alcohol consumption, drinking behavior, and alcohol-related problems. With the exception of the last two items, the questions refer to drinking patterns during the previous year. Items were selected for inclusion in the AUDIT based on their ability to discriminate hazardous or harmful drinkers from those without hazardous/harmful drinking patterns. In the initial testing using a cut point of 8, the sensitivity of AUDIT for hazardous alcohol consumption was 95% to 100%, alcohol problems in the last year was 91% to 100%, and alcohol dependence syndrome was 100%. Interscale reliability of the three conceptual domains had mean alpha coefficients of 0.93 for drinking behavior and 0.81 for adverse psychological reactions (Saunders et al., 1993). In addition, AUDIT scores were found to be significantly correlated ($r = 0.31$; $p < .01$ to $.51$; $p < .001$) with a series of biochemical measures used to predict heavy alcohol use (Bohn, Babor, & Kranzler, 1995).

The first three questions of the AUDIT, those that are associated with the domain of alcohol consumption, are sometimes used to measure quantity, frequency, and variability. The questions are as follows: (1) How often do you have a drink containing alcohol? (response set: never; monthly or less; 2–4 times per month; 2–3 times per week; 4+ times per week); (2) How many drinks containing alcohol do you have on a typical day when you are drinking? (response set: 1 or 2; 3 or 4; 5 or 6; 7–9; 10 or more); (3) How often do you have six or more drinks on one occasion? (response set: never; less than monthly; monthly; weekly; daily or almost daily) (Saunders et al., 1993). The drawback of using these questions rather than more standard questions of quantity, frequency, and variability is that the data are categorical rather than ratio based, reducing the options for statistical analysis and data interpretation. The AUDIT-C uses the three alcohol consumption questions as a brief screening test for heavy drinking and performs as well as the full AUDIT in men but not women (Aertgeerts, Buntinx, Ansoms, & Fevery, 2001; Bush, Kivlahan, McDonell, Fihn, & Bradley, 1998).

The AUDIT is the best instrument to use in clinical populations with a range of alcohol use, from sensible drinking, to hazardous and harmful drinking, to alcohol dependence. Two extensive reviews of research using AUDIT (Allen et al., 1997; Reinert & Allen, 2002) concluded that research supports the use of AUDIT as a means for screening for alcohol use disorders in health care settings across a variety of populations. Additional research is needed to assess the psychometric properties in non-English-speaking populations and other special populations such as adolescents.

CONCLUSION

Taken as a whole, the scientific literature provides certain clear signposts about alcohol consumption. When eliciting self-reports of alcohol consumption, the interviewer would do well to stress the standard drink definition and create a setting where the respondent has a safe and confidential environment for reporting drinking. Quantity and frequency measures are essential, and measures of variability provide additional information about unusual drinking patterns and heavy, episodic drinking. Self-reports in general can be used with confidence if the investigator or clinician uses certain strategies known to enhance the validity of self-reported drinking. Further research is needed to develop strategies to improve the validity of self-report and to understand the role of collateral reports and biological measures.

The blood alcohol concentration with gas chromatography is considered the gold standard to quantify drinking in the early hours after alcohol consumption. Other body fluids and breath can also be analyzed for ethanol content, but each of the techniques has its own drawbacks. Total body water distribution and sex hormones can change the rate of ethanol distribution and metabolism, as can food and gastric transit time. A BAC across all populations cannot be attributed to the same level of drinking. For short-term drinking, particularly among young and middle-aged men, carbohydrate-deficient transferrin has shown the strongest evidence as a sensitive and specific biological marker. For more long-term drinking, the γ-glutamyl transferase level is the most sensitive and specific across all populations. Biological markers require further refinement to identify markers that are more sensitive and specific for mid-range and long-range drinking patterns and in women and special populations.

The science of quantifying alcohol consumption has advanced since the 1930s, when it became a topic of interest. Nurse-scientists use consumption variables for a multitude of reasons, such as outcome measures for clinical trials, inclusion/exclusion criteria, and descriptions of populations in epidemiologic studies. Clinicians use these measurement techniques to make a diagnosis of alcohol dependence, to assess the value of alcohol treatment programs, or to tailor an intervention to reduce risky behavior. Although complex and in need of further research, the quantification of alcohol consumption has become an important strategy for both investigators and clinicians, and by increasing the scientific understanding of alcohol measurement strategies, nurses can move to improve health outcomes for the population we serve.

ACKNOWLEDGMENTS

This work was supported in part by the National Center for Injury Prevention and Control, Centers for Disease Control and Prevention, Grant R49/CCR-523225.

REFERENCES

Adams, W. L., Barry, K. L., & Fleming, M. F. (1996). Screening for problem drinking in older primary care patients. *Journal of the American Medical Association, 276*, 1964–1967.

Aertgeerts, B., Buntinx, F., Ansoms, S., & Fevery, J. (2001). Screening properties of questionnaires and laboratory tests for the detection of alcohol abuse or dependence in a general practice population. *British Journal of General Practice, 51*, 206–217.

Alanko, T. (1984). An overview of techniques and problems in the measurement of alcohol consumption. *Research Advances in Alcohol and Drug Problems, 8*, 209–226.

Alcohol Policies Project, Center for Science in the Public Interest. (2000). Fact sheet: Binge drinking on college campuses. Retrieved October 1, 2004, from http://www. cspinet.org/booze/collfact1.htm

Allen, J. P., Litten, R. Z., Fertig, J. B., & Babor, T. F. (1997). A review of research on the Alcohol Use Disorders Identification Test (AUDIT). *Alcoholism: Clinical and Experimental Research, 21,* 613–619.

Allen, J. P., Maisto, S. A., & Connors, G. J. (1995). Self-report screening tests for alcohol problems in primary care. *Archives of Internal Medicine, 155,* 1726–1730.

Allen, J. P., Sillanaukee, P., & Anton, R. (1999). Contribution of carbohydrate deficient transferrin to gamma glutamyl transpeptidase in evaluating progress of patients in treatment for alcoholism. *Alcoholism: Clinical and Experimental Research, 23,* 115–120.

Alte, D., Ludemann, J., Piek, M., Adam, C., Rose, H., & John, U. (2003). Distribution and dose response of laboratory markers to alcohol consumption in a general population: Results of the study of health in Pomerania. *Journal of Studies on Alcohol, 64,* 75–82.

American Society of Addiction Medicine (ASAM). (2001). The definition of alcoholism. Retrieved October 1, 2004, from http://www.asam.org/ppol/Definition%20of%20 Alcoholism.htm

Anton, R. F. (2001). Carbohydrate-deficient transferrin for detection and monitoring of sustained heavy drinking. *Alcohol, 25,* 185–188.

Anton, R. F., Stout, R. L., Roberts, J. S., & Allen, J. P. (1998). The effect of drinking intensity and frequency on serum carbohydrate-deficient transferrin and γ-glutamyl transferase levels in outpatient alcoholics. *Alcoholism: Clinical and Experimental Research, 22,* 1456–1462.

Babor, T. F., Brown, J., & Del Boca, F. K. (1990). Validity of self-reports in applied research on addictive behaviors: Fact or fiction? *Behavioral Assessment, 12,* 5–31.

Babor, T. F., Stephens, R. S., & Marlatt, G. A. (1987). Verbal report methods in clinical research on alcoholism: Response bias and its minimization. *Journal of Studies on Alcohol, 48,* 410–424.

Banwell, C. (1999). How many standard drinks are there in a glass of wine? *Drug and Alcohol Review, 18,* 99–101.

Barry, K. L., & Fleming, M. F. (1993). The Alcohol Use Disorders Identification Test (AUDIT) and the SMAST-13: Predictive validity in a rural primary care sample. *Alcohol and Alcoholism, 28,* 33–42.

Bates, M. E., & Martin, C. (1997). Immediate, quantitative estimation of blood alcohol concentration from saliva. *Journal of Studies on Alcohol, 58,* 531–538.

Bendtsen, P., Jones, A. W., & Helander, A. (1998). Urinary excretion of methanol and 5-hydroxytryptophol as biochemical markers of recent drinking in the hangover state. *Alcohol and Alcoholism, 33,* 431–438.

Bishop, M. L., Duben-Engelkirk, J. L., & Fody, E. P. (2000). *Clinical chemistry: Principles, procedures, correlations* (4th ed.). Philadelphia: Lippincott.

Bohn, M. J., Babor, T. F., & Kranzler, H. R. (1995). The Alcohol Use Disorders Identification Test (AUDIT): Validation of a screening instrument for use in medical settings. *Journal of Studies on Alcohol, 56,* 423–432.

Bradley, K. A., Bush, K. R., Davis, T. M., Dobie, D. J., Burman, M. L., Rutter, C. M., et al. (2001). Binge drinking among female Veterans Affairs patients: Prevalence and associated risks. *Psychology of Addictive Behaviors, 15,* 297–305.

Brennan, D. F., Betzelos, S., Reed, R., & Falk, J. (1995). Ethanol elimination rates in an ED population. *American Journal of Emergency Medicine, 13,* 276–280.

Burke, V., Puddey, I., Rakic, V., Swanson, N., Dimmitt, S., Beilin, L., et al. (1998). Carbohydrate-deficient transferrin as a marker of change in alcohol intake in men

drinking 20 to 60 g of alcohol per day. *Alcoholism: Clinical and Experimental Research,*
22, 1973–1980.

Bush, K., Kivlahan, D. R., McDonnel, M. B., Fihn, S. D., & Bradley, K. A. (1998). The
AUDIT alcohol consumption questions (AUDIT-C): An effective brief screening test
for problem drinking. *Archives of Internal Medicine, 158*, 1789–1795.

Carey, K. B. (2001). Understanding binge drinking: Introduction to the special issue.
Psychology of Addictive Behavior, 15, 283–286.

Chang, G., Goetz, M. A., Wilkins-Haug, L., & Berman, S. (2000). A brief intervention
for prenatal alcohol use. *Journal of Substance Abuse Treatment,18*, 365–369.

Cherpitel, C. J. (1997). Brief screening instruments for alcoholism. *Alcohol Health and
Research World, 21*, 348–351.

Cho, Y. I., Johnson, T. P., & Fendrich, M. (2001). Monthly variations in self-reports of
alcohol consumption. *Journal of Studies on Alcohol, 62*, 268–272.

Chung, T., Colby, S. M., Barnett, N. P., & Monti, P. (2002). Alcohol use disorders
identification test: Factor structure in an adolescent emergency department sample.
Alcoholism: Clinical and Experimental Research, 26, 223–231.

Clark, W. B. (1982). Frequency of drunkenness in the U.S. population. *Journal of Studies
on Alcohol, 43*, 1267–1275.

Conigrave, K. M., Degenhardt, L. J., Whitfield, J. B., Saunders, J. B., Helander, A., &
Tabakoff, B. (2002). CDT, GGT, and AST as markers of alcohol use: The WHO/
ISBRA collaborative project. *Alcoholism: Clinical and Experimental Research, 26*,
332–339.

Cunningham, J. A., Ansara, D., Wild, T. C., Toneatto, T., & Koski-Jannes, A. (1999).
What is the price of perfection? The hidden costs of using detailed assessment instruments to measure alcohol consumption. *Journal of Studies on Alcohol, 60*, 756–758.

Davies, B. T., & Bowen, C. K. (1999). Total body water and peak alcohol concentration:
a comparative study of young, middle-age, and older females. *Alcoholism: Clinical and
Experimental Research, 23*, 969–975.

Dawson, D. A. (1998a). Measuring alcohol consumption: Limitations and prospects for
improvement. *Addiction, 93*, 965–968.

———. (1998b). Volume of ethanol consumption: Effects of different approaches to
measurement. *Journal of Studies on Alcohol, 59*, 191–197.

Dawson, D. A., Grant, B. F., & Harford, T. C. (1995). Variation in the association of
alcohol consumption with five *DSM-IV* alcohol problem domains. *Alcoholism: Clinical
and Experimental Research, 19*, 66–74.

Duffy, J. C. (1985). Questionnaire measurement of drinking behavior in sample surveys.
Journal of Official Statistics, 1, 229–234.

Dufour, M. C. (1999). What is moderate drinking? Defining "drinks" and drinking levels.
Alcohol Research and Health, 23, 5–14.

Embree, B. G., & Whitehead, P. C. (1993). Validity and reliability of self-reported
drinking behavior: Dealing with the problem of response bias. *Journal of Studies on
Alcohol, 54*, 334–344.

Figlie, N. B., Benedito-Silva, A. A., Monteiro, M. G., & Souza-Formigoni, M. L. (2002).
Biological markers of alcohol consumption in nondrinkers, drinkers, and alcohol-
dependent Brazilian patients. *Alcoholism: Clinical and Experimental Research, 26*,
1062–1069.

Fleming, M. F., Barry, K. L., Manwell, L. B., Johnson, K., & London, R. (1997). Brief physician advice for problem alcohol drinkers: A randomized controlled trial in community-based primary care practices. *Journal of the American Medical Association, 277,* 1039–1045.

Fleming, M., Mihic, S. J., & Harris, R. A. (2001). Ethanol. In J. G. Hardman & L. E. Limbird (Eds.), *Goodman & Gilman's the pharmacological basis of therapeutics* (10th ed., pp. 429–445). New York: McGraw-Hill.

Fuller, R., Lee, K., & Gordis, E. (1988). Validity of self-report in alcoholism research: Results of a Veterans Administration Cooperative Study. *Alcoholism: Clinical and Experimental Research, 12,* 201–205.

Gibb, K., Yee, A., Johnson, C., Martin, S., & Nowak, R. (1984). Accuracy and usefulness of a breath alcohol analyzer. *Annals of Emergency Medicine, 13,* 516–520.

Gill, J. S. (2002). Reported levels of alcohol consumption and binge drinking within the UK undergraduate student population over the last 25 years. *Alcohol and Alcoholism, 37,* 109–120.

Gordon, A. J., Maisto, S. A., McNeil, M., Kraemer, K. L., Conigliaro, R. L., Kelley, M. E., et al. (2001). Three questions can detect hazardous drinkers. *Journal of Family Practice, 50,* 313–320.

Gunzerath, L., Faden, V., Zakhari, S., & Warren, K. (2004). National Institute on Alcohol Abuse and Alcoholism report on moderate drinking. *Alcoholism: Clinical and Experimental Research, 28,* 829–847.

Harasymiw, J. W., & Bean, P. (2001). Identification of heavy drinkers by using the early detection of alcohol consumption score. *Alcoholism: Clinical and Experimental Research, 25,* 228–235.

Hasin, D. (2003). Classification of alcohol use disorders. National Institute on Alcohol Abuse and Alcoholism. Retrieved October 1, 2004, from http://www.niaaa.nih.gov/publications/arh27-1/5-17.htm

Helander, A., & Eriksson, J. P. (2002). Laboratory tests for acute alcohol consumption: Results of the WHO/ISBRA study on state and trait markers of alcohol use and dependence. *Alcoholism: Clinical and Experimental Research, 26,* 1070–1077.

Hingson, R., Heeren, T., Winter, M. R., & Wechsler, H. (2003). Early age of first drunkenness as a factor in college students' unplanned and unprotected sex attributable to drinking. *Pediatrics, 111,* 34–41.

International Center for Alcohol Policies. (1999). What is a standard drink? *Journal of Substance Use, 4*(2), 67–69.

————. (2002). Blood alcohol concentration limits worldwide. ICAP Reports 11. Retrieved October 1, 2004, from http://www.icap.org/pdf/report11.pdf

Intoximeters. (2002). Alco-Sensor. Retrieved October 1, 2004, from http://www.intoximeters.com

Ivis, F. J., Bondy, S. J., & Adlaf, E. M. (1997). The effect of question structure on self-reports of heavy drinking: Closed-ended versus open-ended questions. *Journal of Studies on Alcohol, 58,* 622–624.

Jacobs, D. S., Demott, W. R., Finley, P. R., Horvat, R. T., Kasten, B. L., & Tilzer, L. L. (1994). *Laboratory test handbook* (3rd ed.). Cleveland: Lexi-Comp.

Jones, A. W., & Helander, A. (1999). Time course and reproducibility of urinary excretion profiles of ethanol, methanol, and the ratio of serotonin metabolites after intravenous infusion of ethanol. *Alcoholism: Clinical and Experimental Research, 23,* 1921–1926.

Kadden, R. M., & Litt, M. D. (2004). Searching for treatment outcome measures for use across trials. *Journal of Studies on Alcohol, 65*, 145–152.

Kaplan, A., Jack, R., Opheim, K., Toivola, B., & Lyon, A. (1995). *Clinical chemistry: Interpretation and techniques* (4th ed.). Baltimore: Williams & Wilkins.

Kaskutas, L. A., & Graves, K. (2001). Pre-pregnancy drinking: How drink size affects risk assessment. *Addiction, 96*, 1199–1209.

Kerr, W. C., Fillmore, K. M., & Marvy, P. (2000). Beverage-specific alcohol consumption and cirrhosis mortality in a group of English-speaking beer-drinking countries. *Addiction, 95*, 339–346.

Koch, H., Meerkerk, G., Zaat, J., Ham, M., Scholten, R., & Assendelft, W. (2004). Accuracy of carbohydrate-deficient transferring in the detection of excessive alcohol consumption: A systemic review. *Alcohol and Alcoholism, 39*, 75–85.

Lange, J. E., & Voas, R. B. (2001). Defining binge drinking quantities through resulting blood alcohol concentrations. *Psychology of Addictive Behaviors, 4*, 310–316.

Lapham, S. C., Gregory, C., & McMillan, G. (2003). Impact of an alcohol misuse intervention for health care workers: Frequency of binge drinking and desire to reduce alcohol use. *Alcohol and Alcoholism, 38*, 176–182.

Lintonen, T., & Rimpela, M. (2001). The validity of the concept of "self-perceived drunkenness" in adolescent health surveys. *Journal of Substance Use, 6*, 145–150.

Lucey, M. R., Hill, E. M., Young, J. P., Demo-Dananberg, L., & Beresford, T. P. (1999). The influences of age and gender on blood ethanol concentrations in healthy humans. *Journal of Studies on Alcohol, 60*, 103–110.

Luczak, S. E., Wall, T. L., Shea, S. H., Byun, S. M., & Carr, L. G. (2001). Binge drinking in Chinese, Korean, and White college students: Genetic and ethnic group differences. *Psychology of Addictive Behaviors, 15*, 306–309.

Manwell, L. B., Fleming, M. F., Johnson, K., & Barry, K. (1998). Tobacco, alcohol, and drug use in a primary care sample: 90-day prevalence and associated factors. *Journal of Addictive Diseases, 17*, 67–81.

McClatchy, K. (1994). *Clinical laboratory medicine.* Baltimore: Williams & Wilkins.

Measham, F. (1996). The big bang approach to sessional drinking: Changing patterns of alcohol consumption amongst young people in North West England. *Addiction Research, 4*, 283–289.

Medical Algorithms Project. (2004). Evaluation of patients for alcohol use and abuse. Medical Algorithms Project, urine ethanol levels. Retrieved October 1, 2004, from http://webglimpse.net/cgibin/mfs.cgi?id=6&link=http%3a%2f%2fwww%2emedal reg%2ecom%2fwww%2factive%2fch32%2ephp&file=%2fhome%2fwgdemo% 2f6%2f%2eremote%2f104%2eabra&line=335&highlight=%5cb%28alcohol %29%5cb#mfs

Meerkerk, G. J., Njoo, K. H., Bongers, I. M. B., Trienekens, P., & van Oers, J. A. M. (1999). Comparing the diagnostic accuracy of carbohydrate deficient tranferrin, γ glutamyltransferase, and mean cell volume in a general practice population. *Alcoholism: Clinical and Experimental Research, 23*, 1052–1059.

Midanik, L. T. (1982a). Over-reports of recent alcohol consumption in a clinical population: A validity study. *Drug and Alcohol Dependence, 9*, 101–110.

———. (1982b). The validity of self-reported alcohol consumption and alcohol problems: A literature review. *British Journal of Addiction, 77*, 357–382.

————. (1999). Drunkenness, feeling the effects and 5+ measures. *Addiction, 94,* 887–897.

Midanik, L. T., Tam, T. W., Greenfield, T. K., & Caetano, R. (1996). Risk functions for alcohol-related problems in a 1988 US national sample. *Addiction, 91,* 1427–1437.

Moller, G. (2004). Prenatal alcohol exposure as predictor of attention deficit and other behavioral problems in 6 to 7 year olds. *Danish Medical Bulletin, 51,* 213.

Murgraff, V., Parrott, A., & Bennett, P. (1999). Risky single-occasion drinking amongst young people: Definition, correlates, policy, and interventions: A broad overview of research findings. *Alcohol and Alcoholism, 34,* 3–14.

Musshoff, F. (2002). Chromatographic methods for the determination of markers of chronic and acute alcohol consumption. *Journal of Chromatography B, 781,* 457–480.

Naimi, T. S., Brewer, R. D., Mokdad, A., Denny, C., Serdula, M. K., & Marks, J. S. (2003). Binge drinking among US adults. *Journal of the American Medical Association, 289,* 70–75.

National Institute on Alcohol Abuse and Alcoholism (NIAAA). (1990). Screening for alcoholism. *Alcohol Alert,* 8(April 1990), 1–5.

————. (1995). *The physician's guide to helping patients with alcohol problems* (NIH Pub. No. 95-3769). Bethesda, MD: National Institutes of Health.

————. (1999). Alcohol consumption levels by sex, age, and education: NHIS, 1987 and 1992. Retrieved October 1, 2004, from http://www.niaaa.nih.gov/databases/dkpat17.htm

————. (2002a). Alcohol: What you don't know can harm you. Retrieved October 1, 2004, from http://www.niaaa.nih.gov/publications/harm-al.htm

————. (2002b). *A call to action: Changing the culture of drinking at U.S. Colleges* (NIH Pub. No. 02-5010).

————. (2000c). Quick facts, NIAAA data bases: Percent who drink beverage alcohol, by gender, 1939–1999. Retrieved October 1, 2004, from http://www.niaaa.nih.gov/databases/dkpat1.txt

————. (2000d). *Tenth special report on alcohol and health.* Bethesda, MD: Author.

————. (2003). Helping patients with alcohol problems: A health practitioner's guide. Retrieved October 1, 2004, from http://www.niaaa.nih.gov/publications/Practitioner/HelpingPatients.htm#Note14

————. (2004). Standard drinks chart. Retrieved October 1, 2004, from http://www.niaaa.nih.gov/publications/niaaa-guide/standardDrinksChart.htm

Nielsen, A. L. (1999). Testing Sampton and Laub's life course theory: Age, race/ethnicity, and drunkenness. *Deviant Behavior, 20,* 129–151.

Nine, J. S., Moraca, M., Virji, M. A., & Rao, K. N. (1995). Serum-ethanol determination: Comparison of lactate and lactate dehydrogenase interference in three enzymatic assays. *Journal of Analytical Toxicology, 19,* 192–196.

Oslin, D. W., Pettinati, H. M., Luck, G., Semwanga, A., Cnaan, A., & O'Brien, C. P. (1998). Clinical correlations with carbohydrate deficient-transferrin levels in women with alcoholism. *Alcoholism: Clinical and Experimental Research, 22,* 1981–1985.

Parmahamsa, M., Reddy, K. R., & Varadacharyulu, N. (2004). Changes in composition and properties of erythrocyte membrane in chronic alcoholics. *Alcohol and Alcoholism, 39,* 110–112.

Pelletier, S., Vaucher, E., Aider, R., Martin, S., Perney, P., Balmes, J., et al. (2002). Wine consumption is not associated with a decreased risk of alcoholic cirrhosis in heavy drinkers. *Alcohol and Alcoholism, 37,* 618–621.

Perkins, H. W., Linkenbach, J., & DeJong, W. (2001). Estimated blood alcohol levels reached by binge and nonbinge drinkers: A survey of young adults in Montana. *Psychology of Addictive Behavior, 15*, 317–320.

Pincus, M., & Abraham, N. (2001). Toxicology and therapeutic drug monitoring. In J. B. Henry (Ed.), *Clinical diagnosis and management by laboratory methods* (20th ed., pp. 359–560). Philadelphia: W. B. Saunders.

Ravel, R. (1995). *Clinical laboratory medicine: Clinical application of laboratory data* (6th ed.). St. Louis: Mosby.

Rehm, J. (1998). Measuring quantity, frequency, and volume of drinking. *Alcoholism: Clinical and Experimental Research, 22*(2 Suppl.), 4S–14S.

Reinert, D. F., & Allen J. P. (2002). The alcohol use disorders identification test (AUDIT): A review of recent research. *Alcoholism: Clinical and Experimental Research, 26*, 272–279.

Room, R. (1990). Measuring alcohol consumption in the United States: Methods and rationale. In L. T. Kozlowski, H. M. Annis, H. D. Cappell, F. B. Glaser, M. S. Goodstadt, Y. Israel, H. Kalant, E. M. Sellers, & E. F. Vingilis (Eds.), *Research advances in alcohol and drug problems* (Vol. 10, pp. 39–80). New York: Plenum Press.

Room, R., Bondy, S., & Ferris, J. (1995). The risk of harm to oneself from drinking, Canada 1989. *Addiction, 90*, 499–513.

Rukstalis, M., Lynch, K., Oslin, D., Pettinati, H, Anderson, S., Volpicelli, J., et al. (2002). Carbohydrate-deficient transferrin levels reflect heavy drinking in alcohol-dependent women seeking treatment. *Alcoholism: Clinical and Experimental Research, 26*, 1539–1544.

Sacher, R. A., & McPherson, R. A. (1991). *Widmann's clinical interpretation of laboratory tests* (10th ed.). Philadelphia: F. A. Davis.

Salaspuro, M. (1999). Carbohydrate-deficient transferrin as compared to other markers of alcoholism: A systemic review. *Alcohol, 19*, 261–271.

Sarkola, T., Eriksson, C. J. P., Niemela, O., Sillanaukee, P., & Halmesmaki, E. (2000). Mean cell volume and gamma-glutamyl transferase are superior to carbohydrate-deficient transferrin and hemoglobin-acetaldehyde adducts in the follow-up of pregnant women with alcohol abuse. *Acta Obstetricia et Gynecologica Scandinavica, 79*, 359–366.

Saunders, J. B., Aasland, O. G., Babor, T. F., de la Fuenta, J. R., & Grant, M. (1993). Development of the Alcohol Use Disorders Identification Test (AUDIT): WHO collaborative project on early detection of persons with harmful alcohol consumption. *Addiction, 88*, 791–804.

Saunders, J. B., & Lee, N. K. (2000). Hazardous alcohol use: Its delineation as a subthreshold disorder, and approaches to its diagnosis and management. *Comprehensive Psychiatry, 41*(S1), 95–103.

Scottish Executive Online. (2004). The definition of alcohol misuse. Retrieved on October 1, 2004, from http://www.scotland.gov.uk/cru/kd01/red/tpamwr-04.asp

Serdula, M., Mokdad, A. H., Byers, T., & Siegel, P. Z. (1999). Assessing alcohol consumption: Beverage-specific versus grouped-beverage questions. *Journal of Studies on Alcohol, 60*, 99–102.

Shalala, D. (1995). Message from secretary of health and human services. *Alcohol Alert, 29*, 1–4.

Sharpe, P. C. (2001). Biochemical detection and monitoring of alcohol abuse and abstinence. *Annals of Clinical Biochemistry, 38*, 652–664.

Sillanaukee, P., Massot, N., Jousilahti, P., Vartiainen, E., Poikolainen, K., Olsson, U., et al. (2000). Enhanced clinical utility of γ-CDT in a general population. *Alcoholism: Clinical and Experimental Research, 24,* 1202–1206.

Sillanaukee, P., Ponnio, M., & Seppa, K. (1999). Sialic acid: New potential marker of alcohol abuse. *Alcoholism: Clinical and Experimental Research, 23,* 1039–1043.

Sillanaukee, P., Strid, N., Allen, J. P., & Litten, R. Z. (2001). Possible reasons why heavy drinking increases carbohydrate-deficient transferrin. *Alcoholism: Clinical and Experimental Research, 25,* 34–40.

Smart, R. (1996). Behavioral and social consequences related to the consumption of different beverage types. *Journal of Studies on Alcohol, 57,* 77–84.

Smith, G. T., McCarthy, D. M., & Goldman, M. S. (1995). Self-reported drinking and alcohol-related problems among early adolescents: Dimensionality and validity over 24 months. *Journal of Studies on Alcohol, 56,* 383–394.

Sobell, L. C., Brown, J., Leo, G. I., & Sobell, M. B. (1996). The reliability of the Alcohol Timeline Followback when administered by telephone and by computer. *Drug and Alcohol Dependence, 42,* 49–54.

Sobell, L. C., Maisto, S. A., Sobell, M. B., & Cooper, A. M. (1979). Reliability of alcohol abusers' self reports of drinking behavior. *Behavioral Research Therapy, 17,* 157–160.

Sobell, L. C., & Sobell, M. B. (1990). Self-report issues in alcohol abuse: State of the art and future directions. *Behavioral Assessment, 12,* 77–90.

———. (1992). Timeline follow-back. In R. Litten & J. Allen (Eds.), *Measuring alcohol consumption.* Totowa, NJ: Humana Press.

Sobell, L. C., Sobell, M., Leo, G. I., & Cancilla, A. (1988). Reliability of a timeline method: Assessing normal drinkers' reports of recent drinking and a comparative evaluation across several populations. *British Journal of Addiction, 83,* 393–402.

Sobell, L. C., Toneatto, T., & Sobell, M. B. (1994). Behavioral assessment and treatment planning for alcohol, tobacco, and other drug problems: Current status with an emphasis on clinical applications. *Behavioral Therapy, 25,* 533–580.

Sobell, L. C., Toneatto, T., Sobell, M. B., Leo, G. I., & Johnson, L. (1992). Alcohol abusers' perceptions of the accuracy of their self-reports of drinking: Implications for treatment. *Addictive Behavior, 17,* 507–511.

Sokol, R. J., Martier, S. S., & Ager, J. W. (1989). The T-ACE questions: Practical prenatal detection of risk-drinking. *American Journal of Obstetrics and Gynecology, 160,* 868–870.

Sommers, M. S., Dyehouse, J. M., Howe, S. R., Lemmink, J., Volz, T., & Manharth, M. (2000). Validity of self-reported alcohol consumption in non-dependent drinkers with unintentional injuries. *Alcoholism: Clinical and Experimental Research, 24,* 1406–1413.

Sommers, M. S., Dyehouse, J. M., Howe, S. R., Wekselman, K., & Fleming, M. (2002). "Nurse, I only had a couple of beers": Validity of self-reported drinking before serious injury. *American Journal of Critical Care, 11,* 106–114.

Sommers, M. S., Savage, C., Wray, J., & Dyehouse, J. M. (2003). Laboratory measures of alcohol (ethanol) consumption: Strategies to assess drinking patterns with biochemical measures. *Biological Research for Nursing, 4,* 203–217.

Sommers, M. S., Wray, J., Savage, C., & Dyehouse, J. M. (2003). Assessing acute and critically patients for problem drinking. *Dimensions of Critical Care Nursing, 22,* 76–88.

Stibler, H. (1991). Carbohydrate-deficient transferrin in serum: A new marker of potentially harmful ethanol consumption reviewed. *Clinical Chemistry, 37,* 2029–2037.

Stoler, J. M., Huntington, K. S., Peterson, C. M., Peterson, K. P., Daniel, P., Aboagye, K. K., et al. (1998). The prenatal detection of significant alcohol exposure with maternal blood markers. *Journal of Pediatrics, 133*, 346–352.

Substance Abuse and Mental Health Services Administration (SAMHSA). (2001). Binge drinking in adolescents and college students. National Clearinghouse for Alcohol and Drug Information, SAMHSA. Retrieved October 1, 2004, from http://www.health.org/govpubs/rpo995/

————. (2004). Results from the 2002 National Survey on Drug Use and Health: National findings. Retrieved October 1, 2004, from http://www.oas.samhsa.gov/NHSDA/2k2NSDUH/Results/2k2results.htm#chap3

Taproom. (2004). Alcohol content of beer. Retrieved October 1, 2004, from http://www.taproom.com/beer/beerprf.htm

Taylor, D., Drew, C., Waiters, W., & Bluthenthal, R. (2003). What the public doesn't know: Alcohol beverage type advertising and classifications systems. *Proceeding of the 131st Annual Meeting, American Public Health Association* (Abstract 70388). Retrieved October 1, 2004, from http://apha.confex.com/apha/131am/techprogram/paper_70388.htm

Thomas, G., Reifman, A., Barnes, G. M., & Farrell, M. P. (2000). Delayed onset of drunkenness as a protective factor for adolescent alcohol misuse and sexual risk taking: A longitudinal study. *Deviant Behavior, 21*, 181–210.

Turner, C. (1990). How much alcohol is in a "standard drink"? An analysis of 125 studies. *British Journal of Addiction, 85*, 1171–1175.

van Pelt, J., Leusink, G. L., van Nierop, P. W. M., & Keyzer, J. J. (2000). Test characteristics of carbohydrate-deficient transferrin and γ-glutamyltransferase in alcohol-using perimenopausal women. *Alcoholism: Clinical and Experimental Research, 24*, 176–179.

Venes, D. (2001). *Taber's cyclopedic medical dictionary* (19th ed.). Philadelphia: F. A. Davis.

Walitzer, K. S., & Connors, G. J. (1999). Treating problem drinking. *Alcohol Research and Health, 23*, 138–143.

Wallach, J. (2000). *Interpretation of diagnostic tests* (7th ed.). Philadelphia: Lippincott Williams & Wilkins.

Wechsler, H., Dowdall, G. W., Davenport, A., & Castillo, S. (1995). Correlates of college student binge drinking. *American Journal of Public Health, 85*, 921–926.

White, A. M., Kraus, C. L., McCracken, L. A., & Swartzwelder, H. S. (2003). Do college students drink more than they think? Use of a free-pour paradigm to determine how college students define standard drinks. *Alcoholism: Clinical and Experimental Research, 27*, 1750–1756.

Wikipedia. (2004). Alcoholic beverage. Retrieved October 1, 2004, from http://www.wikipedia.org/wiki/Alcoholic_beverage

Yersin, B., Nicolet, J., Dercrey, H., Burnier, M., van Melle, G., & Pecoud, A. (1995). Screening for excessive alcohol drinking. *Archives of Internal Medicine, 155*, 1907–1911.

Chapter 3

Moderate Drinking and Cardiovascular Disease

Joan A. Masters

ABSTRACT

The adverse consequences of heavy alcohol use are well known. However, recent media reports of a possible cardiovascular benefit associated with moderate drinking have revived public interest in the use of alcohol for "medicinal purposes." Knowledge development regarding guidelines for moderate alcohol use has lagged behind public interest in the possible health benefits of moderate alcohol use. At this time, evidence-based primary health promotion interventions related to the risks and benefits of moderate alcohol use are lacking in the health care literature. This chapter reviews 22 reports describing the relationship between moderate drinking and cardiovascular disease. The reports are classified by the level of evidence and critiqued on seven aspects of method. Conclusions related to the strength of the evidence that moderate drinking is a useful primary health promotion intervention are presented.

Keywords: moderate drinking, cardiovascular disease, health promotion

The adverse consequences of heavy drinking and alcohol abuse on the cardiovascular system are well documented (for reviews, see Anderson, Cremona, Paton,

Turner, & Wallace, 1993; Crabb, Matsumoto, & You, 2004; Spies et al., 2001). However, some researchers suggest that moderate drinking, compared to both abstinence and higher levels of consumption, is associated with decreased rates of morbidity and mortality that are mostly attributable to lower rates of cardiovascular disease. Specifically, individuals who drink moderately have lower rates of coronary artery disease, congestive heart failure, sudden cardiac death, myocardial infarction, embolic stroke, and peripheral artery disease. The variety of clinical conditions found to be inversely correlated with alcohol consumption has led to speculation that a common cardiovascular mechanism may be responsible for the decreased rates of both cardiac disease and vascular disease documented among moderate drinkers. Current knowledge about the association between moderate alcohol use and cardiovascular disease is based on numerous studies using multiple cardiovascular end points rather than one specific clinical outcome variable such as coronary artery disease or stroke. Therefore, this review will consider the relationship between moderate alcohol use and the broader phenomenon of cardiovascular disease rather than one specific clinical condition.

Authors, writing on the topic of cardiovascular disease, frequently use more than one word to signify the same pathological process. A familiar example is the use of the terms *coronary artery disease, coronary heart disease, coronary vessel disease, ischemic heart disease,* and *atherosclerotic heart disease* to indicate a narrowing of the coronary arteries, usually related to atherosclerosis, that results in a decreased delivery of oxygen to the myocardium. In such cases, in order to clarify comparisons across articles, the most commonly used term will be used in this review. In this chapter, the term used is *coronary artery disease.*

Media reports of the possible cardiovascular benefit of moderate alcohol use have revived public interest in the use of alcohol for "medicinal purposes" (Klatsky, 1999). This has led to a novel problem. Researchers and clinicians have historically responded to concerns about alcohol-related risk and developed interventions aimed at curtailing alcohol use. Now nurses and other health care professionals are confronted with patient concerns that they may not be drinking enough. However, knowledge development regarding guidelines for moderate alcohol use has lagged behind public interest in the possible health benefits of moderate alcohol use. At this time, evidence-based, primary health promotion interventions related to the risks and benefits of moderate alcohol use are lacking in the health care literature.

The purpose of this chapter is to present and critique the accessible English language research literature related to moderate drinking and cardiovascular disease. The review will answer the following question: What is the strength of the evidence that moderate drinking is a useful primary health promotion intervention?

METHOD

The following search strategy was used to select the articles included in this review. First, a computerized search of Medline, the Cumulative Index of Nursing and Allied Health Literature (CINAHL), and ETOH, a database of alcohol research maintained by the National Institute on Alcohol Abuse and Alcoholism (NIAAA; http://www.niaaa.nih.gov/databases/databases.htm) was completed. The search terms *moderate alcohol* and *moderate drinking* were used independently and then in conjunction with each of the following terms: *disease, health, heart, benefit, risk, harm, cardiovascular, coronary artery disease, myocardial infarction, stroke,* and *peripheral vascular disease.* The literature exploring the relationship of moderate drinking and cardiovascular system has burgeoned over the last 30 years, and this search technique identified over 1,000 articles. The titles of these articles were scanned, and the abstracts of databased articles in which moderate alcohol and a cardiovascular end point were the major variables of interest were extracted.

Representative articles for review were selected from the array of abstracts based on the following criteria: (1) the population of interest was specified as adult nonpregnant females and/or adult males, (2) description of the relationship between moderate alcohol and cardiovascular disease was the primary focus of the report, (3) the reported research introduced a novel variable or generalized previous findings to a new population, (4) the reported research contributed to knowledge development by asking a new question about the relationship between moderate alcohol and cardiovascular disease (e.g., the mechanism, pattern of drinking, or type of alcohol). Because a bias against publishing smaller studies examining the association between moderate alcohol use and cardiovascular disease and studies with nonsignificant findings has been documented in two recent meta-analyses (Corrao, Bagnardi, Zambon, & Arico, 1999; Corrao, Rubbiati, Bagnardi, Zambon, & Poikolainen, 2000), adequate representation of these studies was a priority during the selection process. Finally, 22 articles were selected for review in this chapter.

The search method provided the following rough timeline of the evolution of research describing the relationship between moderate alcohol use and cardiovascular disease. Early articles were broad ecological and histological reports of an inverse relationship between alcohol use and cardiovascular disease and were mostly specific to coronary artery disease. These studies were followed by a series of mid-sized and large-scale prospective cohort and cross-sectional survey studies conducted primarily by researchers in the United Kingdom and the United States. Many of these publications were secondary analyses of alcohol data that was collected during general lifestyle surveys. In these cases, the original studies did not have stated objectives that pertained to alcohol. Sample composition was mostly limited to Caucasian subjects. Next came a period of normal science in which researchers designed smaller alcohol-dedicated survey studies. The samples in these smaller studies were more diverse, and multiple cardiovascular end points were identified. Some researchers assessed the benefit of initiating moderate drinking after a lifetime of light drinking or abstinence. Others tested the hypotheses that the reduction in cardiovascular disease among moderate drinkers was mediated by the type of alcoholic drink, or by a psychosocial or lifestyle variable. Additionally, laboratory work was conducted to identify a possible physiological substrate for the reduction in cardiovascular disease seen among moderate drinkers. For the purposes of this review, this body of literature will be designated as the moderate alcohol literature.

LITERATURE RATING SYSTEM

The designs of the studies reviewed here were rated according to a seven-level system developed by the Agency for Health Care Research and Policy (AHRQ) and slightly modified to fit the designs of the studies in this review. Modifications are included in parentheses. This system was used to develop evidence-based guidelines for the Clinical Practice Guidelines series published by the U.S. Department of Health and Human Services. The seven levels, arranged in descending order according to the strength of the evidence produced by the study design, are:

I: Evidence from large, well-conducted clinical trials
II: Evidence from small, well-conducted clinical trials
III: Evidence from well-conducted (prospective) cohort studies
IV: Evidence from well-conducted (retrospective) case controlled (and cross-sectional) studies
V: Evidence from poorly controlled or uncontrolled studies
VI: Conflicting evidence but tending to favor the recommendation
VII: Expert opinion

The quality of the studies was also assessed on seven aspects of method: sample selection and composition, response rate and response bias, exclusion criteria, measurement of alcohol use, definition of abstainers, specification of the comparison group, and data analysis and interpretation.

DEFINITION OF TERMS

Standard Drink

The definition of a standard drink varies across countries, settings, alcohol categories, and research studies and poses a major barrier to synthesis of the literature. Throughout the rest of the chapter, in order to facilitate comparisons across studies, alcohol intake will be reported as standard drinks per unit of time rather than in the rates or measures peculiar to each article. One standard drink will be defined according to the U.S. standard of 12 g of ethanol. This is the amount of alcohol contained in 1.5 fl oz 80-proof distilled spirits, 5 fl oz wine, or 12 oz of beer (Dufour, 1999). In addition, because a significant portion of the moderate alcohol literature originates in Great Britain, the British standard of 1 unit = 8 g of ethanol will be considered the equivalent to 0.66 of a standard drink.

Moderate Drinking

Moderate drinking will be defined according to current age- and gender-based federal guidelines. The fifth edition of *Nutrition and Your Health: Dietary Guidelines for Americans*, a joint publication of the Department of Health and Human Services and the Department of Agriculture, defines drinking in moderation to be no more than two standard drinks per day for men. Drinking in moderation for women is defined as no more than one standard drink per day (U.S. Department of Agriculture, 2000). Further, moderate drinking for individuals over age 65 will be more narrowly defined according to the U.S. Department of Health and Human Services low-risk drinking guidelines for older adults as specified in *Treatment Improvement Protocol Series Number 26: Substance Abuse in Older Adults*. Moderate drinking for men over age 65 will be considered to be one drink per day on most days and two drinks on special occasions (weddings, New Year's). "Somewhat lower" limits will be accepted as moderate for women over age 65 (U.S. Department of Health and Human Services, 1998).

The problems associated with defining moderate drinking have particular relevance for this review. Researchers, clinicians, and patients do not share a common definition of moderate drinking. Researchers have used the term *moderate* to describe alcohol consumption levels between 3.0 and 5.7 standard drinks per day (Karhunen, Erkinjuntii, & Laippala, 1994), fewer than 3.0 standard drinks per day (Iso et al., 1995), and 1.0 to 2.0 standard drinks per day (Mills & Graubard, 1987). Yet consumption at all of these levels incurs increased risk. For example, women, in general, experience increased rates of breast cancer and liver disease at rates as low as one to two standard drinks per day (U.S. Department of Health and Human Services, 2000).

Additionally, when surveyed, young and middle-aged adults quantified moderate drinking between 2.1 and 3.0 drinks per day. The stipulated threshold for moderate drinking increased with age, male gender, tolerance, and level of self-reported intake (Able & Kruger, 1995). Nearly all adults report exceeding current federal guidelines at least once (Dawson, 2000). A survey of middle-aged and older adults found that the definition of moderate drinking may also vary as a function of ethnicity. Older Caucasian subjects defined moderate drinking at a higher level (2.5 ± 1.2 standard drinks per day) than Latino (2.1 ± 1.6 standard drinks per day and African American (1.3 ± 1.4 standard drinks per day) subjects (Masters, 2003). Physicians exhibit less variability in the operationalization of drinking terms than other groups. A sample of practicing physicians defined moderate drinking as 2.2 (± 0.9) standard drinks per day (Able, Kruger, & Friendl, 1996). Thus, many adults, as well as researchers and clinicians define and consume alcohol at levels that incur significant risk and exceed federal guidelines. The lack of consensus on the definition of moderate drinking among researchers, clinicians, and patients is a barrier to the development of effective primary health promotion interventions related to the risks and benefits of moderate drinking.

REVIEW OF THE LITERATURE

Historical Background

In 1926, Richard Pearl reported an inverse correlation between moderate drinking and cardiovascular disease. This was the first research-based assertion that moderate drinking could be a useful primary health promotion intervention. Published during Prohibition, Pearl's report was quickly disregarded. Twenty-five years later, necropsy studies described dissociation between alcoholic cirrhosis and coronary artery disease. These findings revived interest in the cardiovascular benefits of alcohol consumption. Later, two seminal ecological studies of geographic populations stimulated current interest in the possible cardiovascular benefit of alcohol (Laport, Cresanta, & Kuller, 1980; Renaud, & deLorgeril, 1992). These projects revealed that France had the highest alcohol consumption rate and lowest rate of coronary artery disease morbidity of any country studied. The additional findings that the French diet was high in animal fat and that Frenchmen had high serum cholesterol levels was dubbed the "French paradox" and became the catalyst for multiple programs of research.

Mid-Sized and Large Population-based Survey Studies

Prospective cohort and cross-sectional survey studies from only a few mid-sized and large research projects dominate the corpus of studies that make up the moderate alcohol literature. Although many of these projects were not originally designed to answer alcohol-related questions, secondary data analyses have generally revealed inverse relationships between moderate drinking and various cardiovascular end points. It is important to note that all of the reports from any given project are based on data gathered from one sample and thus share many aspects of method. Therefore, multiple reports based on data from one large population-based study will be reviewed and critiqued in clusters.

Surveys of Male British Physicians

Reports from the Imperial Cancer Research Fund's Cancer Studies Unit in Oxford are based on data from 34,439 British physicians who originally replied to a survey about smoking in 1951. Subjects, who were 48 to 78 years of age at the time of enrollment, provided data over a period of 40 years. Health histories were recorded and coded for each subject, but no health-related exclusion criteria were applied in subject selection. The major objective of the study was to evaluate the relationship between smoking and mortality.

In 1978, all subjects were queried about the frequency and quantity of alcohol they consumed. Specifically, subjects were asked if they "never or almost never," "less often than weekly," "in most weeks, but less often than daily," or "on most days" consumed alcohol. Subjects were also asked to indicate the quantity and type of alcohol consumed. Reported alcohol consumption in the sample ranged from abstinence to more than 30 drinks per week. Chi-square analysis of the data from the 12,321 subjects who provided complete answers to these questions revealed that subjects who drank six to nine standard drinks per week had the lowest rates of cardiovascular disease and all-cause mortality. Death due to coronary artery disease was more frequent among subjects reporting abstinence and among subjects reporting more than nine standard drinks per week compared to subjects reporting six to nine standard drinks per week. For most causes of mortality assessed, mortality was higher among abstainers compared to light and moderate drinkers (Doll, Peto, Hall, Wheatley, & Gray, 1994).

Surveys of Scottish Men

The original objective of this study of 5,766 employed men between the ages of 35 and 65 living in three areas in Scotland was to assess the association between several socioeconomic and lifestyle variables and health (Hart, Smith, Hole, & Hawthorne, 1999). Between 1970 and 1973, subjects reported alcohol use across six categories of consumption (none, 0.1–5, 5–9, 9–14, 14–20, and 20+ drinks per week). Cox proportional hazards modeling was used to estimate the relative risk of coronary artery disease across categories of consumption. This statistical method reveals the level of alcohol use associated with the lowest relative risk for specific cardiovascular diseases (i.e., the nadir), and specifies the lowest level of alcohol consumption that carries a decreased relative risk (RR) of cardiovascular disease (i.e., level of onset) (see Table 3.1). The frequent use of this statistical approach in the moderate-alcohol literature facilitates comparisons across studies.

The investigators reported that consumption rates of up to nine drinks per week were not significantly associated with risk for coronary artery disease. Subjects who reported higher levels of consumption had increased relative risk of coronary artery disease. Risk of stroke was increased at all levels of consump-

TABLE 3.1   Studies from Great Britain

Author(s) (year), literature rating level	Sample, additional exclusion criteria	Design (follow-up period), statistically controlled variables, end point(s)		1. Findings 2. shape of association 3. nadir; onset of effect
Doll et al. (1994) III	12,321 males None	Prospective cohort (13 years) Smoking, aspirin use Mortality from various causes	1. 2. 3.	Subjects who drank 6 to 9 drinks per week had lower rates of cardiovascular disease compared to abstainers. U-shaped 6–9 drinks per week; 0.6–4.2 drinks per week
Hart (1999) III	5,766 males None	Prospective cohort (21 years) All-cause mortality	1. 2. 3.	Up to 9 drinks per week, physiologically neutral RR mortality at 10–14 drinks per week was 1.34 (95% confidence interval 1.14–1.58) Positive linear Not applicable; not applicable
Wannamethee & Shaper (1997) III	7,167 males Recall of coronary artery disease	Prospective cohort (9.8 years) Age, social class, physical activity, body mass index, diabetes, angina, smoking, and use of regular medications Coronary artery disease	1. 2. 3.	RR coronary artery disease .79 (0.63–0.99) No dose response relationship among regular drinkers Not applicable 0.6–0.9 drinks per week; 0.6–0.9 drinks per week
Wannamethee et al. (1998) III	7,142 males Recall of coronary artery disease	Prospective cohort (15 years) Age, social class, physical activity, body mass index, diabetes, angina, smoking	1. 2. 3.	RR coronary artery disease 0.84 (0.74–0.96) No dose response relationship among regular drinkers 0.6–0.9 drinks per week; 0.6–0.9 drinks per week

RR = relative risk

tion (Hart et al., 1999). The study is noteworthy for two reasons. First, this is one of only a few studies to include socioeconomic variables, as well as physiological variables, in the design of the study. Second, the failure to find a relationship between moderate alcohol use and coronary artery disease contradicts the findings of most other studies.

The British Regional Heart Study

The British Regional Heart Study was a prospective cohort study of male primary-care patients between the ages of 40 and 59 living in 24 towns in England, Scotland, and Wales. In 1978, 7,735 subjects were purposefully selected to represent the social-class distribution of English men. The major objective of the study was to assess the relationship between modifiable lifestyle variables and both cardiovascular disease and all-cause mortality.

Subjects were queried about the frequency and quantity of alcohol use. Six drinking categories were identified: lifelong teetotalers, ex-drinkers, occasional drinkers (< 1 per week), light drinkers (1–10 drinks per week), moderate (11–28 drinks per week), and heavy (> 42 drinks per week). Cox proportional hazards modeling was used to calculate relative risks associated with selected lifestyle variables. Light drinkers had a small but statistically significant decrease in relative risk of cardiovascular disease compared with all other groups. Occasional, moderate, and heavy drinkers had similar relative risks for all-cause and cardiovascular mortality when occasional drinkers were specified as the comparison group (Wannamethee & Shaper, 1997). A later publication from the British Regional Health Study indicated that other modifiable behaviors (e.g., smoking, body mass index, and physical activity) have a much greater impact on the odds of developing cardiovascular disease than moderate alcohol use (Wannamethee, Shaper, Walker, & Ebrahim, 1998).

Reports from this project are important because the study design allowed for the risks of ex-drinkers and lifelong teetotalers to be examined separately. Ex-drinkers were found to have the highest risk for cardiovascular and noncardiovascular death. Lifelong teetotalers had the lowest risk for overall cardiovascular mortality, but an increased risk for coronary artery disease related death and all noncardiovascular causes of mortality. The investigators speculated that inclusion of ex-drinkers in the abstainer group artificially increases the relative risk of abstinence and causes the apparent decreased relative risks in the moderate drinking group. Wannamethee and colleagues recommended that in addition to separating ex-drinkers from abstainers in the analysis, future researchers should consider using light drinkers rather than abstainers as the comparison group. This recommendation was based on their belief that light drinking, and not abstinence, is the norm in most Western societies.

The Physicians' Health Study

The Physicians' Health Study (PHS) is the single most influential project reviewed in this chapter. A convenience sample of 22,071 healthy male physicians between the ages of 40 and 84 was recruited for the project. Exclusion criteria specific to the goals of the original study were stroke, transient ischemic attack, myocardial infarction, cancer, hepatic or renal disease, gout, and peptic ulcer disease. The original project was a clinical trial designed to evaluate the use of beta-carotene and aspirin for the prevention of cancer and cardiovascular disease (Ridker, Manson, Buring, Muller, & Hennekens, 1990). The clinical trial phase of the study ended in 1995, but sample subjects continue to complete biannual surveys on many health-related issues, including alcohol consumption.

An "abbreviated food frequency questionnaire" was the sole source of all the information garnered about alcohol consumption in this study. Self-reported consumption among the sample ranged from abstinence to 6+ standard drinks per day. The distribution was right-skewed, as 97% of the physicians were coded as drinking one or fewer standard drinks per day.

Secondary analyses of alcohol use data collected during this project have been used to refine findings from the earlier necropsy and ecological studies (for a detailed review of this early literature, see Moore & Pearson, 1986). Cox proportional hazards modeling was used to calculate relative risks for specific cardiovascular end points as a function of reported level of alcohol use. Reports from the PHS have uniformly documented that moderate alcohol use is associated with lower risks of cardiovascular disease compared with all other levels of drinking, including abstinence. Specific end points of these reports have been angina and myocardial infarction (Camargo, 1997a), peripheral arterial disease (Camargo, Stampfer, Glynn, Gaziano, Mason, Goldhaber, et al., 1997b), stroke and ischemic stroke (Berger et al., 1999), sudden cardiac death (Alpert et al., 1999), and total mortality, as well as mortality due to coronary artery disease, myocardial infarction, stroke, and cancer (Gaziano et al., 2000). Details of these secondary analyses, including additional exclusion criteria, other controlled variables, relative risks, shape of the relationship, level of onset of effect, and nadir, are summarized in Table 3.2.

Reports from the Channing Laboratory

The Health Care Professionals Follow-up Study (HCPFS) and the Nurses Health Study (NHS) are two large prospective cohort studies designed by researchers in the Channing Laboratory at the Harvard Medical School. The reports from these studies complement and extend the reports from the PHS. The HCPFS is an ongoing observational prospective cohort survey study designed to describe the relationship between dietary variables and both cardiovascular disease and cancer. A sample comprised of 44,059 healthy male physicians, dentists, optome-

TABLE 3.2   The Physicians' Health Study: Selected Moderate-Alcohol Publications

Author(s) (year), literature rating level	Sample, additional exclusion criteria	Design (follow-up period), statistically controlled variables, end point(s)	1. Findings: relative risk and 95% confidence interval at nadir 2. shape of association 3. nadir; onset of effect
Alpert et al. (1999) III	21,537 males None	Prospective cohort (12 years) Not applicable Sudden cardiac death	1. RR sudden cardiac death 0.21 (0.22–0.75) 2. Not applicable 3. 5–6 drinks per week; 2–4 drinks per week
Berger et al. (1999) III	21,870 males None	Prospective cohort (12.2 years) Age, systolic blood pressure, smoking, diabetes, body mass index, exercise, hypertension Stroke	1. RR ischemic stroke 0.77 (0.63–0.94) RR hemorrhagic stroke 0.92 (0.55–1.54) Stroke, risk reduced only if SBP > 140 or exercised 2. U-shaped 3. 1 drink per week; 1 drink per week
Camargo et al. (1997a) III	22,071 males Peripheral arterial disease	Prospective cohort (11) Age, smoking, exercise, diabetes, family history myocardial infarction New onset peripheral arterial disease	1. RR peripheral arterial disease 0.74 (0.57–0.97); smoking overwhelmed alcohol effect 2. Inverse linear 3. ≥ 7 drinks per week; 1 drink per week
Camargo et al. (1997b) III	21,530 males Angina, coronary artery bypass graft surgery	Prospective cohort (10) Age, smoking, diabetes, exercise, and family history of myocardial infarction Angina, myocardial infarction	1. RR angina 0.69 (0.59–0.81) RR myocardial infarction 0.65 (0.52–0.81) 2. Inverse 3. 2+ drinks per day; 5–6 drinks per week
Gaziano et al. (2000) III	89,299 males None	Prospective cohort (5.5) Hypertension and elevated All-cause and specific-cause mortality	1. RR total mortality 0.74 (0.65–0.85) RR total cancer 0.77 (0.60–0.93) 2. Inverse 3. 1 drink per week; 1 drink per week (total mortality)

RR = relative risk; SBP = systolic blood pressure

trists, pharmacists, podiatrists, and veterinarians between the ages of 45 and 75 in 1985 was recruited for the study. Exclusion criteria, which pertained to the goals of the original study, included a diagnosis of cancer, myocardial infarction, stroke, angina, and a history of coronary artery surgery.

In contrast to the PHS, alcohol intake was evaluated as part of a semiquantitative food frequency questionnaire. Specifically, subjects were provided with a definition of a standard drink, asked questions about quantity as well as frequency of consumption, and type of alcoholic beverage consumed. These changes were made in an effort to increase the validity of self-reported alcohol intake. Alcohol intake ranged between abstinence and more than four drinks a day. Approximately 12% of the sample reported drinking more than two drinks per day. This range of alcohol intake permitted examination of the relationship between alcohol and cardiovascular disease at higher levels of consumption than was possible in the PHS.

Reports from the HCPFS indicated that the inverse association between alcohol consumption and coronary artery disease persisted up to levels exceeding 2.5 drinks per day. This level exceeds all government guidelines for moderate drinking. Cox proportional hazard modeling revealed that men who reported drinking 3 or 4 days per week had a lower relative risk of developing coronary artery disease than men who drank an equal amount of alcohol but drank only on 1 day per week. This finding was the initial indication that pattern as well as quantity of consumption was an important predictor of cardiovascular risk (Rimm et al., 1991). The importance of both quantity and frequency of consumption to relative risk was clarified by a later report that individuals who drank lesser quantities on a regular basis had the greatest reduction in relative risk of myocardial infarction across all levels of consumption. In fact, when frequency was added to the model, the significant association between quantity and relative risk of myocardial infarction disappeared. Additionally, the type of alcohol or timing of drinking with respect to meals did not change the relative risk for myocardial infarction (Mukamal et al., 2003).

The NHS, established in 1976, used a design analogous to the HCPFS to assess risk factors for major diseases in a sample of 85,709 healthy registered nurses. Subjects were between the ages of 34 and 59 years of age at the time of enrollment. The nurses reported alcohol consumption rates that varied between abstinence and more than four standard drinks per day. Potential subjects were excluded from the sample if they had a history of cancer, angina, myocardial infarction, or stroke. Similar to the HCPFS, subjects were provided with a definition of a standard drink, and a semiquantitative food-frequency questionnaire was used to assess the frequency, quantity, and type of alcohol consumed.

The NHS expanded research exploring the association between moderate drinking and cardiovascular disease to include women. The researchers hypothesized that the risks and benefits of moderate drinking for women would be different from those previously documented in men. The basis for this hypothesis was that women experience alcohol-related morbidity and mortality at lower levels of consumption than men and that middle-aged women experience lower rates of coronary artery disease compared with men.

Study subjects who drank between one and three drinks per week had a lower risk of all-cause mortality that was primarily due to a lower risk of mortality due to cardiovascular disease. However, the relative risks were highly age dependent. For example, women between the ages of 34 and 39 who drank between one standard drink per week and two standard drinks per day had an increased relative risk of death (RR 2.08, CI 0.92–4.71) compared with abstainers. Women 60 years of age and older who consumed the same level of alcohol had a reduced relative risk of death (RR 0.79, CI 0.68–0.91) compared with abstainers. Further, among the subset of women over 60 years of age, only those with multiple cardiac risk factors exhibited an alcohol-related reduced relative risk of death (Fuchs et al., 1995). That is, alcohol helped those at highest cardiac risk.

In a separate analysis of the data, researchers reported that women who consumed between three and nine standard drinks per week had a decreased risk for coronary artery disease and ischemic stroke but a significantly increased risk of subarachnoid hemorrhage (RR. 3.7, CI 1.0–13.8) (Stampfer, Colditz, Willett, Speizer, & Hennekens, 1988). However, other reports from the NHS, not reviewed in this chapter, have documented that alcohol intake of approximately one to two drinks per day was associated with an increased risk of hypertension (Thadhani et al., 2002) and breast cancer, especially in women with low folate levels (Colditz & Rosner, 2000; Jiang et al., 2003). Thus, the hypothesis that the balance of risks and benefits associated with moderate alcohol consumption in women is different from that in men was substantiated. Details of reports from the Women's Health Study, including additional exclusion criteria, other controlled variables, relative risks, shape of the relationship, nadir, and level of onset, are summarized in Table 3.3.

The Framingham Heart Study

The overarching goal of the Framingham Heart Study (FHS) was to identify behaviors or characteristics that contribute to cardiovascular disease in a group of subjects over a long time period. The study, which began in 1948, currently continues to follow members of the original cohort of 5,209 men and women as well as 5,124 of their offspring. At the time of enrollment, original subjects were between the ages of 30 and 62 and free of clinical symptoms of cardiovascular disease. The FHS investigators are generally credited with being the first scientists to recognize that smoking, cholesterol, hypertension, and decreased physical activity increase the risk of heart disease and stroke.

FHS researchers also examined the association between alcohol use and heart disease. Information about alcohol use was collected biannually, and later

TABLE 3.3   Reports from the Channing Laboratory: The Health Care Professionals Follow-up Study and the Nurses Health Study

Author(s) (year), literature rating level	Sample, additional exclusion criteria	Design, follow-up period, statistically controlled variables, end point(s)		Findings: relative risk and 95% confidence interval at nadir; shape of association; nadir; onset of effect
			1.	Findings: relative risk and 95% confidence interval at nadir
			2.	shape of association
			3.	nadir; onset of effect
Fuchs et al. (1995) III	85,709 females None	Prospective cohort (12 years) Age, smoking Death	1.	RR death from all causes 0.83 (0.74–0.93) RR death from cardiovascular death 0.57 (0.43–0.76)
			2.	U-shaped
			3.	1–3 drinks per week; 1–3 drinks per week
Mukamal et al. (2003) III	38,007 males None	Prospective cohort (4 years) Age, smoking, diet, body mass index, physical exertion, HTN, diabetes, parental history of myocardial infarction Fatal and nonfatal myocardial infarction	1.	RR nonfatal myocardial infarction 0.55 (035–0.85) RR fatal myocardial infarction 0.50 (0.31–0.79) RR any myocardial infarction at frequency 5–7 days per week = 0.62 (0.48–0.78)
			2.	Inverse
			3.	For quantity ~4 drinks per day; ~1 drink per day For frequency 5–7 days per week; 1–2 days per week
Stampfer et al. (1988) III	87,526 females	Prospective cohort None Coronary artery disease Ischemic stroke Subarachnoid hemorrhages	1.	RR coronary artery disease 0.4 (0.2–0.8) RR ischemic stroke 0.3 (0.1–0.7) RR subarachnoid hemorrhage 3.7 (1.0–13.8)
			2.	Inverse
			3.	2.5 drinks per day; 3.9 drinks per week 0.5 to 1.0 drink per day; 0.5 to 1.0 drink per day Not applicable; 0.5 to 1.0 drink per day
Rimm et al. (1991) III	44,059 males None	Prospective cohort (2 years) Age, smoking, diet Fatal coronary disease, nonfatal myocardial infarction, CABG, and PCTA	1.	RR coronary artery disease .53 (0.35–0.79)
			2.	Inverse
			3.	≥ 2.5 drinks per day; 0.5–2.5 drinks per day

CABG = coronary artery by pass graft; HTN = hypertension; PCTA = percutaneous transluminal angioplasty; RR = relative risk annually, by a standardized questionnaire. Subjects were asked if they drank alcohol in the last 12 months, and if so, the average number of drinks per week of beer, wine, and spirits. In some, but not all, reports from the Framingham study, subjects who reported alcohol intake at year 2 of the study and denied intake at year 7 were categorized as former drinkers.

After 22 years of follow-up, men who drank alcohol were found to have lower all-cause mortality rates than those who did not drink. Among women subjects, alcohol use was protective from mortality (Gordon & Kannell, 1984). However, a subsequent analysis of the data revealed that men who drank alcohol also had lower levels of function. Alcohol use did not predict function in women (Pinsky, Leaverton, & Stokes, 1987). Data from the FHS also revealed that alcohol intake was positively associated with both left ventricular hypertrophy and left ventricular dilation among men. Again, the association was not found among women (Manolio, Levy, Garrison, Castelli, & Kannell, 1991). Increased ventricular mass is a documented risk factor for heart failure. Paradoxically, Framingham researchers have recently reported that the risk of congestive heart failure among men was lower at all levels of alcohol consumption and lowest among men who drank between 8 and 14 drinks per week. For women, the risk of congestive heart failure was also reduced and lowest among women drinking three to seven drinks per week, but this relationship was insignificant in the multivariate model (Walsh et al., 2002). In these studies, relative risk was calculated by Cox proportional hazards modeling. Nondrinkers were used as the comparison group. Cox proportional hazards modeling also revealed a decreased risk of intermittent claudication among both men and women participating in the FHS (Djousse, Levy, Murabito, Cupples, & Ellison, 2000). Thus, reports of findings generally reinforced the inverse association between moderate drinking and heart disease in men who consume alcohol. FHS reports also supported the hypothesis that the balance of risks and benefits of alcohol consumption is different for women than men.

FHS investigators (Djousse et al., 2002) recently reported that the relative risk of ischemic stroke is unrelated to alcohol use in either men or women, except in the subset of males age 60 to 69. This new analysis is notable for two reasons. First, this finding is in contradiction to the findings of most studies of ischemic stroke in the moderate-alcohol literature. Second, lifelong teetotalers were designated as the comparison group, and the relative risks for ischemic stroke were analyzed separately for former light and former heavy drinkers. This technique identified a threefold increase in risk of ischemic stroke among current nondrinking subjects who previously consumed one or more drinks per day compared with current nondrinking subjects who previously consumed less than one drink per day (Djousse et al., 2002). Whereas other researchers have argued that including both former drinkers and lifelong teetotalers in the drinking group artificially inflates the risks of abstinence, the findings of this study can be used to argue that including both light drinkers and heavy drinkers in the former drinking group artificially decreases the risks associated with former drinking. Details of reports from the FHS, including additional exclusion criteria, other controlled variables, relative risks, shape of the relationship, nadir, and level of onset, are summarized in Table 3.4.

The American Cancer Society Volunteer Study

The American Cancer Society Volunteer Study (ACSVS) is a prospective cohort study of 1.2 million adults over age 30 who were recruited by American Cancer Society volunteers. Subjects completed a questionnaire on alcohol, tobacco, diet, and other potential correlates of mortality (from cancer) in 1982. The analysis reviewed here was based on data from the 490,000 subjects who provided alcohol and smoking data. Alcohol consumption was assessed by the question How many cups, glasses, or drinks of these beverages do you usually drink a day, and for how many years? Type of alcohol (wine, beer, and spirits) was assessed separately. The study is notable for two reasons. First, this is by far the largest sample studied in the moderate-alcohol literature. One of every 180 adults living in the United States participated in this study. Second, one of the original aims of the study was to quantify the relationship between alcohol use at baseline and causes of death expected to be related to alcohol use. No previous study began with alcohol as a stated variable of interest.

The range of alcohol consumption reported was abstinence to more than six drinks per day. Cox proportional hazards analysis was used to calculate relative risks. The relative risks for cancers of the mouth, esophagus, pharynx, larynx, liver and breast were higher for subjects who drank any amount of alcohol compared with abstainers. The relative risk of breast cancer for women who drank one drink per day was 1.2 (CI 1.0–1.6). The relative risk of cardiovascular disease in general, and coronary artery disease death in particular, was decreased among all drinkers compared with abstainers. The largest reduction in heart disease occurred among older subjects with preexisting heart disease and subjects with multiple risk factors for heart disease. Women younger than 60 years of age or free of cardiovascular disease at baseline derived no benefit from alcohol use. Moderate drinkers had a decreased risk of diseases believed to be unrelated to alcohol as well as decreased rates of all-cause mortality (Thun et al., 1997). This latter finding was unexpected and may indicate that the reductions in relative risk associated with alcohol are actually mediated by an intervening variable such as socioeconomic status, access to health care, or lifestyle.

Studies in Ethnically Diverse Samples

A significant number of middle-aged and older Americans believe that news stories about the benefits of moderate drinking apply to most people (Masters,

TABLE 3.4   Reports from the Framingham Heart Study

Author(s) (year), literature rating level	Sample, additional exclusion criteria	Design and rating (Follow-up period), statistically controlled variables, end point(s)	1. Findings: lowest relative risk and 95% confidence interval at nadir 2. shape of association 3. nadir; onset of effect
Djousse et al. (2000)	18,339 males and females Intermittent claudication	Prospective Cohort (6.8 years) Age, diabetes, tobacco, systolic blood pressure, congestive heart failure Intermittent claudication	1. RR in males 0.67 (0.42–0.99) RR in females 0.44 (0.23–0.80) 2. J-shaped 3. Males 1–2 drinks per day; 1–2 drinks per day Women 0.5–1.0 drink per day; 0.5–1.0 drink per day
Djousse et al. (2002) III	5,209 males and females None	Prospective cohort (10 years) Tobacco use, blood pressure, diabetes mellitus, body mass index, and age Stroke	1. In the multivariate model, alcohol intake was not associated with ischemic stroke in either men or women 2. Not applicable 3. Not applicable
Manolio et al. (1991) IV	2,491 males and females None	Cross-sectional Not applicable Age, height, body mass index, systolic blood pressure, hypertension, tobacco Not applicable	1. Alcohol use was independently associated with left ventricular mass in men but not in women 2. Direct 3. Not applicable
Pinsky et al. (1987) IV	1,474 males and females None	Cross-sectional Not applicable Age, alcohol intake, tobacco use, ventricular rate, and education	1. Alcohol intake inversely related to function in men but not in women 2. Inverse 3. Not applicable
Walsh et al. (2002) III	6,289 males and females Congestive heart failure, coronary artery disease	Prospective cohort Not reported Age, smoking body mass index, diabetes, vascular heart disease, hypertension Heart failure	1. RR heart failure men: 0.46 (0.22–0.81) 2. No association in women in multivariate model 3. 8–14 drinks per week; 1–7 drinks per week

RR = relative risk

2003). This belief may be based on the sweeping generalizations about the possible cardiovascular benefits commonly provided by the popular media (Klatsky, 1999). However, sample composition of the studies reviewed up to this point predominantly has been limited to middle- and upper-class Caucasian subjects. Research in non-Caucasian populations is sparse. This section will describe the few reports extant about Japanese, Japanese American, African American, and Hispanic samples.

Japanese Men

Men from three rural Japanese communities between the ages of 40 and 69 without a history of stroke or coronary artery disease participated in the first of these studies (Iso et al., 1995). Subjects reported a range of alcohol intake from abstinence to more than six drinks per day. This distribution of intake was higher than for most Caucasian samples and allowed examination of the association of alcohol and cardiovascular disease and stroke at higher levels of consumption. The results revealed that the risk of all types of cardiovascular disease, except coronary artery disease, increased across all levels of alcohol consumption. Heavy alcohol consumption (more than 3.5 standard drinks per day) was associated with increased risk of ischemic stroke, hemorrhagic stroke, and sudden cardiac death. Although the data include a nonsignificant suggestion of a J-shaped relationship between drinking and coronary artery disease, Iso and colleagues were unable to identify a clear dose-response relationship between alcohol use and coronary artery disease.

Japanese American Men

The Honolulu Heart Study collected data on 8,006 Japanese American men between 1965 and 1962 (Goldberg, Burchfiel, Reed, Wergowske, & Chiu, 1994). Subjects were free of coronary artery disease, cerebrovascular disease, and cancer at baseline. The purpose of the original project was to verify observations that Japanese men who migrated to Hawaii had higher rates of coronary artery disease and lower rates of stroke compared with Japanese men who remained in their native country. Alcohol consumption among the Japanese American subjects ranged from abstinence to more than 3.5 standard drinks per day. Several studies have examined the relationship between alcohol use and cardiovascular disease among these Japanese American subjects. In the most prominent of the studies, data from men age 51 through 64 and men 65 through 75 were analyzed separately. Analysis of Variance (ANOVA) and a chi-square test for trends were used to analyze these data. The authors reported a small but nonsignificant trend toward lower rates of coronary artery disease among moderate drinkers. Intake of approximately one standard drink per day carried the lowest risk in subjects under 65 years of age. Intake of 2.0 to 3.5 standard drinks per day was associated with the lowest risk in older men (Goldberg et al., 1994). However, rates of cerebrovascular disease increased directly across all levels of consumption. This finding has important implications for primary prevention of stroke among Japanese American men. Japanese American men have 6 times the rate of hemorrhagic stroke compared with Caucasian Americans and much lower rates of coronary artery disease. Thus, the balance of risks and benefits of moderate alcohol consumption is very different among Japanese American men compared with Caucasian men living in the United States.

African American Men and Women

The National Health Interview Follow-up Study is a national longitudinal study that was designed to investigate the relationships among clinical, nutritional, and behavioral factors. A secondary analysis of these data addressed the relationship between average alcohol intake and all-cause mortality in 2,054 African American men and women. Alcohol intake was estimated by quantity and frequency questions. The investigators failed to show any cardioprotective effect of moderate alcohol consumption. In general, African American subjects experienced increased mortality at all levels of alcohol intake above an average of one drink per day. The authors speculated that this result was due to a less regular pattern of drinking among African Americans compared with Caucasians. In other words, if both groups drank the same absolute amount of alcohol, but Caucasians drank small amounts frequently and African Americans drank larger amounts infrequently, African American drinkers may be at greater risk due to inconsistent exposure to higher blood alcohol levels (Sempos, Rehm, Wu, Crespo, & Trevisan, 2003). However, this speculation contradicts the findings of an earlier secondary analysis of data from the 1988 National Health Interview Survey. The purpose of that analysis was to specify precisely the amount of alcohol associated with an improvement in cardiovascular health. Data from 43,763 men and women from diverse ethnic groups were included in the analysis. Lifestyle, sociodemographic, and biological variables were included in the analysis. The threshold for increased frequency of self-reported heart disease in the total sample was five drinks per day, but the threshold for increased frequency of self-reported heart disease in African-American men was one drink per day (Hanna, Shou, & Grant, 1997).

Latino Men and Women

The last study in this series determined the association between alcohol consumption and coronary artery disease in subjects from the New Mexico Elder Health Survey. The data reviewed here were collected from 833 subjects almost equally divided into four groups by gender and Hispanic or non-Hispanic ethnicity. Hispanic males and non-Hispanic White males had comparable average daily alcohol intakes (about 1.5 standard drinks per day), and Hispanic women had slightly lower average daily intake than non-Hispanic White women (0.75 drink per day and 0.9 drink per day, respectively). Multivariate adjusted odds ratios were calculated for drinkers and nondrinkers within each of the four gender/ethnic groups. Only male Caucasian subjects had decreased alcohol consumption–associated odds ratios for coronary artery disease. The authors speculated that the lack of significant findings among Hispanic males may be due to the fact that Hispanics enjoy a lower overall incidence of coronary artery disease compared with Caucasians (Lindeman et al., 1999).

In summary, many of the prospective cohort and cross-sectional studies reviewed substantiate an inverse association between moderate drinking and cardiovascular disease in some populations but not others (see Table 3.5). Outcomes from different studies and occasionally from the same study are divergent and conflicting. For example, analyses of data from the PHS clearly demonstrated an association between moderate drinking and decreased risk for cardiovascular disease among healthy (mostly Caucasian) male subjects who were free of angina, stroke, myocardial infarction, transient ischemic attacks, cancer, and renal, gastric, or liver disease at baseline. Similar findings were reported in smaller studies of healthy older adults not included in the 22 studies of this review (Abramson, Williamson, Krunholz, & Vaccarino, 2001; Colditz, 1985). These findings are difficult to reconcile with the report from the ACSVS (Thun et al., 1997) that the benefits of moderate drinking are restricted to older, sicker subjects with more cardiac risk factors at baseline. Further, multiple analyses of data from the same sample have produced inconsistent findings. Alcohol was positively related to left ventricular mass in men participating in the FHS (Manolio et al., 1991) but negatively related to heart failure in the same data (Djousse et al., 2000). Finally, the balance of the risk and benefit of moderate alcohol consumption appears to be different for women and minorities than for middle-class Caucasian males. These findings mandate a critical review of the quality of the studies before any conclusions about the efficacy of moderate drinking as a primary health promotion intervention can be made.

CRITIQUE OF THE LITERATURE

None of the 22 studies reviewed could be classified at level I or II (large or small clinical trials) according to the AHRQ criteria described earlier. However, 17 studies were classified as level III (prospective cohort studies), and 5 studies were classified as level IV (retrospective case control or cross-sectional studies). The quality of the implementation of the studies was evaluated in terms of

TABLE 3.5   Studies in Diverse Populations

Author(s) (year), literature rating level	Sample, additional exclusion criteria	Design (follow-up period), statistically controlled variables, end point(s)	1. Findings 2. shape of association 3. nadir; onset of effect
Iso et al. (1995) III	2,890 Japanese men None	Prospective cohort (10.5 years) Cholesterol, blood pressure, BMI, tobacco, diabetes, hypertension, ophthalmic changes, and ECG Coronary artery disease	1. No dose response relationship for coronary artery disease at any level of alcohol consumption 2. Slight suggestion of a J shape (not significant) 3. Not applicable; not applicable
Goldberg et al. (1994) III	6,069 Japanese American males Cancer, coronary artery disease, stroke	Prospective cohort (15 years) None Coronary artery disease Cerebrovascular disease	1. Slight decrease in coronary artery disease for a middle-aged man at 1 drink per day and for older men at 3.5 drinks per day 2. Not applicable 3. Benefits offset by increase in cerebrovascular disease
Lindeman et al. (1999) IV	220 Hispanic males 195 Hispanic females 245 Caucasian males 224 Caucasian females	Cross-sectional Age, blood pressure, diabetes, body mass index, waist to hip ratio, lipids, smoking, and education Coronary artery disease	1. Multivariate odds ratios indicated that only Caucasian males had an alcohol-associated decreased risk of coronary artery disease (OR 0.37 95%, CI 0.65–0.77) 2. Not applicable 3. Not applicable; not applicable
Hanna et al. (1997) IV	18,323 African American males 25,440 African American females	Cross-sectional Age, BMI, smoking, ex-drinker, ex-smoker, SES Self-reported heart disease	1. Caucasian men reported more heart disease at 5 drinks per day Black men reported more heart disease at 2 drinks per day 2. Women reported more heart disease at 2 drinks per day 3. Former drinkers more likely to have heart disease

(continued)

TABLE 3.5   *(continued)*

Author(s) (year), literature rating level	Sample, additional exclusion criteria	Design (follow-up period), statistically controlled variables, end point(s)	1. Findings 2. shape of association 3. nadir; onset of effect
Sempos et al. (2003) IV	768 males 1,286 females	Prospective cohort (19 years)	1. No beneficial effect was seen; mortality increased at intake levels above 1 drink per day 2. Positive linear 3. Not applicable; not applicable

BMI = body mass index; CI = confidence interval; ECG = electrocardiogram; OR = odds ratio; SES = socioeconomic status

sample composition and external validity, response rate and response bias, exclusion criteria, validity of the measurement of alcohol use, definition of abstainers, specification of the comparison group, and data analysis and interpretation. This evaluation will be discussed in the following sections.

Sample Composition and External Validity

Six of the 22 studies reviewed herein used data collected from practicing physicians (Alpert et al., 1999; Berger et al., 1999; Camargo et al., 1997a,b; Doll, 1997; Gaziano et al., 2000), two studies based findings on the responses of female registered nurses (Fuchs et al., 1995; Stampfer et al., 1988), and two studies used data collected from male health care professionals (Mukamal et al., 2003; Rimm et al., 1991). One other study enrolled friends and acquaintances of American Cancer Society volunteers (Thun et al., 1997). Another six studies enrolled residents of an upscale mid-sized city in the far suburbs of Boston (Djousse et al., 2000, 2002; Gordon & Kannell, 1984; Manolio et al., 1991; Pinsky et al., 1987; Walsh et al., 2002). In all, 17 of these studies enrolled subjects who were almost exclusively middle- and upper-middle-class individuals who were Caucasian, well-educated, and privately insured, with adequate access to health care and a documented interest in health.

Interestingly, although the findings of these large national survey studies generally supported an inverse association between moderate drinking and cardiovascular disease, the findings of several smaller studies that focused on minority subjects (Iso et al., 1995; Lindeman et al., 1999; Sempos et al., 2003) or on women (Djousse et al., 2000; Walsh et al., 2002) did not.

To summarize the contrary studies, a prospective cohort study of 6069 Japanese American men living in Hawaii reported a nonsignificant decreased risk for coronary artery disease (CAD) among light drinkers but an increased risk for stroke, cancer, and cirrhosis (Goldberg et al., 1994). A prospective cohort study of 2,890 Japanese males living in rural Japan also reported a nonsignificant decreased risk of CAD among drinkers but an increased risk of hemorrhagic stroke and cancer among moderate drinkers (Iso et al., 1995). These finding have important subpopulation-specific clinical implications. Unlike male Caucasian populations, Japanese Americans and indigenous Japanese subjects had mortality rates for cancer that were twice their rates for CAD; in addition, the number of deaths due to intracerebral hemorrhage also outnumbered the CAD-related deaths (Goldberg et al., 1994). Thus, the population level risks of moderate drinking may overwhelm any possible cardiovascular benefit among individuals of Japanese ancestry.

Similar reservations apply to women. Findings from the NHS of 85,709 female nurses documented that women consumed one to three standard drinks per week had the lowest risk for total mortality. However, these results were totally attributable to reduced relative risk among women over age 50 with at least one risk factor for CAD. Women drinking two standard drinks per day were at increased risk for death from all causes and from breast cancer in particular (Fuchs, 1997). Findings from the 251,420 women enrolled in the Cancer Prevention Study were worse; breast cancer risk increased at one standard drink per day (Thun et al., 1997). A small cross-sectional study of Hispanic women failed to find any evidence of an alcohol-related cardiovascular benefit, but breast cancer rates were not reported (Lindeman et al., 1999). Hence, sample composition of the largest and most influential of the studies reviewed here have severe sample limitations and cannot be generalized to women, minority groups, or groups defined by other socioeconomic characteristics.

Another problem with the big surveys is that the samples are so large. The ACSVS study enrolled nearly a half-million subjects. Such massive sample sizes lead to statistically significant associations or between group differences that are in fact very small. It is reasonable to hypothesize that any conclusion drawn from these studies that moderate drinking has cardioprotective properties is overreaching the data. Small associations (even if they become statistically significant by virtue of an enormous sample size) frequently hide an unrecognized mediator variable that is actually driving the relationship (Gorden & Kannell, 1983). In this case, genetic makeup of Caucasian males or some other variable may be operating.

Response Rates and Response Bias

In many studies, low response rates and response bias in favor of an inverse relationship between alcohol and cardiovascular disease undermine the validity of findings. Researchers in the PHS initially contacted all 261,248 male physicians age 40 to 84 who were members of the American Medical Association and living in the United States. Approximately 20% of these potential subjects agreed to participate in the study. Almost 33,000 of those willing to participate were eliminated by the exclusion criteria or failure to complete a pilot study. Finally, only 22,071 subjects, or less than 10% of the original subject pool, participated in the study (http://phs.bwh.harvard.edu/; accessed October 19, 2004). This series of reductions in the numbers of potential subjects can produce systematic bias. People do not volunteer to participate in research studies randomly. Volunteers tend to be healthier and more health-conscious than nonvolunteers. The physicians who volunteered to participate in this project were more likely to be healthier and have healthier lifestyle behaviors than physicians who did not respond to the initial invitation to participate in the project. Thus, the generalizability of subsequent secondary analyses focused on the alcohol questions must be called into question. This limitation could have been attenuated by a comparison of a random percentage of the responders and nonresponders. If these groups were shown to be comparable, it could have been argued that the final sample represented the target population. However, none of the studies reviewed here attempted to compare responders to nonresponders.

Decisions about the interpretation of missing data on alcohol items in the large surveys may have produced selection bias. In the ACSV study, 600,120 subjects who indicated that they consumed alcohol did not answer subsequent questions about quantity and were eliminated from the alcohol-focused analyses. Although the authors argued that these subjects were most likely light to moderate drinkers and their elimination did not affect the study findings, it seems equally plausible that many problem drinkers did not respond to the quantity question and were eliminated from the study. If true, their elimination created a bias in favor of an inverse relationship between alcohol and cardiovascular disease, as well as total mortality. Future studies with the large data sets should compare findings with the drink/no quantity subjects in and out of the analyses. Until that happens, concluding that the inverse relationships are valid is inappropriate.

Exclusion Criteria

As stated before, the secondary analyses were conducted on data originally collected in studies with objectives unrelated to alcohol. In several of the surveys, the goals of the original study mandated that subjects with potential alcohol-related diseases be excluded from the study. For example, the PHS examined the association between low-dose aspirin therapy and myocardial infarction, so anyone with a history of gout (a disease often associated with and exacerbated by alcohol use) were excluded. Alcohol is known to be a risk factor for several of the other diseases (hypertension, myocardial infarction, stroke, and liver and peptic ulcer disease) that were exclusionary criteria in the parent studies. In the PHS, 33,000 potential subjects with possible alcohol-related diseases were excluded from the original sample; this number actually outnumbered the subjects included in the final sample. Again, this source of systemic error would create a bias in favor of an inverse association between alcohol and cardiovascular disease in the chosen subjects. Other large-scale projects, such as the HCPFS and the NHS, employed similar exclusion criteria.

Measurement of Alcohol Use

Accurate measurement of alcohol consumption is a critical step in a valid study of the association between moderate drinking and cardiovascular disease. All of the studies discussed in this review used self-report to measure alcohol intake. Although self-reported alcohol consumption is considered to be reliable and valid (for a review, see Dawson, 1998), several factors must be taken into account to ensure the validity of self-reported data. Some examples include the assessment setting and interpersonal situation, respondent characteristics, cognitive recall strategies mandated by the questions, mode of administration, assurance of confidentiality, perception of the availability of corroborating information, clarity of the instructions, and respondent burden. When alcohol data are collected as part of a lengthy survey instrument developed for non-alcohol-related purposes, one cannot know whether the alcohol questions were given adequate consideration either by the instrument designer or by the respondents. These questions raise the concern that the reported alcohol data are suspect (Del Broca & Darkes, 2003).

The variety of items that gathered information about alcohol intake in the 22 studies makes it very difficult to compare instrument-related issues across studies. Researchers frequently classified alcohol consumption empirically, based on clusters of subject responses, rather than from any theoretical base. In some of the studies, self-reported alcohol intake was transformed from categorical data into standard drinks and from standard drinks into grams of ethanol per unit of time. This conversion gives an illusion of measurement precision that misrepresents the original data.

Although the general validity of appropriately gathered self-report data has been established (Del Boca & Darkes, 2003), some researchers misuse this approach. In the PHS, alcohol data were gathered as part of a food frequency questionnaire. Subjects were asked how frequently they consume alcoholic beverages. Frequency choices were "2 times per day," "daily," "5 or 6 times per week," "2 to 4 times per week," "1 time per week," "1 to 3 times per month," and "never/rarely." This set of choices does not elicit definitive information about the quantity of alcohol consumed on each drinking occasion. The never/rarely category could include infrequent binge drinkers, lifelong abstainers, former alcohol abusers, and subjects who drink only one drink on special occasions. The authors translated frequency data into quantity and reported that 97% of the physicians enrolled in the study drank fewer than two drinks per day. This translation overinterprets the data. The PHS study, in particular, is the source of so many publications showing the inverse relationship of moderate alcohol consumption and disease that it is the predominant force for this point of view in the United States. Thus, it is imperative that questions about the validity of alcohol measurement in the original study and decision rules used in coding these items for secondary analyses be addressed in future research.

Finally, the conclusion that 97% of the PHS sample drank fewer than two drinks per day implies that sample selection was biased in favor of moderate drinkers. The National Institute on Alcohol Abuse and Alcoholism (NIAAA, 2004) estimated that between 15.9% and 25.8% of middle-aged men in the United States consume more than five drinks per day at least once a month, and between 8.2% and 12.9% of middle-aged men consume five or more drinks on 12 or more days per month. Under the assumption that male physicians consume alcohol at rates similar to the general male public, the low rates reported from the PHS are suspect.

Definition of an Abstainer

The shape of the relationship between alcohol use and cardiovascular end points has been reported to be U-shaped (nondrinkers and heavy drinkers at equal risk, light and moderate drinkers at less risk), J-shaped (nondrinkers at lower risk than heavy drinkers but at greater risk than moderate drinkers), negative linear (inverse), positive linear (direct), and nonsignificant. Some of the variability in findings can be explained by the methods used to define the abstainer group. Early studies and some later studies included all individuals who reported no current alcohol consumption in the abstainer group. Both lifelong teetotalers and individuals who had stopped drinking because of alcohol-augmented and other illnesses were categorized as abstainers. However, male former drinkers are known to be older, more likely to be unmarried, cigarette smokers, obese, and hypertensive compared with abstainers. Male former drinkers also have greater comorbidity, including angina, myocardial infarction, diabetes, and bronchitis, and are more likely to label their health as poor when compared with lifelong abstainers. In some studies up to 70% of male abstainers were former drinkers (Shaper, 1990; Wannamethee & Shaper, 1988). Similarly, abstinent former-drinking female subjects showed an increased risk of death from both cardiovascular and noncardiovascular causes compared with lifelong abstainers (Fuchs et al., 1995). Thus, putting former drinkers with lifelong abstainers in the comparison group increases morbidity and mortality rates in the comparison group and gives the appearance of reduced risk in the moderate drinker group.

Investigators have attempted to solve the "sick-quitter problem" in two ways. In some studies, all subjects reporting any possible alcohol-augmented cardiovascular disease at baseline were excluded from the study. In other instances, subjects who developed cardiovascular morbidity and mortality during the first few years of follow-up were excluded from the analysis. These strategies effectively remove sick former drinkers from the abstainer group. However, potential subjects, at all levels of consumption, with any existing alcohol-related cardiovascular disease also are excluded. The result is a selection bias that underestimates the risk for cardiovascular disease at all levels of consumption. Additionally, assuming that cardiovascular disease develops over a long period of time, excluding subjects with prodromal stages of disease limits sample composition to middle-aged and older men, who may be resistant to cardiovascular disease because of a genetic predisposition or lifestyle characteristics.

Other investigators addressed the issue by separating former drinkers from abstainers based on responses to questions about past drinking practices. One of the most often cited studies exemplifies the difficulty of constructing questions that achieve this purpose. Thun and colleagues (1997) described the association between alcohol and mortality among 490,000 middle-aged and older adults in the ACSVS. Subjects who reported "zero" for current consumption of any alcoholic beverage and "zero or blank" for previous drinking were considered lifelong abstainers. Certainly it could be argued that interpreting a blank (no response) as no lifelong consumption is suspect and may mean that some number of ex-drinkers was counted in the abstainer group.

Specification of the Comparison Group

Several researchers have argued that even when lifelong abstainers can be identified accurately and separated from currently abstinent ex-drinkers, they are different from the general population in important ways and are not an appropriate choice for the comparison group. Lifelong abstainers are a minority group in Western countries and have reduced rates of cardiovascular mortality but increased rates of noncardiovascular and total mortality compared with other groups. In fact, when occasional drinkers in the British Health Study were used as the comparison group, lifelong abstainers, occasional drinkers, and light drinkers were at equal risk for cardiovascular events. This was true for subjects with and without previously existing heart disease.

Data Analysis and Interpretation

The most common statistical methods used in the data analyses were simple correlations and correlation-based procedures, most notably the Cox proportional hazards model. These procedures describe a relationship between or among variables. Correlations cannot be used to establish cause and effect. However, interpreting correlations as cause and effect is a common practice throughout the moderate-alcohol literature. Researchers frequently adopted the language of causality and reported the "effect of" moderate drinking on risk for coronary artery disease, the "cardioprotective effect" of moderate alcohol use, or the "benefit" of drinking in moderation. One author even wrote that the "evidence for a beneficial effect is massive" (Doll, 1997). All of these statements overstate the statistical evidence. Although there may be a causal relationship between moderate drinking and decreased rates of cardiovascular disease, it cannot be verified from correlation-based studies. Statements of causality can only be derived from true experimental designs. Randomized clinical trials would be necessary to establish a causal link between moderate drinking and decreased rates of cardiovascular disease. Such studies may not be feasible, because alcohol is a risk factor for many diseases and giving it to subjects as part of an intervention would have ethical implications. In addition, the intervention would need to go on for decades. Nevertheless, researchers should strive to design new studies with alcohol consumption as a primary focus and with rigorous attention to overcoming the weaknesses of the studies critiqued in this review.

CONCLUSION

Twenty-two articles were reviewed in this chapter. In general, the studies support an inverse relationship between moderate drinking and cardiovascular disease. An alcohol-associated decrease in incidence, relative risk, or odds of cardiovascular disease was reported in 15 studies. Relative risks of some type of cardiovascular disease ranged between RR = 0.21 (CI 0.22–0.75) for sudden cardiac death and RR = 0.79 (CI 0.63–0.99) for coronary artery disease. However, in 3 of these 15 studies, the imputed benefit of moderate alcohol use was offset, either partially or completely, by increases in cerebrovascular accidents. In 6 of the 22 studies, moderate drinking was physiologically neutral either in all subjects or in women. Non-Caucasian subjects and women experienced more alcohol-related harm at lower levels than Caucasian men. Among studies reporting an inverse association between moderate drinking and cardiovascular disease, the lowest level of consumption at which a significant relationship could be detected was 0.6 to 0.9 standard drinks per week for men. It seems questionable that a dose of alcohol this small can produce a significant physiological effect. This finding supports the hypothesis that the inverse association between moderate alcohol and cardiovascular disease is mediated by an unrecognized third variable, such as genetic protection, diet, socioeconomic status, exercise, or access to health care. The variability of the findings reported here calls into question the oft-drawn conclusion that moderate drinking could have broad efficacy as a primary health promotion intervention.

None of the studies reviewed met the criteria of a clinical trial, 5 were retrospective cross-sectional studies, and 17 were prospective cohort studies. Such studies are useful for generating hypotheses that can be tested in clinical trials but do not provide evidence adequate to recommend changing clinical practice. Finally, the studies were evaluated on several aspects of methodology: sample composition and external validity, response rate and response bias, exclusion criteria, measurement of alcohol use, definition of abstainers, specification of the comparison group, and data analysis and interpretation. Significant concerns were identified in each of these areas.

In conclusion, moderate alcohol is associated with decreased rates or relative risks of cardiovascular disease in some populations. However, the studies are flawed in many components of methodology, and evidence for a causal relationship is lacking. Based on this review, the strength of the available evidence for the proposition that moderate alcohol has broad-based efficacy as a primary health promotion intervention is inadequate, and any clinical recommendations to that effect are premature.

REFERENCES

Able, E. L., & Kruger, M. L. (1995). Hon v. Stroh Brewery Company: What do we mean by "moderate" and "heavy" drinking? *Alcoholism: Clinical and Experimental Research, 19*, 1034–1031.

Able, E. L., Kruger, M. L., & Friendl, J. (1996). How do physicians define "light," moderate, and "heavy" drinking? *Alcoholism: Clinical and Experimental Research, 22*, 979–984.

Abramson, J. L., Williams, S. A., Krunholz, H. M., & Vaccarino, V. (2001). Moderate alcohol consumption and risk of heart failure among older persons. *Journal of the American Medical Association, 285*, 1971–1977.

Alpert, C. M., Manson, J. E., Cook, N. R., Ajani, U. A., Gaziano, J. M., & Hennekens, C. H. (1999). Moderate alcohol consumption and the risk of sudden cardiac death among US male physicians. *Circulation, 100*, 944–950.

Anderson, P., Cremona, A., Paton, A., Turner, C., & Wallace P. (1993). The risk of alcohol. *Addiction, 88*, 1493–14508.

Berger, K., Ajani, U. M., Kase, C. S., Gaziano, J. M., Buring, J. E., Glynn, R. B., et al. (1999). Light-moderate alcohol consumption and the risk of stroke among U.S. male physicians. *New England Journal of Medicine, 34*, 1557–1564.

Camargo, C. A., Stampfer, M. J., Glynn, R. J., Grodstein, F., Gaziano, J. M., Manson, J. E., et al. (1997a). Moderate alcohol consumption and risk for angina pectoris or myocardial infarction in U.S. male physicians. *Annals of Internal Medicine, 126*, 364–371.

Camargo, C. A., Stampfer, M. J., Glynn, R. J., Grodstein, F., Gaziano, J. M., Manson, J. E., et al. (1997b). Prospective study of moderate alcohol consumption and risk of peripheral arterial disease in US male physicians. *Circulation, 95*, 577–580.

Chen, W. Y., Colditz, G. A., Rosner, B., Hankinson, S. E., Hunter, D. J., Manson, J. E., et al. (2002). Use of postmenopausal hormones, alcohol and risk for invasive breast cancer. *Annals of Internal Medicine, 137,* 798–804.

Colditz, G. A., Branch, L. G., Lipnick, R. J., Willett, W. C., Rosner, B., Posner, B., et al. (1985). Moderate alcohol and decreased cardiovascular mortality in an elderly cohort. *American Heart Journal, 109,* 886–889.

Colditz, G. A., & Rosner, B. (2000). Cumulative risk of breast cancer to age 70 years according to risk factor status: Data from the Nurses' Health Study. *American Journal of Epidemiology, 152,* 950–964.

Corrao, G., Bagnardi, V., Zambon, A., & Arico, S. (1999). Exploring the dose response relationship between alcohol consumption and the risk of several alcohol-related conditions: A meta-analysis. *Addiction, 94,* 1551–1573.

Corrao, G., Rubbiati, L., Bagnaredi, V., Zambon, A., & Poikolainen, K. (2000). Alcohol and coronary heart disease: A meta-analysis. *Addiction, 95,* 1505–1523.

Crabb, D. W., Matsumoto M., & You, M. (2004). Overview of the role of alcohol dehydrogenase and aldehyde dehydrogenase and their variants in the genesis of alcohol related pathology. *Proceedings of the Nutrition Society, 63,* 49–63.

Dawson, D. A. (1998). Measuring alcohol consumption: Limitations and prospects for improvement. *Addiction, 93,* 965–968.

————. (2000). US low-risk drinking guidelines: An examination of four alternatives. *Alcoholism: Clinical and Experimental Research, 24,* 1820–1829.

Del Boca, F. K., & Darkes, J. (2003). The validity of self-reports of alcohol consumption: State of the science and challenges for research. *Addiction, 98*(Supp. 2), 1–72.

De Lorgeril, M., Dalen, P., Martin, J. L., Boucher, F., Pillard, F., & deLeiris, J. (2002). Wine drinking and risks of cardiovascular complications after recent acute myocardial infarction. *Circulation, 106,* 1465–1470.

Djousse, L., Ellison, T. C., Beiser, A., Scaramucci, A., D'Agostino, R. B., & Wolf, P. A. (2002). Alcohol consumption and risk of ischemic stroke: The Framingham Study. *Stroke, 33,* 907–912.

Djousse, L., Levy, D., Murabito, J. M., Cupples, L. A., & Ellison, C. (2000). Alcohol consumption and risk of intermittent claudication in the Framingham heart study. *Circulation, 102,* 3092–3097.

Doll, T. (1997). One for the heart. *British Medical Journal, 315,* 1664–1668.

Doll, T., Peto, R., Hall, E., Wheatley, K., & Gray, R. (1994). Mortality in relation to consumption of alcohol: 13 years' observations on male British doctors. *British Medical Journal, 309,* 911–918.

Dufour, M. C. (1999). What is moderate drinking defining "drinks" and drinking levels. *Alcohol Research and Health, 23,* 5–14.

Fuchs, C. S., Stampfer, M., Colditx, G. A., Giovannucci, E., Manson, J. W., Kawachi, I., et al. (1995). Alcohol consumption and mortality among women. *New England Medical Journal, 332,* 1245–1250.

Gaziano, J. M., Gaziano, T. A., Glynn, R. J., Sesso, H. D., Ajani, U. A., Stampfer, M. J., et al. (2000). Light to moderate alcohol consumption and mortality in the physicians' health study enrollment cohort. *Journal of the American College of Cardiology, 35,* 96–105.

Goldberg, R. J., Burchfiel, C. M., Reed, D. M., Wergowske, G., & Chiu, D. (1994). Valvular and myocardial heart disease: A prospective study of health effects of alcohol consumption in middle-aged and elderly men—the Honolulu heart program. *Circulation, 89,* 651–659.

Gordon, T., & Kannell, W. B. (1983). Drinking habits and cardiovascular disease: The Framingham study. *American Heart Journal, 105,* 667–673

———. (1984). Drinking and mortality: The Framingham study. *American Journal of Epidemiology, 120,* 97–107.

Hanna, E. Z., Shou, S. P., & Grant, B. F. (1997). The relationship between drinking and heart disease morbidity in the United States: Results from the National Health interview survey. *Alcoholism: Clinical and Experimental Research, 21,* 111–118.

Hart, C. L., Smith, G. D., Hole, D. J., & Hawthorne, V. M. (1999). Alcohol consumption and mortality from all causes, coronary heart disease, and stroke: Results from a prospective cohort study of Scottish men with 21 years follow-up. *British Medical Journal, 318,* 1725–1729.

Herrington, D. M., & Klein, K. P. (2003). Randomized clinical trials of hormone replacement therapy for treatment or prevention of cardiovascular disease: Review of the findings. *Atherosclerosis, 166,* 203–212.

Hersh, A. L., Stefanick, M. L., & Stafford, R. S. (2004). National use of postmenopausal hormone therapy: Annual trends and response to recent evidence. *Journal of the American Medical Association, 291,* 104–106.

Iso, H., Kitamura, A., Shimamoto, T., Sankai, T., Naito, Y., Sato, S., et al. (1995). Alcohol intake and the risk of cardiovascular disease in middle-aged Japanese men. *Stroke, 26,* 767–773.

Jiang, R., Hu, F. B., Giovannucci, E. L., Rimm, E. B., Stampfer, M. J., Spiegelman, D., et al. (2003). Joint association of alcohol and folate intake with risk of major chronic disease in women. *American Journal of Epidemiology, 158,* 760–761.

Karhunen, P. J., Erkinjuntii, T., & Laippala, P. (1994). Moderate alcohol consumption and loss of cerebellar Purkinje cells. *British Medical Journal, 308,* 1663–1667.

Klatsky, A. R. (1999). Moderate drinking and reduced risk of heart disease. *Alcohol Research and Health, 23,* 15–23.

Laporte, R. E., Cresanta, J. L., & Kuller, L. H. (1980). The relationship between alcohol consumption and atherosclerotic heart disease. *Preventive Medicine, 9,* 22–40.

Lindeman, R. D., Romero, L. J., Allen, A. S., Liang, H. C., Baumgartner, R. N., Koehler, K. M., et al. (1999). Alcohol consumption is negatively associated with the prevalence of coronary heart disease in the elder health survey. *Journal of the American Geriatrics Society, 47,* 396–401.

Manolio, T. A., Levy, D., Garrison, R. J., Castelli, W. P., & Kanell, W. B. (1991). Relation of alcohol intake to left ventricular mass: The Framingham study. *American Journal of Cardiology, 17,* 717–721.

Masters, J. A. (2003). Moderate alcohol consumption and unappreciated risk for alcohol-related harm among ethnically diverse, urban-dwelling elders. *Geriatric Nursing, 24,* 155–161.

Mills, J. L., & Graubard, B. I. (1987). Is moderate drinking during pregnancy associated with an increased risk for malformations? *Pediatrics, 80,* 309–314.

Moore, R. D., & Pearson, T. A. (1986). Moderate alcohol consumption and coronary artery disease. *Medicine, 65,* 242–267.

Mukamal, K. J., Conigrave, K. M., Mittleman, M. A., Camargo, C. A., Stampfer, M. J., Willett, W. C., et al. (2003). Roles of drinking pattern and type of alcohol consumed and coronary heart disease in men. *New England Journal of Medicine, 348,* 109–118.

National Institute on Alcohol Abuse and Alcoholism (NIAAA). (2004). NHIS 1997–
    2002 data table of heavy drinking by males 18 years of age and older. Retrieved on
    October 24, 2004, from http://www.niaaa.nih.gov/databases/dkpat28.htm
Pearl, R. (1926). *Alcohol and longevity.* New York: Knopf.
Pinsky, J. L., Leaverton, P. E., & Stokes, J. (1987). Predictors of good function: The
    Framingham study. *Journal of Chronic Disease, 40*(1 Supp.), 159S–167S, 181S–2.
Renaud, S., & deLorgeril, M. (1992). Wine, alcohol, platelets, and the French paradox
    for coronary artery disease. *Epidemiology, 3339,* 1523–1526.
Ridker, P. M., Manson, J. E., Buring, J. E., Muller, J. E., & Hennekens, C. H. (1990).
    Circadian variation of acute myocardial infarction and the effect of low-dose aspirin
    in randomized trial of physicians. *Circulation, 82,* 897–902.
Rimm, E. B., Giovannucci, E. L., Willett, W. C., Colditz, G. A., Ascherio, A., Rosner,
    B., et al. (1991). Prospective study of alcohol consumption and risk of coronary artery
    disease in men. *Lancet, 338,* 1073–1074.
Romelsjo, A., & Leifman, A. (1999). Association between alcohol consumption and
    mortality, myocardial infarction, and stroke in a 25-year follow-up of 49,618 young
    Swedish men. *British Medical Journal, 319,* 821–822.
Rossouw, J. E., Anderson, G. L., Prentice, R. L., LaCroix, A. Z., Koope, C., Stefanick,
    M. L., et al. Writing Group for the Women's Health Initiative Investigators. (2002).
    Risks and benefits of estrogen plus progestin in healthy postmenopausal women: Princi-
    pal results from the Women's Health Initiative randomized controlled trial. *Journal of
    the American Medical Association, 288,* 321–333.
Sempos, C. T., Rehm, J. W. T., Crespo, C. J., & Trevisan, M. (2003). Average volume
    of alcohol consumption and all cause mortality in African Americans: The NHEFS
    cohort. *Alcoholism: Clinical and Experimental Research, 27,* 88–92.
Sesso, H. D., Stampfer, M. J., Rosner, B., Hennekens, C. H., Manson, J. E., & Gaziano,
    J. M. (2000). Seven-year changes in alcohol consumption and subsequent risk of
    cardiovascular disease in men. *Archives of Internal Medicine, 160,* 2605–2612.
Shaper, A. G. (1990). Alcohol and mortality: A review of prospective studies. *British
    Journal of Addiction, 85,* 837–847.
Shaper, A. G., & Wannamethee, S. G. (2000). Alcohol intake and mortality in middle-
    aged men with diagnosed coronary heart disease. *Heart, 83,* 394–399.
Spies, C. D., Sander, M., Stangl, K., Fernandez-Sola, J., Preedy, V. R., Rubin, E., Andreas-
    son, S., Hanna, E. Z., & Kox, W. J. (2001). Effects of alcohol on the heart. *Current
    Opinions in Critical Care, 7,* 337–343.
Stampfer, M. J., Colditz, G. A., Willlett, W. C., Speizer, F. E., & Hennekens, C. H.
    (1988). A prospective study of moderate alcohol consumption and the risk of coronary
    disease and stroke in women. *New England Journal of Medicine, 319,* 267–273.
Tanasescu, M., Hu, F. B., Willett, W. C., Stampfer, M. J., & Rimm, E. B. (2001). Alcohol
    consumption and risk of coronary heart disease among men with type 2 diabetes
    mellitus. *Journal of the American College of Cardiology, 38,* 1836–1842.
Thadhani, T., Carmargo, C. A., Stampfer, M. J., Curhan, G. C., Willett, W. C., &
    Rimm, E. B. (2002). Prospective study of moderate alcohol consumption and risk of
    hypertension in young women. *Archives of Internal Medicine, 162,* 569–570.
Thun, M. J., Peto, R., Lopez, A. D., Monaco, J. H., Henley, J., Heath, C. W., & Doll,
    R. (1997). Alcohol consumption and mortality among middle-aged and elderly U.S.
    adults. *New England Journal of Medicine, 337,* 1705–1714.

U.S. Department of Agriculture. (2000). *Nutrition and your health: Dietary guidelines for Americans*. Washington, DC: Author.

U.S. Department of Health and Human Services. (1998). Substance abuse among older adults, treatment improvement protocol series. Washington, DC: Author.

———. (2000). *10th special report to the U.S. Congress on alcohol and health*. Washington, DC: Author.

Walsh, C. R., Larson, M. G., Evans, J. C., Djousse, L., Elison, R. C., Vasan, R. S., et al. (2002). Alcohol consumption and risk for congestive heart failure in the Framingham heart study. *Annals of Internal Medicine, 136*, 247–249.

Wannamethee, S. G., & Shaper, A. G. (1988). Men who do not drink: A report from the British regional heart study. *International Journal of Epidemiology, 17*, 307–316.

———. (1997). Lifelong teetotallers, ex-drinkers, and drinkers: Mortality and the incidence of major coronary heart disease events in middle-aged British men. *International Journal of Epidemiology, 26*, 523–531.

Wannamethee, S. G., Shaper, A. G., Walker, A., & Ebrahim, B. (1998). Lifestyle and 15 year survival free of heart attack, stroke, and diabetes in middle aged British men. *Archives of Internal Medicine, 158*, 2433–2440.

White, I. R. (1999). The level of alcohol consumption at which all-cause mortality is the least. *Journal of Clinical Epidemiology, 52*, 537–540.

PART II

Research on Alcohol
Use, Misuse, Abuse,
and Dependence
through the Life Span

Chapter 4

Alcohol Consumption During Pregnancy

Cara J. Krulewitch

ABSTRACT

Alcohol is a potent teratogen in humans, and prenatal alcohol exposure is a leading preventable cause of birth defects and developmental disabilities. The term fetal alcohol syndrome (FAS) refers to a pattern of birth defects found in children of mothers who drank during pregnancy. FAS has four criteria: maternal drinking during pregnancy, a characteristic pattern of facial abnormalities, growth retardation, and brain damage (often manifested by intellectual difficulties or behavioral problems). As surveillance and research have progressed, it has become clear that FAS is but a rare example of a wide array of defects that can occur from exposure to alcohol in utero. At least 1 in 10 women will continue to consume alcohol during pregnancy, putting their fetuses at risk for the effects of alcohol exposure.

Nurses are in a key position to provide care and conduct research that will contribute to the prevention of the adverse effects of prenatal alcohol exposure during the preconception and perinatal periods, as well as deal with the negative outcomes of exposure in the developing infant. Many areas have yet to be evaluated. Screening tools and interventions have been developed and tested, mostly in majority cultures. Culturally sensitive instruments must be generated and validated for high-risk groups such as Native Americans. Fetal alcohol biomarkers and genetic research are new and need considerably more work. Effective "no drinking during pregnancy" campaigns for high-risk groups must be created and tested. Nurses are well placed to conduct

101

research that will describe the effects at social, behavioral, and biological levels; develop middle-range theories targeted at preventing the drinking behavior and optimizing care of affected children after birth; and generate and test effective interventions that enhance prevention strategies in the 21st century.

Keywords: pregnancy, prenatal care, alcohol use in pregnancy, drinking in pregnancy, fetal alcohol syndrome, fetal alcohol effects, infant outcome, alcohol consumption

Alcohol is a potent teratogen (an agent that interferes with normal embryonic development) in humans (Adams et al., 2002; Burd & Wilson, 2004; Eustace, Kang, & Coombs, 2003). For this reason, prenatal alcohol exposure has been identified as one of the leading preventable causes of birth defects and developmental disabilities (Jacobs, Cooperman, Jeffe, & Kulig, 2000; Weber, Floyd, Riley, & Snider, 2002). Within this context, Healthy People 2010 objectives for pregnant women are dedicated to reducing this problem: The goal is abstinence in 94% (16-17a) of pregnant women and elimination of binge drinking in 100% of pregnant women (16-17b) (U.S. Department of Health and Human Services [USDHHS], 2000b). Alcohol use during the childbearing years, as well as during pregnancy, is a major public health challenge.

Effects of prenatal alcohol exposure are mentioned in the Bible, and references in medical and nursing literature date to 1885 (Ismail & Moawad, 1984). Nearly three decades ago, researchers coined the term *fetal alcohol syndrome* to describe a pattern of birth defects found in children of mothers who drank during pregnancy. A diagnosis of FAS requires meeting four criteria: maternal drinking during pregnancy, a characteristic pattern of facial abnormalities, growth retardation, and brain damage (often manifested by intellectual difficulties or behavioral problems) (Stratton, Howe, & Battaglia, 1996). The evolution of terminology and progress in the research are summarized in Table 4.1.

Nurses have had a long and active involvement in the investigation of prevalence, etiology, prevention strategies, and health services research for low birth weight and birth defects. Nurse-researchers broke new ground with their work on the role of alcohol during pregnancy shortly after it was first described (Anderson, Anderson, & Smith, 1986; Barbour, 1990; Burns, Kruckeberg, Stibler, Cerven, & Borg, 1984; Dowdell, 1981; Marbury et al., 1983) and also played a key role in developing the earliest preconception and prenatal education programs (Davis & Frost, 1984; Jessup, 1988; Rowe, 1989).

This chapter includes a discussion on alcohol use and pregnancy and a critique of the relevant research. It is organized around two major topics: drinking during pregnancy and alcohol effects on infants. The review covers prevalence, screening, measurement, prevention, and treatment.

TABLE 4.1   A Historical Overview of Events Related to Prenatal Exposure to Alcohol

Description	Citation or date of event	Comments and importance
Association between prenatal drinking and the rate of infant mortality	Sullivan (1899)	First reported association between alcohol use and infant outcome
Directly linked maternal alcohol consumption and fetal growth restriction	Rouquette (1957)	First reports noted in the 1950s
Described characteristics, including growth deficit, mental retardation	Lemoine et al. (1968)	First to describe an association between alcohol consumption and birth defects in 127 children born to alcoholic mothers
First description of physical growth and intellectual and social performance	Ulleland (1972)	Identified abnormalities, including slow growth, deficient intellectual and social performance, structural abnormalities of face in 8 out of 12 children born to alcoholic mothers
Fetal alcohol syndrome (FAS) introduced	Jones & Smith (1973)	First use of the term
Animal research on the effects of alcohol and pregnancy funded by NIH and reported	Abel (1974)	CRISP database search reveals first studies funded by NIH in 1977
USDHHS and USDT prepare report to Congress	1980	Initial public awareness of problem
First Surgeon General's report on FAS	1981	Recommendation to study the problem
Introduction of term *fetal alcohol effects* (FAE)	Sokol & Clarren (1989)	This term was vague and often became "possible FAE." To date, alcohol effects focused on heavy drinking (> 14 standard drinks per day)

(continued)

TABLE 4.1 *(continued)*

Description	Citation or date of event	Comments and importance
Section 705 of Public Law 102-321 (the AD-AMHA Reorganization Act)	Stratton et al. (1996)	Mandated Institute of Medicine to conduct a study of FAS and related birth defects
Expansion of terminology	Sokol, Delaney-Black, & Nordstrom (2003)	Including prenatal alcohol effects (PAE), alcohol-related birth defects (ARBD), and alcohol-related neurodevelopment defects (ARND). Confusion develops in diagnosis of the prenatal effects of alcohol consumption
Research begins to look at lower levels of drinking and binge drinking	May 1996	20 years after FAS first identified, several thousand articles published, most focusing on biochemical mechanisms. Newer research begins to look at social, behavioral, and psychological influences. (see Baer et al., 2003, Day et al., 2002 and Autti-Ramo et al., 2002)
National Task Force on Fetal Alcohol Syndrome and Fetal Alcohol Effects (FAE) formed	Weber et al. (2002)	Established in 2000, delegated to Centers for Disease Control and Prevention National Center on Birth Defects and Developmental Disabilities (NCBDDD)
Landmark agreement between National Organization on Fetal Alcohol Syndrome (NOFAS), government agencies (including NCBDDD, and NIH) and private experts meet and develop a consensus statement	Bertrand et al. (2004)	Provides researchers and clinicians with an umbrella term when discussing the problem; the term is not intended for clinical diagnoses

ADAMHA = Alcohol, Drug Abuse, and Mental Health Administration; CRISP = Computer Retrieval of Information on Scientific Projects; NIH = National Institutes of Health; USDHHS = U.S. Department of Health and Human Services; USDT = U.S. Department of Treasury

METHOD

An electronic search was completed using the Medline and Cumulative Index of Nursing and Allied Health Literature (CINAHL) and PsychINFO databases from January 1, 1966, to September 14, 2004, for all studies using the terms *alcohol consumption*. The search engine recommended the use of the term *alcohol drinking*. In addition, searches were completed on the terms *pregnancy, prenatal care, pregnancy outcome, fetal alcohol syndrome,* and *infant outcome*. The search engine recommended using the terms *infant, newborn, biological markers alcohol, genetics,* and *alleles*. All subheadings were used for each term. Additional searches included the Computerized Retrieval of Information on Scientific Projects (CRISP) database for studies funded by the National Institutes of Health (NIH) from 1971 to 1975 to find the earliest studies of animal research. The ETOH Archival Database, Medline in Process, and other nonindexed citations were also searched.

EPIDEMIOLOGY

Alcohol Consumption during Pregnancy: National Estimates

Current data on alcohol use in pregnancy are limited by a dearth of national surveys specifically evaluating pregnancy behavior and outcomes. Floyd and Sidhu (2004) described rates of alcohol use among women of childbearing age using general health survey datasets. Even with limitations in these data, they found that rates of alcohol use remained unchanged over the past decade. One in eight pregnant women consume alcohol (i.e., 500,000 women) during pregnancy, and about 80,000 of them are binge drinkers (i.e., heavy, episodic drinkers; see chapter 2, Table 2.1, for definitions of drinking terms).

Three primary data systems—the Pregnancy Risk Assessment Monitoring System (PRAMS), the National Survey on Drug Use and Health (NSDUH, formerly known as the National Household Survey on Drug Abuse, NHSDA), and the Behavioral Risk Factors Surveillance Survey (BRFSS)—are used for these estimates. They all use self-reported alcohol consumption data and thus are subject to bias due either to recall errors or to reluctance to disclose. Potential subjects receive questionnaires by mail or telephone, so pregnant women are missed who have no telephone, are institutionalized, or are homeless.

PRAMS

This is an ongoing, state- and population-based surveillance system designed to monitor selected self-reported maternal behaviors and experiences that occur before, during, and after pregnancy among women who deliver a live-born infant. PRAMS began in 1987, and currently 31 states and New York City participate. Survey data are linked to birth certificate information and can be used to produce statewide estimates of perinatal health behaviors, including alcohol consumption. Because it covers only about 62% of the U.S. population, national estimates cannot be extrapolated accurately (Williams et al., 2003). The most recent PRAMS estimates of alcohol consumption during pregnancy included eight states where 2000–2001 weighted data were available. Estimates of alcohol use in pregnancy ranged from 3.4% to 9.9%, with an increase in reported consumption in all eight states. The highest prevalence of alcohol use during the last trimester occurred among older, higher income, non-Hispanic women with more than a high school education (Phares et al., 2004).

National Survey on Drug Use and Health

National estimates of alcohol consumption in childbearing women and during pregnancy are contained in two national surveys. The National Survey on Drug Use and Health is conducted annually by the Office of Applied Studies within the Substance Abuse and Mental Health Services Administration (SAMHSA). Data have been collected annually by face-to-face interviews of noninstitutionalized civilians 12 years or older since 1971. Respondents are asked about substance use in the past month, and women of childbearing age are asked if they are currently pregnant (SAMHSA, 2004). In 2002 several improvements were made to the procedures and weighting rules, so comparisons with earlier surveys are risky (SAMHSA, 2002, 2003a,b). Nevertheless, the estimated proportion of pregnant women drinkers in 1999–2000 was 12%, and in 2002 it was 9%. Binge drinking dropped from 4.6% to 3% overall, but it was 7% in the 15 to 17 age group, compared with 3.1% among women ages 25 to 44.

BRFSS

The Centers for Disease Control and Prevention (CDC) conducts the BRFSS, which is a monthly telephone survey of adults 18 years and older. This surveillance system began in 1984 with 15 states, and by 1994 all 50 states, the District of Columbia, Puerto Rico, Guam, and the Virgin Islands were participating. The telephone survey includes detailed questions on many health behaviors including alcohol intake (CDC, 2004).

Early reports of alcohol use in pregnancy came from the BRFSS; data showed a decline from 32% in 1985 to 20% in 1988 (Stratton et al., 1996). Ebrahim et al. (1998) reviewed BRFSS data from 1988 to 1995 and found that any alcohol use during pregnancy continued to drop until 1992, when the rate was 9.5%. After 1992, rates rose to a high of 16.3% in 1995 (CDC, 1997). This change was significant at $p < .01$ and persisted after controlling for selected sociodemographic characteristics, including age, income, marital and employment status, education, smoking, and race. A similar pattern occurred in frequent drinking (seven or more drinks per week or five or more drinks per occasion); it reached a high of 3.5% in 1995. Consumption rates were lower in married women, women ages 18 to 24, and White women. Although rates of any drinking dropped to 12.8% in 1999, there was no drop in rates of binge or frequent drinking (CDC, 2002a).

Critique of National Databases

Although the NSDUH and the BRFSS provide the most comprehensive estimates of national alcohol use during pregnancy, the telephone sampling approach is subject to potential bias. A better design was used in 1992 by the National Institute on Drug Abuse (NIDA) in a study called the National Pregnancy and Health Survey (NPHS). This survey included a randomized sample of pregnant women and was weighted to represent all women with live-born infants in the 48 contiguous United States for the subject year (NIDA, 1996). Drinking estimates reported from this study were 23% among White women and 19% overall. These figures were much higher than estimates from other national studies and suggest underestimation in the convenience sample surveys described above (Drews, Coles, Floyd, & Falek, 2003).

Other problems with the NHSDA and BRFSS data include the relatively small numbers of pregnant women plus nonresponse that is as high as 22% in the NHSDA. Furthermore, women without phones, homeless women, and institutionalized women are not represented in the data, but such women may be pregnant and at risk for alcohol consumption (CDC, 2002a; Floyd & Sidhu, 2004). Even with these limitations, the samples are weighted to represent population samples and provide the most comprehensive data available on alcohol use in pregnant and childbearing women. Clearly, a population-based surveillance system that includes alcohol consumption information, possibly using biochemical markers as well as self-report, would provide more accurate estimates.

Alcohol Consumption in Women of Childbearing Age: National Estimates

Understanding drinking patterns of women of childbearing age is important because alcohol-related birth defects occur early in pregnancy before a woman knows or confirms the pregnancy. In addition, half of all pregnancies are unintended (Henshaw, 1998). Naimi, Lipscomb, Brewer, and Gilbert (2003) evaluated the risk and found that women with unintended pregnancies were 1.43 times (CI 1.13–1.54) more likely to report binge drinking compared with those with intended pregnancies. Also, the proportion of unintended pregnancies increased with the number of episodes of binge drinking. Women with four or more episodes of binge drinking were 2.3 (CI 2.12–2.57) times more likely to experience an unintended pregnancy. These findings persisted among White women after adjustments for race, sociodemographic, and pregnancy risk factors. The association was not significant for Black respondents.

The BRFSS was used to evaluate drinking patterns in nonpregnant women of childbearing age. Rates were 50.6% for any drinking, 12.6% for frequent drinking (7–14 drinks per week), and 1% for heavy drinking (> 14 drinks per week); these 1997 findings were not significantly different from 1991 (CDC, 1997). The 1995–1999 data showed some pattern differences. Although any drinking changed only from 11.2% (1991) to 12.3% (1999), binge drinking was 1.7 (CI 1.6–1.8) times greater for younger women (ages 18 to 30) compared with women ages 31 to 44. Frequent drinking was 1.4 (CI 1.4–1.5) times greater in younger women (CDC, 2002a). Thus, the group most likely to become pregnant drinks more heavily.

Special Populations

Some investigators studied small samples of women in vulnerable or clinic populations. A recent study in northeastern Maine evaluated predominantly Caucasian women from a rural health clinic. Rate of pre-pregnancy alcohol use was 25%, with significant decreases during pregnancy (Hayes et al., 2002). In a group of pregnant prison inmates, 50% had used alcohol during their current pregnancy (Fogel & Melyea, 2001). Data from the Metropolitan Atlanta Congenital Defects Program (MACDP) showed that 35% of women in public hospitals and 28% of women in private hospitals drank during the first trimester of pregnancy. Among these women, 85% abstained during the second trimester and less than 10% drank in the third trimester (Drews et al., 2003).

Critique of Data on Alcohol Use during the Childbearing Years

Expansion of PRAMS to all 50 states and territories and a targeted study of pregnant women would provide more accurate estimates of the actual extent of drinking during pregnancy. This targeted survey should evaluate women during pregnancy and/or immediately following delivery; it should ask about specific timing (in relation to pregnancy onset), quantity, and frequency of consumption, timing, and patterns of binging, and length of time that alcohol was ingested over the trimesters. Further, a longitudinal follow-up that tracked children through age 5 would help fill in some of the unknowns about the effects of different quantities of alcohol during critical periods of fetal development. Because contextual factors can affect this relationship, a detailed data collection approach that includes sociodemographic factors, stressors, living conditions, and other potential cofactors should be included in the data collection tool.

Special populations merit scientific scrutiny, because there are alarming data about drinking patterns in minority and vulnerable populations of pregnant women. Larger scale studies of diverse populations would provide a more comprehensive description of the patterns of alcohol use and the cultural, social, and behavioral characteristics that may be associated with any use, persistent use, and heavy use in these populations.

SCREENING FOR ALCOHOL CONSUMPTION DURING PREGNANCY AND THE CHILDBEARING YEARS

Screening can be achieved with interview tools, laboratory tests, or physical examinations. Early work on alcohol screening tools focused on the White male population (Ewing, 1984; Selzer, 1971). The field still has no valid and reliable instrument for childbearing-age and pregnant women. There is also need for one or more instruments that are appropriate for culturally diverse groups of women in a variety of settings.

During pregnancy, screening has many purposes; some are directed at evaluating the mother, and others seek to evaluate the fetus. Savage et al. (2003) noted that there are two separate patients when screening for alcohol consumption in pregnancy, and each may suffer from a different disorder. Screening intended to evaluate the mother is focused on identifying alcohol dependence and a need for intervention for the addiction. Evaluation of the fetus is for alcohol exposure that may create risk for FAS or other negative developmental sequelae.

Nurses are in a primary position to screen for alcohol use because they have the first contact with the client and conduct other screenings and assessments during an office or hospital visit. Unfortunately, there is no national guideline for alcohol screening of pregnant women (Savage et al., 2003). Alcohol consumption tools have only been available for 2 decades, and most focus on the woman's dependence, not her developing fetus's exposure. Indirect fetal assessment requires the number of drinks consumed per day, together with reports of sporadic binge drinking episodes and the trimester of pregnancy. Timing and blood alcohol concentration (BAC) are more predictive of fetal risk than weekly intake (Cornelius, Goldsmith, Taylor, & Day, 1999; Gladstone, Levy, Nulman, & Koren, 1997; Livy, Miller, Maier, & West, 2003; Lundsberg, Bracken, & Staftlas, 1997).

Self-Report Screening Instruments

Screening tools for women are finally being evaluated. The 4-question CAGE (Ewing, 1984) and the 25-question Michigan Alcohol Screening Test (MAST)

(Seltzer, 1971) are less valid in women, who have different patterns of alcohol consumption than men (Babor & Grant, 1989), but instrument refinements and new tools specific to women did not occur until the 1990s (Allen, Litten, Fertig, & Babor, 1997; Chang, 2001). The purpose of newer tools continued to be detection of alcohol dependence rather than specific consumption patterns (Bradley, Boyd-Wickizer, Powell, & Burman, 1998). In pregnancy, heavy drinking associated with alcohol dependence is rare, but moderate drinking occurs in 1 in 10 pregnant women.

Questions about quantity and frequency pose challenges for pregnant women because of the stigma associated with alcohol consumption (Ernhart, Marrow-Tlucack, Sokol, & Martier, 1988; Jacobson, Chiodo, Sokol, & Jacobson, 2002). Women may alter their drinking when they discover they are pregnant; so it is important to determine consumption patterns during the first few weeks before pregnancy was confirmed. Newer tools have been developed to account for these issues. Jacobson et al. (2002) demonstrated that women who reported the absolute alcohol consumption of 0.9 oz per day at conception decreased their drinking to 0.2 oz per day in the second and third trimesters. The first instrument developed to test for risky drinking during pregnancy (in 1989 defined as 1 oz of absolute alcohol or more per day, 14 or more drinks per week) was the four-question T-ACE (Chang, 2001; Sokol, Martier, & Ager, 1989). This tool and the five-question TWEAK (Russell et al., 1994) included questions from the MAST or CAGE, along with a question about tolerance to alcohol (Russell et al., 1996). Earlier versions of both tools asked the woman how many drinks it took to feel the effects of alcohol (How many drinks does it take to make you feel high?); this item became the maximum number of drinks it takes to feel sleepy or pass out (How many can you hold?) (Russell et al., 1996). The new item removes the stigma of consumption during pregnancy and is quite sensitive in African American women (Chang, 2001; Dawson et al., 2001). Tolerance is an important measure, because as tolerance increases, consumption during one drinking episode (binging) often increases. The addition of the tolerance question allows the TWEAK and T-ACE to identify infrequent heavy intake, such as binge drinking, as well as moderate levels of drinking in pregnant women (Dawson et al., 2001).

Chang, Goetz, Wilkins-Haug, and Berman (1999) tested the T-ACE to predict alcohol dependence in pregnant women alone and with the addition of clinical covariates (age, early pregnancy recognition, routine obstetric care, and craving alcohol in the past week). The T-ACE correctly identified 65% of current prenatal drinkers when used alone and 75% with the addition of the clinical indicators. Based on these findings, Chang et al. (1999) identified the T-ACE plus additional clinical questions as an effective means of identifying women who consume alcohol while pregnant. Russell et al. (1996) evaluated the CAGE, MAST, TWEAK, and T-ACE, along with the "hold" (tolerance) question against the T-ACE alone. A positive response to the tolerance question was defined as six or more drinks. Sensitivity increased as cut points decreased, with relatively small decreases in specificity. The TWEAK correctly identified 90% of women, and the T-ACE correctly identified 89%. The reported sensitivity of the T-ACE administered alone was lower than when included in the larger set of questions. The "hold" version of the tolerance question produced higher rates of sensitivity compared with the "high" version used in earlier years (79% for TWEAK, 70% for T-ACE).

The Alcohol Use Disorders Identification Test (AUDIT), a 10-question screen that may be self- or interviewer-administered, was designed to distinguish between early versus late-stage alcohol abuse in male and female populations (Allen et al., 1997; Babor & Grant, 1989). The AUDIT has high sensitivity (80%–100%) and specificity (95%–100%) in a variety of populations (Bradley et al., 1998; Savage et al., 2003). Chang et al. (1999) found that the AUDIT identified 70% of current drinkers, increasing to 75% with the addition of clinical indicators. These three tools—AUDIT, T-ACE, and TWEAK—are effective in identification of women at risk for alcohol consumption during pregnancy. Although they do focus on alcohol dependence, not consumption, either four-item tool with the tolerance question included (T-ACE or TWEAK), plus the specific quantity question in the AUDIT, can identify binge and moderate drinking in pregnant women.

Critique of Self-Report Screening Instruments

There is no gold standard to measure sensitivity and specificity. Currently, screening tools are measured against the longer MAST and detailed questions by trained interviewers on actual quantity and frequency of alcohol consumption. This makes accumulation of evidence difficult across studies. Replicated studies using a consistent gold standard, perhaps determined by a consensus of experts, would further knowledge development.

In light of measurement challenges, new approaches were proposed. Computer-assisted interviewing was introduced by Thornberry et al. (2002). It uses an enhanced version of TWEAK in an audio-computerized self-report interview. Women in an urban clinic population found it easy to use. Findings for alcohol use (30%) during pregnancy were similar to reports in other urban areas (Chang et al., 1999; Russell, 1994). These rates are higher than the national estimates of 9% to 12%, possibly reflecting urban influences, the effectiveness of the approach, or the anonymity provided by the technique. Results showed good sensitivity and specificity of 70.6% and 73.2%, respectively, for heavy drinking and 65.6% and 63.7%, respectively, for any drinking during pregnancy. This study did not ascertain trimester or pattern of consumption.

Savage et al. (2003) proposed a two-step approach to address the dual screening necessary in obstetric populations: First, do alcohol dependence detection in women, then fetal alcohol exposure risk in infants. This approach uses the timeline followback method (Sobel, Brown, Leon, & Sobel, 1996) (see chapter 2 in this volume for an explanation of this method). The two steps would be repeated at each prenatal visit. Because this data collection strategy has not been tested for validity and reliability, it will be necessary to determine the psychometrics, feasibility, and cost effectiveness prior to its institution as standard practice.

The most serious gap in measurement is the absence of tools to detect alcohol exposure of the fetus. Negative alcohol effects might derive from frequent low-volume drinking, one binge session, or other drinking patterns depending on the timing of the fetus's brain-growth status (Burns, 1990). Considering the variety of patterns that constitute risk for the developing fetus, no tool currently exists that meets the requirement. An ideal tool would detect sporadic binge drinking and the timing of consumption over the course of the three trimesters. Timing of drinking and blood alcohol concentrations are more predictive of negative fetal outcome than total volume of alcohol consumed over a number of days (Cornelius et al., 1999; Gladstone et al., 1997; Gladstone, Nulman, & Koren, 1996; Livy et al., 2003; Lundsberg et al., 1997).

In conclusion, the several screening tools that have demonstrated high sensitivity and specificity in detecting alcohol dependence do not detect lower levels of risk drinking, yet lower levels can pose a risk to the fetus. Nurse-researchers and others have proposed newer approaches to screening, including a two-step approach and the use of computer-assisted interviewing. These approaches may increase the identification of low-volume fetal exposure to alcohol and in so doing minimize fetal risk. Further testing of these and development of new tools to capture fetal risk are warranted. Ideally, there would be a comprehensive instrument that would address both alcohol dependence in the mother and the risk for effects of alcohol exposure on the fetus.

Biological Markers as Screening Tools

Biochemical markers address the concerns of many researchers that self-report underestimates alcohol consumption (Ernhart et al., 1988; Russell et al., 1996). In the pregnant woman, biochemical analysis can be used to screen for current alcohol consumption by measuring the concentration in blood, saliva, urine, or the breath. These measures are relatively accurate, and several have sensitivities and specificities of 99% (Sommers, Savage, Wray, & Dyehouse, 2003). (For a review of biomarkers, see chapter 2 in this volume.)

The most popular biologic marker to detect earlier exposure to alcohol in the newborn infant is fatty acid ethyl esters (FAEEs), a product formed by the esterfication of ethanol that can be found in blood, hair, placenta, cord blood, and meconium (Bearer, 2001; Moore, Jones, Lewis, & Buchi, 2003). Its presence in serum has been detected up to 24 hours following ingestion (Soderberg et al., 1999). Hair may indicate the timing of the exposure, but it is not always available and cutting the infant's hair may be unacceptable to the parents (Bar-Oz, Klein, Karaskov, & Koren, 2003). Meconium has been identified as having the greatest promise for evaluation of prior alcohol exposure. FAEEs have a longer half-life and have been detected in meconium at 48 to 72 hours of age (Bearer, 2001). Bearer et al. (1999) compared FAEEs in meconium with maternal self-report of alcohol consumption and found that the presence of ethyl linoleate, an FAEE, in meconium was significantly associated with maternal reports of a higher mean number of drinks per week in the month before pregnancy and during the first trimester. The sensitivity and specificity of the test to distinguish mothers who had one or more drinks per week in the third trimester compared with those who denied use were 72% and 51%, respectively. Accuracy was lower for predicting one or more drinks per day in the month before pregnancy (68% and 48%, respectively). Quality of meconium analysis is dependent on the testing method used.

Moore, Lewis, and Leikin (1995) evaluated the three published procedures and found false-positive rates as high as 43%. Bearer et al. (2003) carefully outlined a method of FAEE isolation and tested it in a group of South African women; it detected heavy drinking (14 drinks per week before pregnancy), with specificity 83%, sensitivity 84%, and positive predictive value 94%. Chan et al. (2003) conducted a population-based study to identify the levels of a variety of FAEEs (stearate, oleate, linoleate, laurate, palmitate, and mysristate) in meconium of infants from nondrinking women and found that using a cutoff score of 2 nmol total FAEE per gram of meconium yielded a sensitivity of 100% and specificity of 98.4%, regardless of the ethyl ester evaluated. Moore et al. (2003) noted that the degradation of specimens is high (up to 86%) and must be frozen for best stability (11% loss over 6 days and more than 50% over 43 days).

Required now is further refinement of testing and storage methods, population-based studies in nondrinking women (as well as case-control studies), and replication in diverse populations. If this work continues to show promise, it may be the best method to determine fetal exposure during late pregnancy. The problem is that it is then too late to prevent the problem.

Critique of Biomarkers in Pregnancy

The accuracy of biological measures in women generally and during pregnancy differs from accuracy in men. The sensitivity of hemoglobin acetaldehyde (HAA) was reported at 67%, with a specificity of 77% at an area of 0.030% in chronic heavy alcohol users of both sexes (Hazelett et al., 1998). Although HAA levels in males are higher than in females, pregnant women with the highest concentrations of HAA subsequently delivered an infant with fetal alcohol effects (Cook, 2003). Therefore, this measure has been identified as the most sensitive measure of binge drinking in pregnant women (Stoler et al., 1998). The combination of markers increased sensitivity and the risk of having an affected infant significantly increased when there were two or more positive markers. Risk was 8.83 times (CI 3.1–25.03) higher with two or more positive biomarkers and 10.97 times (CI 3.18–37.86) higher when adjusting for toxicology screens (Stoler et al., 1998). Although sample sizes were small, this relatively new approach is fertile ground for further research. Nurses skilled in screening tool administration are well placed to conduct research that evaluates the efficacy of a combined marker and self-report approach. The cost effectiveness of biochemical markers to augment self-report has not been investigated. This is another important area for investigation.

INTERVENTIONS FOR ALCOHOL USE DURING PREGNANCY

Methods to decrease alcohol consumption in pregnant women were investigated by Rosett and colleagues in 1980. Several approaches have been tried, including brief intervention (Chang, Goetz, Wilkins-Haug, & Berman, 1997, 2000), motivational interviewing (Handmaker, Miller, & Manicke, 1999), and the "one-stop shop" approach without (Whiteside-Mansell, Crone, & Conners, 1999) and with home visits from paraprofessionals (Dunnagan, Haynes, Christopher, & Leonardson, 2003; Grant, Ernst, Pagalilauan, & Streissguth, 2003).

Brief Intervention

Brief intervention (BI) involves one to three short sessions comprised of personalized feedback on alcohol-related health problems and risk, as well as advice, options of treatment, and self-help options (Chang et al., 1999, 2000; Handmaker & Wilbourne, 2001). Most BI studies have not included pregnant women. Manwell, Fleming, Mundt, Staffacher, and Barry (2000) reanalyzed data from the Fleming (1997) randomized clinical trial (RCT) (482 men and 292 women) who received care from community-based physicians in 10 Wisconsin counties. Experimental group women who became pregnant after the intervention were 1.93 times (CI 1.07–3.46) more likely to reduce drinking by 20% or more. However, 20% reduction is probably not enough to prevent negative fetal effects.

Only two dedicated clinical trials have evaluated the use of brief intervention in pregnant or postpartum women (Chang et al., 1999, 2000; Hankin & Sokol, 2003). Chang and colleagues (1999) screened 886 (76% of those approached) women using a health habits survey that included the T-ACE and identified 532 (60%) women as positive. The first 250 positives who met inclusion criteria were entered. Subjects were randomized to receive comprehensive alcohol assessment only (AO) or BI. More than half (143, or 57%) of subjects did not drink alcohol during pregnancy and were reportedly abstinent prior to the assessment. The remainder (107, or 43%) consumed alcohol prior to the study assessment. The return rate for follow-up was 99% and averaged 57 days postdelivery. No significant differences between groups were found for decreased number of drinks per episode or number of episodes during their pregnancies. The control group improvement may have been due to the extensive pretest assessment conducted by Chang and colleagues (1999, 2000) in both groups. The pretest probably became a confounder.

Hankin and Sokol (2003) conducted an RCT to evaluate BI as a prevention strategy to prevent alcohol-related neurodevelopmental defects (ARNDs) in future children exposed to alcohol during pregnancy. Women received BI in the postpartum period, with the goal of improving neurodevelopmental outcomes in subsequent siblings. A total of 96 women were randomly assigned either to a BI group or usual care. Women were followed through a subsequent pregnancy, and infants were tested using the Psychomotor Developmental Index (PDI) and the Mental Developmental Index (MDI) at 15 months of age. A significant protective effect on developmental delay ($p < .03$) was demonstrated for those who received BI postpartum.

These two studies represent the only evaluations of BI during pregnancy or the postpartum period. Although limited by small sample sizes and clinical convenience sampling, these data suggest that BI may show promise for childbearing age and pregnant women. Further research on BI before and during pregnancy is warranted.

Motivational Interviewing

Motivational interviewing (MI) goes beyond BI strategies; it involves more comprehensive counseling and guides the recipients to explore their ambivalence about changing behavior while focusing on the perceived discrepancy between current behaviors and overall goals (Miller & Rollnick, 2002). Motivational interviewing was tested in two prenatal settings (Handmaker et al., 1999; Ingersoll, Floyd, Sobell, & Velasquez, 2003). Handmaker and colleagues tested MI in 42 pregnant women who reported recent alcohol consumption. After administration of a comprehensive alcohol use assessment, subjects were randomized to a 1-hour motivational interview session or an information-only session that included a personalized letter informing them of the risks of drinking during pregnancy. Both groups of women decreased alcohol consumption during pregnancy, but MI was more effective in women with high blood alcohol concentrations initially.

Ingersoll et al. (2003) used MI in women of childbearing age to reduce alcohol consumption during pregnancy and to increase contraceptive use. Six high-risk community-based settings were included. Subjects had to have reported drinking more than seven standard drinks per week or consuming five or more standard drinks in a single day within the past 3 months. Women received four MI sessions and one contraceptive counseling session. Women who completed the intervention and 6-month reassessment were compared with those who dropped out. A total of 190 women agreed to participate in the study, and 143 completed the 6-month assessment. Among the completers, 98 (68.5%) satisfied the criteria for success. There were no differences in demographic or treatment history between the groups. At 6-month reassessment, the predictors for successful change were the AUDIT ($p > .011$) and the Brief Situational Confidence Questionnaire ($p = .016$). The authors concluded that women who felt least able to control their drinking and experienced more temptation were the least likely to be successful.

"One-Stop Shop" of Services

Another intervention is called the "one-stop shop" of services (Grant et al., 2003; Whiteside-Mansell et al., 1999; Dotson, Henderson, & Magraw, 2003; Dunnagan et al., 2003; Struck, 2003). Each experimental program included home visits, social services linked to health services, and alcohol treatment. Except for Grant et al., these projects are still undergoing evaluation. The Grant et al. program included home visiting by paraprofessionals annually for 3 years after enrollment (2+ years postpartally). Subjects were heavy drinkers (more than five drinks per occasion 1 or more times per month) or illicit drug users. Women were recruited immediately before giving birth. Every third eligible woman was assigned to the control group. A total of 103 women were enrolled, with 65 in the experimental group, where paraprofessional advocates supported them to obtain treatment, encouraged them to provide a safe environment, and linked families to community and health services. Structured interviews were done at exit and 1.6 to 3.6 years after the program. At the end of 3 years, 60 (92%) were located, and 45 (74%) were interviewed at all three points. A significantly higher number of experimental group women reported current abstinence of at least 6 months (0% at baseline vs. 31% at exit, $p < .001$).

Critique of Treatment Research

Treatment research in pregnant populations is still in the early stages of science building. A few quasi-experimental studies and RCTs showed effective treatment outcomes for some but not all women. Samples were small, and investigators did not separate the effects of treatment from the effect of the pregnancy itself in reducing alcohol consumption. Although the BI trials were not being evaluated for long-term effects on the fetus, a 9-month period of abstinence would protect the fetus from harm (Handmaker & Wilbourne, 2001; Miller, 2000; Morse & Hutchins, 2000). Therefore, BI may hold promise as a prenatal approach, given that pregnancy is a time-limited phenomenon. This said, there are still the issues of abstinence in childbearing age women who might become pregnant and postpartum mothers who are breastfeeding. Hence, randomized controlled trials must be conducted that focus on preconceptional, prenatal, and breastfeeding women, and these trials should evaluate potential motivators, separate out the natural effects of pregnancy, evaluate the dosage and content of the interventions, and compare the skill levels of interventionists. Postprogram follow-ups such as ones by Grant et al. (2003) and Ingersoll et al. (2003) and Hankin and Sokol's (2003) focus on women interconceptionally may show promise in addressing some of these issues.

Handmaker and Wilbourne (2001) recommended a stepped approach to intervention: screening (using TWEAK); comprehensive assessment, combined with advice for those who screen positive; brief intervention and monitoring for those identified at risk for moderate drinking; and motivational intervention with additional social service referrals for those identified as heavy drinkers. This intervention model should be coupled with a focus on motivators for change. Also, the influences of age, education, and intention to breastfeed need further exploration since Chang et al. (1999) found that intention to breastfeed among older, more educated mothers was associated with increased alcohol consumption.

ALCOHOL TERATOGENICITY IN HUMANS

There is compelling evidence that alcohol use is a potent organ system and behavioral teratogen in humans (Adams et al., 2002; Burd & Wilson, 2004; Eustace et al., 2003; Livy et al., 2003; Polygenis et al., 1998; Weber et al., 2002). Gaps in knowledge about fetal alcohol effects remain about specific timing and amount of alcohol consumed, contextual risk factors, and effective prevention strategies. The Public Affairs Committee of the Teratology Society on Fetal Alcohol Syndrome (FAS) has categorized these gaps into five areas of focus: (1) improved recognition of FAS, (2) identification of neurobehavioral effects associated with prenatal exposure to alcohol, (3) determining risks of heavy alcohol consumption during early pregnancy, (4) risk factors for and prevention of FAS, and (5) social and economic factors associated with the prevalence of FAS (Adams et al., 2002). Nurses and nurse-researchers have the experience to evaluate all of these areas in both animal and human models.

Investigators have evaluated many of the physical, neurobehavioral, and direct effects of alcohol on the fetus. Alcohol use in pregnancy can result in prenatal developmental problems, such as intrauterine growth restriction (Abel & Hannigan, 1996; Shu, Hatch, Mills, Clemens, & Susser, 1995; Sokol, 1981) and in poor postnatal development, including full-blown FAS (Abel, 1984; Jones & Smith, 1973). Alcohol consumption has also been associated with an increased rate of spontaneous abortions (Coleman, Rearson, Rue, & Cougle, 2002; Rasch, 2003; Windham, Fenster, Hopkins, & Swan, 1995), congenital anomalies (Day et al., 1989; Ernhart et al., 1987; Martinez-Frias, Bermejo, Rodriguez-Pinilla, & Frias, 2004), problems in childhood development (Coles, Smith, Fernhoff, & Falek, 1985; Coles et al., 1991; Day & Richardson, 1991; Hindemarch, Kerr, & Sherwood, 1991), sudden infant death syndrome (Iyasu et al., 2002), and other causes of fetal, infant, and child mortality (Burd & Wilson, 2004; Rasch, 2003).

Studies have also examined the direct effects of alcohol on perinatal survival. A French team demonstrated a strong association between stillbirth and alcohol consumption even after adjustment for sociodemographic factors (Kaminski, Rumeau, & Schwartz, 1978). Kesmodel, Wisborg, Olsen, Henriksen, and Secher (2002) noted similar findings in Denmark. Sokol (1981) found that women who drank reported higher rates of prior spontaneous abortions and low-birth-weight babies. Burd and Wilson (2004) reviewed this corpus of studies and noted that, in addition to mortality, impaired parenting and multigenerational alcohol abuse led to a circle of vulnerability that can produce negative effects through entire life cycles and over several generations.

Fetal Response to Alcohol in Utero

There are several factors that affect fetal response to alcohol effects. These factors include timing of exposure or critical periods, susceptibility to alcohol exposure, and threshold and pattern of drinking.

Critical Periods of Fetal Development

There is a gap in knowledge linking the timing of exposure to alcohol and the gestational age of the infant. Given the ethical issues, no studies exist wherein pregnant women actively consumed alcohol in a controlled experiment. Only case-control studies and prospective observational studies have been conducted.

Variations in definitions of quantity and frequency make comparisons across studies difficult. In particular, there is little agreement on the definitions of moderate intake. Two drinks per day in pregnancy is defined as risk drinking (Abel, Kruger, & Friedl, 1998). Although most study teams measured alcohol exposure by a day-by-day diary of alcohol consumption over a period of time once or twice during the pregnancy or the 3 months prior to pregnancy, the intake amount was averaged over the measurement period. This obfuscates precise intake in critical fetal periods because it does not account for the timing of alcohol consumption, and it levels out the number of drinks across the week and misses binges. But when binging episodes are specifically examined, timing is seldom evaluated. Both parameters are necessary.

When using self-report, all the above problems are confounded by the definition of a standard drink. Although researchers identify a standard drink as 0.5 oz of absolute alcohol, women have identified a variety of quantities as one drink, depending on how questions are asked (Serdula, Mokdad, Byers, & Siegel, 1999). Many investigators provided the subjects with definitions of a standard drink (Thornberry et al., 2002). Considering the drawbacks to human studies, it seems that animal studies may offer the best promise for learning about the relationship between low levels of daily alcohol intake, sporadic high levels of consumption, and phase of fetal development.

FETAL ALCOHOL SYNDROME AND FETAL ALCOHOL EFFECTS

Intrauterine growth restriction (IUGR) due to alcohol occurs primarily during the third trimester. By contrast, functional damage can occur at any time during development once organs have formed. The full spectrum of FAS is more likely to occur when drinking has persisted during all three trimesters, but individual anomalies may occur as a result of drinking at relatively high levels during more discrete periods. There appears to be no "safe" time to drink during pregnancy. Extremely early alcohol exposure often leads to nonviability of the fetus and spontaneous abortion (Coles, 1994). The effects associated with specific amounts of consumption are unknown (Eustace et al., 2003). More current research indicates that specific genotypes are associated with susceptibility to alcohol exposure. An allele of interest has been alcohol dehydrogenase 2 (ADH2) (Stoler, Ryan, & Holmes, 2002). Chambers and Jones (2002) argued that the presence of this gene may actually alter drinking behavior as opposed to creating a protective effect on alcohol consumption. Eustace et al. (2003) concluded that there has been little systematic empirical work on determining factors for adverse effects of alcohol consumption in human infants.

Incidence and Prevalence Rates of FAS and FAE

FAS is the most severe form of fetal damage from alcohol and refers to a distinct disorder with clinical features. The Fetal Alcohol Study Group of the Research Society on Alcoholism proposed formal criteria for the diagnosis of FAS in 1980

(Rosett et al., 1980). National estimates of the prevalence of FAS through the 1990s ranged from 0.2 to 1.0 per 1,000 live-born infants (CDC, 2002a). A study conducted by the Fetal Alcohol Syndrome Surveillance Network (FASSNet) evaluated rates in Alaska, Arizona, Colorado, and New York and found rates of 0.3 to 1.5 per 1,000 live births. The study found that rates varied by ethnicity, with rates highest in Alaska. Researchers noted that rates in American Indians/ Alaska Natives was 3.0 per 1,000 live births compared with other Alaska residents, with a rate of 0.2 per 1,000 live births. Rates were also higher among Blacks (CDC, 2002b). May (1996) evaluated 16 studies that estimated the prevalence of FAS, FAE, and total alcohol related birth defects (ARBD) between 1977 and 1993. FAS rates for clinic-based studies ranged from 0.4 to 3.1 per 1,000 live births.

The incidence of FAS in sites serving low-income women and African Americans is about 10 times higher than at sites serving middle-class women (Abel, 1995). Sokol et al. (1986) compared 25 FAS and 50 non-FAS infants in a synthetic case-control study to examine factors related to FAS. The mothers of FAS children were older, were more likely to be Black, had higher gravidity and parity, and were more likely to screen positive on the MAST. For women who drank heavily and who were in all four of the above categories, the probability of having a child with FAS was 85.2% (Whitty & Sokol, 1996). The risk for Black infants appears to be 7 times greater than for White infants, after adjusting for frequency of maternal alcohol intake (Iosub, 1985; Sokol et al., 1986).

Registry-based studies ranged from 0.2 to 0.37 per 1,000 live births overall. A study by Chavez, Cordero, and Becerra (1988) reported rates by ethnicity. The highest rate was among Native Americans (2.97 per 1,000 live births), and the lowest rate was among Asians (0.03 per 1,000 live births). Population-based studies focused on specific populations. Among Southwest and Plains Native Americans, rates varied from 2.0 to 8.5 per 1,000 live births. In British Columbia, rates were 1.4 to 6.5 per 1,000 live births. Rates for ARBD, FAE, and FASD are higher than assessed, but these less severe variations are not often calculated because of the lack of standardized criteria for diagnosis and delay in discovery of the condition. Sampson, Streissguth, and Bookstein (1997) estimated that the rates of these less severe conditions are about 3 times higher than rates of FAS. Surveillance of these less severe conditions is absent from the prevalence data, but they are necessary to form a complete picture of alcohol effects and for early treatment purposes.

Effects of Heavy Alcohol Use

Heavy alcohol consumption during pregnancy is associated with a characteristic facial dysmorphology that includes midfacial hypoplasia, long, smooth philtrum, thin upper lip, small widely spaced eyes, and inner epicanthal folds (Hannigan &

Armant, 2000; Polygenis et al., 1998; Sokol, Delancey-Black, & Nordstrom, 2003). Because facial development occurs during the embryonic period, craniofacial anomalies due to maternal drinking probably result from drinking during this earliest stage of pregnancy (Wolfgan, 1997), when the mother is unaware of her pregnant state. This assumption has not been fully supported. After statistically analyzing craniofacial anomalies in children exposed to alcohol prenatally, some investigators reported a relationship between these anomalies and first-trimester exposure. They found greater dysmorphia (associated with lower intelligence quotient, IQ) a relationship between heavy maternal drinking in the periconceptual period and the first 2 months of pregnancy (Day et al., 1989; Ernhart et al., 1987; Graham, Hanson, Darby, Barr, & Streissguth, 1988). But a recent case-control study noted that eye abnormalities occurred during sporadic higher doses of alcohol (Martinez-Frias et al., 2004) across all trimesters of pregnancy.

A variety of abnormal parameters, including head circumference, height, weight (in varying severity levels—25th percentile, 10th percentile, etc.), and growth restriction, consistently have been documented when alcohol exposure is in the high range (> 14 drinks per day) (Day et al., 2002; Day, Richardson, Geva, & Robles, 1994; Windham et al., 1995). Infants that were exposed to heavy drinking in utero do not catch up to other infants. Small brain size and other brain abnormalities have been confirmed at autopsy. In addition, intellectual and behavioral abnormalities and increased risk of seizures result (Wekselman, Spiering, Hetteberg, Kenner, & Flandermeyer, 1995).

Effects of prenatal alcohol exposure on full-body growth appear to be related to exposure later in pregnancy. Coles et al. (1991) demonstrated that alcohol exposure that continues throughout pregnancy produces fetal growth deficiencies that can be observed at birth. When alcohol is discontinued by the beginning of the second trimester, growth may approach that in children of nondrinkers (Coles et al., 1985; Rosett et al., 1980). This suggests that the growth deficit associated with alcohol occurs in the third trimester. Day et al. (1991), in a large longitudinal study, found that alcohol-related stunting appeared to be related to second- and third-trimester exposure. Also, they found adverse effects on growth from first-trimester alcohol exposure; thus, there may be more than one mechanism for alcohol effects on growth. The exact mechanisms and the timing of the effect remain unanswered, and further research, including long-term follow-up studies, is warranted.

Longitudinal studies that have followed children for up to 21 years have documented all stages of development and identified a variety of neurobehavioral and growth distortions that persisted throughout childhood and adolescence. The Maternal Health Practices and Child Development Project (Day et al., 2002) followed alcohol-exposed (light [< 0.2 drinks per day], moderate [0.2–0.89 drinks per day], heavy [> 0.89 drinks per day]) and non-alcohol-exposed children for 16 years. The researchers identified an association between growth deficits and prenatal alcohol exposure in the first trimester. Deficits continued through at least 14 years of age and were accompanied by short- and long-term learning and memory deficits. The effects demonstrated a dose–response pattern and were significant at levels below one drink (0.5 oz absolute alcohol) per day. Reaction time also is affected by prenatal alcohol exposure; children ages 5 to 10 years were tested on simple and choice reaction times. Those who had been exposed to alcohol had significantly slower reaction times compared with controls (Simmons, Wass, Thomas, & Riley, 2002).

Brain abnormalities were observed on magnetic resonance imaging (MRI) in 17 school-aged children exposed to differing amounts of alcohol (Autti-Ramo et al., 2002). Long-term studies of social outcome (Dorris & Lindley, 1968) indicate that young adults with FAS have difficulty finding and holding jobs because of unreliability, lack of social skills, and functional illiteracy. They also have difficulty maintaining lasting interpersonal relationships and are at higher risk for becoming involved in substance abuse and criminal behavior. Other associated conditions include higher rates of young adult drinking (Baer, Sampson, Barr, Connor, & Streissguth, 2003), disrupted school experiences, trouble with the law, inappropriate sexual behavior, mental health problems, dependent living, and problems with parenting (Streissguth et al.,1996). Because FAS was defined as a specific condition just 30 years ago, more longitudinal studies are necessary to get a full description of the implications of prenatal alcohol exposure throughout the life cycle.

Effects of Moderate Alcohol Use

Streissguth, Bookstein, Sampson, and Barr (1989) found that moderate drinking either before pregnancy recognition or at mid-pregnancy was associated with relatively mild deficits on neuropsychological tests. The mild forms are referred to as fetal alcohol effects (Sokol & Clarren, 1989), but clear diagnostic criteria have not been developed.

Yang et al. (2001) conducted an epidemiologic study of maternal alcohol consumption, including levels less than 1 oz of absolute alcohol per day, and found no effect on intrauterine growth restriction (IUGR). Lundsberg et al. (1997) identified a relationship between preterm delivery and alcohol consumption in month 7 of pregnancy. There was an increased risk of preterm delivery with light consumption (0.1 oz of absolute alcohol per day) (adjusted RR = 2.1, CI = 1.26–3.54) and mild consumption (0.1–0.25 oz of absolute alcohol per day) (adjusted RR = 2.15, CI = 1.03–4.52), as well as an increased risk of low birthweight (adjusted RR = 1.89, CI = 1.21–2.94); however, there was no significant increase in IUGR.

Currently, it is not possible to specify critical periods of alcohol exposure for behavioral effects. However, varying levels of exposure during gestation seem to produce negative behavioral outcomes. The severe central nervous system damage associated with microencephaly probably results from maternal drinking patterns that are different from those that cause milder effects. Although heavy early exposure results in the most severe outcomes of mental retardation, sensory deficits, and motor problems, subtler behavioral effects, such as learning disabilities and attention deficits, can result from less extensive exposure (Coles, Kable, Drews-Botsch, & Falek, 2000; Wilford, Richardson, Leech, & Day, 2004).

Larssen, Bohlin, and Tunell (1985) found that preschool children who were exposed to alcohol throughout pregnancy tended to be hyperactive and have language problems and motor deficits compared with children whose mothers stopped drinking by the second trimester. Coles et al. (1991) showed that alcohol exposure during any part of pregnancy was associated with poor academic achievement. Aptitude deficits associated with third-trimester exposure are probably the result of the cumulative effect of alcohol exposure throughout pregnancy. Other deficits seen in children exposed through the third trimester of pregnancy (e.g., poor attention, sequencing, and motor problems) are consistent with those seen in people with damage to the hippocampus and the cerebellum (Mirsky, 1987). These are the same brain structures that Livy et al. (2003) and others identified as affected by third-trimester alcohol exposure in rats.

Stopping alcohol intake during pregnancy has a beneficial effect, even on many of the functions (e.g., growth and behavior) that were affected by earlier drinking. As with knowledge development about heavy exposure, animal studies about light alcohol exposure over various pregnancy phases may clarify effects on specific brain structures and resulting patterns of behavior (Livy et al., 2003; West & Goodlett, 1990) in humans.

Susceptibility

FAS occurs only in children born to women who drink heavily; however, relatively few women who drink heavily give birth to children with FAS. May, Hymbaugh, Aase, and Samet (1983) found that about one third of babies born to Native American mothers who drank heavily during pregnancy had FAS, whereas almost half appeared entirely normal. Approximately 20% had some combination of mental deficit, growth delay, and maladaptive behavior, all of which could be caused by agents other than alcohol or be due to genetics. Abel and Hannigan (1995a) reported that only 4% of alcoholic women gave birth to children with FAS. This relatively small attack rate may be due to variations in timing of exposure during critical fetal periods, differences in the amount and pattern of alcohol ingestion, or specific (maternal or fetal) genetic vulnerabilities and protective factors.

Critique of Human Studies about FAS

Although longitudinal studies have followed children into adulthood, measurement of alcohol quantity is not consistent across studies. The current state of the science derived from animal studies may inform the development of better questions framed around pregnancy phase for human studies. Studies in humans that use the timeline followback or daily diary approach would gather details on quantity and frequency by day. The resulting data should not be averaged into weekly or monthly totals, but instead should be analyzed using time series or other time-associated analyses from the last menstrual period (or estimated date of conception) to identify actual alcohol consumption in relation to gestational period.

Unless severe, identification of FASD is often difficult until 4 years of age because developmental delays are often not observed until children enter the school system (Adams et al., 2002). Thus, more sensitive diagnostic techniques are necessary to fully evaluate the relationship between quantity and frequency of exposure and outcome. Computer-based analysis of facial photos is being used to quantitatively define the characteristics of 7-year-old children (Wolfgan, 1997). Further development of this and other tools, such as the Fetal Alcohol Behavior Scale (FASB), developed by Streissguth et al. (1998), merit further work. The FABS demonstrated high item-to-scale reliability (Cronbach's alpha = .91) and acceptable test–retest reliability (r = .69) over an average interval of 5 years. Development and psychometric testing of additional scales are vital to creating a standardized diagnostic definition of FAS and FAE that will allow researchers to conduct larger scale studies using the same criteria.

CONCLUSION

At least 1 woman in 10 continues to consume alcohol during pregnancy, putting their fetuses at risk for the effects of alcohol exposure. Self-report appears to be an accurate measure of alcohol consumption, but if self-report could be validated by biochemical markers in pregnant respondents, it would strengthen conclusions drawn from population-based surveys. Development of better analysis of peak blood alcohol concentrations and possibly using these measures to validate self-report would also enhance measurement approaches in smaller studies. The T-ACE and TWEAK have been found to identify both heavy drinking and binge drinking in samples of pregnant women. However, there are no tools that measure moderate or lower level drinking during pregnancy, and timing tools (targeted to the pattern of drinking during each phase of pregnancy) are still lacking.

Also remaining to be clarified is the role of contextual variables that seem to affect women's choice to drink during pregnancy. Perhaps qualitative studies would be useful to develop a better understanding of the motivators and barriers to alcohol abstinence during pregnancy. New research findings about genetic predispositions and protection will increase understanding of susceptibility and allow clinicians to target those at greatest risk.

The recommendation can be made to pregnant women that there is no safe time to drink, because there is not adequate evidence to establish guidelines about safe alcohol consumption during pregnancy. Drinking behavior and metabolism of alcohol vary greatly among women, and there are differences in genetic susceptibility of fetuses, so it is currently impossible to determine when quantity and frequency begin to be dangerous for a particular developing fetus.

Nursing research and educational programs in nursing should focus on alcohol use and its potential effects during pregnancy. To do broad-spectrum assessments, accurate but simple tools are needed. Screening in pregnant women is complex because it must cover both the drinking of the mother and the potential negative effect on the fetus; so tools that measure alcohol abuse/dependence must be augmented by tools that measure quantity and frequency. Future opportunities abound for the development and testing of theory-based intervention protocols to increase abstinence rates among pregnant women or to at least curtail drinking during the critical first and third trimesters.

Evidence-based screening guidelines are necessary to promote screening in primary care, obstetric, and gynecologic practices that care for women of childbearing age. Evaluation of the two-step screening model proposed by Savage et al. (2003) will be an important step in development of these guidelines. Both brief interventions and motivational interviewing show promise in decreasing alcohol use during pregnancy; these should be evaluated in both private practices and, perhaps using one-stop shopping methods, in clinics and other settings that serve low-income and vulnerable groups of women. Nurse-researchers and clinicians have extensive expertise and are in excellent positions to participate in the unfolding plethora of science work that still lies ahead if the spectrum of fetal alcohol–related disorders is to be eradicated during the 21st century.

REFERENCES

Abel, E. L. (1974). Alcohol ingestion in lactating rats: Effects on mothers and offspring. *Archives of Internal Pharmacodynamic Therapy, 210,* 121–127.

———. (1984) *Fetal alcohol syndrome and fetal alcohol effects.* New York: Plenum Press.

———. (1995). Update on incidence of FAS: FAS is not an equal opportunity birth defect. *Neurotoxicology and Teratology, 17*(4), 437–443.

Abel, E. L., & Hannigan, J. H. (1995a). Maternal risk factors in fetal alcohol syndrome: Provocative and permissive influences. *Neurotoxicology and Teratology, 17,* 445–462.

Abel, E. L., & Hannigan, J. H. (1995b)."J-shaped" relationship between drinking during pregnancy and birth weight: Reanalysis of prospective epidemiological data. *Alcohol Alcohol, 30,* 345–355.

Abel, E. L., & Hannigan, J. H. (1996). Risk factors and pathogenesis. In H. L. Spohr & H. C. Steinhausen (Eds.), *Alcohol, pregnancy, and the developing child*. Cambridge, England: Press Syndicate of the University of Cambridge.

Abel, E. L., Kruger, M. L., & Friedl, J. (1998). How do physicians define "light," "moderate," and "heavy" drinking? *Alcoholism: Clinical and Experimental Research, 22*(5), 979–984.

Abel, E. L., & Sokol, R. J. (1986). Fetal alcohol syndrome is now the leading cause of mental retardation. *Lancet, 85,* 171–222.

Adams, J., Bittner, P, Buttar, H. S., Chambers, C. D., Collins, T. F. X., Daston, P., et al. (2002). Statement of the Public Affairs Committee of the Teratology Society on the fetal alcohol syndrome. *Teratology, 66,* 344–347.

Allen, J. P., Litten, R. Z., Fertig, J. B., & Babor, T. (1997). A review of research on the Alcohol Use Disorders Identification Test (AUDIT). *Alcohol: Clinical and Experimental Research, 21,* 613–619.

Anderson, P. (2002). Brief interventions over the long term: Unfinished business. *Addiction, 97,* 619–620.

Anderson, R. C., Anderson, K. E., & Smith, A. O. (1986). Effects of alcohol consumption during pregnancy. *Journal of the American Association of Occupational Health Nurses, 34*(2), 88–91.

Autti-Ramo, I., Autti, T., Korkman, M., Kettunen, S., Salonen, O., & Valanne, I. (2002). MRI findings in children with school problems who had been exposed prenatally to alcohol. *Developmental Medicine and Child Neurology, 44,* 98–106.

Babor, T. F., & Grant, M. (1989). From clinical research to secondary prevention: International collaboration in the development of the Alcohol Consumption Disorders Identification Test (AUDIT). *Alcohol Health and Research World: International Perspectives, 13,* 371–374.

Baer, J. S., Sampson, P. D., Barr, H. M., Connor, P. D., & Streissguth, A. P. (2003). A 21-year longitudinal analysis of the effects of prenatal alcohol exposure on young adult drinking. *Archives of General Psychiatry, 60,* 377–385.

Barbour, B. G. (1990). Alcohol and pregnancy. *Journal of Nurse-Midwifery, 35,* 78–85.

Bar-Oz, B., Klein, J., Karaskov, T., & Koren, G. (2003). Comparison of meconium and neonatal hair analysis for detection of gestational exposure to drugs of abuse. *Archives of Diseases Child Fetal Neonatal Education, 88,* F98–F100.

Bearer, C. F. (2001). Markers to detect drinking during pregnancy. *Alcohol Research and Health, 25,* 210–218.

Bearer, C. F., Jacobson, J. L., Jacobson, S. W., Barr, D., Croxford, J., & Molteno, C. D. (2003). Validation of a new biomarker of fetal exposure to alcohol. *Journal of Pediatrics, 143,* 463–469.

Bearer, C. F., Lee, S., Salvator, A. E., Minnes, S., Swick, A., Yamashita, T., et al. (1999). Ethyl linoleate in meconium: A biomarker for prenatal ethanol exposure. *Alcoholism: Clinical and Experimental Research, 23,* 487–493.

Bertrand, J., Floyd, R. L., Weber, M. K., O'Connor, M., Riley, P., Johnson, K. A., & Cohen, D. E. (2004). *National Task Force on FAS/FAE: Fetal alcohol syndrome—guidelines for referral and diagnosis.* Atlanta: Centers for Disease Control and Prevention.

Bradley, K. A., Boyd-Wickizer, J., Powell, S. H., & Burman, M. L. (1998). Alcohol screening questionnaires in women: A critical review. *Journal of the American Medical Association, 280*(2), 166–171.

Burd, L., & Wilson, H. (2004). Fetal, infant and child mortality in a context of alcohol use. *American Journal of Medical Genetics, 127C*, 51–58.

Burns, E. M. (1990). The effect of stress during the brain growth spurt. In *Annual Review of Nursing Research: Research on Nursing Practice* (Vol. 8, pp. 57–82). New York: Springer.

Burns, E. M., Kruckeberg, T. W., Stibler, H., Cerven, E., & Borg, S. (1984). The effects of ethanol exposure during the brain growth spurt in rats. *Teratology, 29*, 251–258.

Centers for Disease Control and Prevention (CDC). (1997). Alcohol consumption among pregnant and childbearing-aged women—United States, 1991 and 1995. *Morbidity and Mortality Weekly Review, 46*(16), 346–350.

———. (2002a). Alcohol use among women of childbearing-age—United States, 1991–1999. *Morbidity and Mortality Weekly Review, 51*(13), 273–276.

———. (2002b). Fetal alcohol syndrome—Alaska, Arizona, Colorado, and New York, 1995–1997. *Morbidity and Mortality Weekly Review, 51*(20), 433–435.

———. (2004). Behavioral risk factor surveillance system technical data and information. Retrieved September 7, 2004, from http://www.cdc.gov/brfss/technical_infodata/surveydata.htm

Chambers, C. D., & Jones, K. L. (2002). Is genotype important in predicting fetal alcohol syndrome? *Pediatrics, 141*, 751–752.

Chan, D., Bar-Oz, B., Pellerin, B., Paciorek, C., Klein, J., Kapur, B., et al. (2003). Population baseline of meconium fatty acid ethyl esters among infants of nondrinking women in Jerusalem and Toronto. *Therapeutic Drug Monitoring, 25*(3), 271–278.

Chang, G. (2001). Alcohol-screening instruments for pregnant women. *Alcohol Research and Health, 25*(3), 204–209.

Chang, G., Goetz, M. A., Wilkins-Haug, L., & Berman, S. (1997). Alcohol use in pregnancy: Intervention. *Alcoholism, Clinical and Experimental Research, 21*, 363A.

———. (1999). Identifying prenatal alcohol use: Screening instruments versus clinical predictors. *American Journal of Addictions, 8*(2), 87–93.

———. (2000). A brief intervention for prenatal alcohol use: An in-depth look. *Journal of Substance Abuse Treatment, 18*, 365–369.

Chavez, G. F., Cordero, J. F., & Becerra, J. E. (1988). Leading major congenital malformations among minority groups in the U.S., 1981–1986. *Morbidity and Mortality Weekly Review, 37*, 4–24.

Coleman, P. K., Reardon, D. C., Rue, V. M., & Cougle, J. (2002). A history of induced abortion in relation to substance use during subsequent pregnancies carried to term. *American Journal of Obstetrics and Gynecology, 187*, 1673–1678.

Coles, C. (1994). Critical periods for prenatal alcohol exposure: Evidence from animal and human studies. *Alcohol and Research World, 18*(1), 22–29.

Coles, C. D., Brown, R. T., Smith, I. E., Platzman, K. A., Erickson, S., & Falek, A. (1991). Effects of prenatal alcohol exposure at school age: Physical and cognitive development. *Neurotoxicology and Teratology, 13*(4), 1–11.

Coles, C. D., Kable, J. A., Drews-Botsch, C., & Falek, A. (2000). Early identification of risk for effects of prenatal alcohol exposure. *Journal of Studies on Alcohol, 61*(4), 607–616.

Coles, C. D., Smith, I. E., Fernhoff, P. M., & Falek, A. (1985). Neonatal neurobehavioral characteristics as correlates of maternal alcohol use during gestation. *Alcohol: Clinical and Experimental Research, 9*(5), 1–7.

Cook, J. D. (2003). Biochemical markers of alcohol use in pregnant women. *Clinical Biochemistry, 36*, 9–19.

Cornelius, M. D., Goldsmith, L., Taylor, P. M., & Day, N. L. (1999). Prenatal alcohol consumption among teenagers: Effects on neonatal outcomes. *Alcoholism, Clinical and Experimental Research, 23*, 1238–1244.

Davis, J. H., & Frost, W. A. (1984). Fetal alcohol syndrome: A challenge for the community health nurse. *Journal of Community Health Nursing, 1*(2), 99–110.

Dawson, D. A., Das, A., Faden, V. B., Bhaskar, B., Krulewitch, C. J., & Wesley, B. (2001). Screening for high and moderate risk drinking during pregnancy: A comparison of several TWEAK-based screeners. *Alcohol: Clinical and Experimental Research, 25*, 1342–1349.

Day, N. L., Cottreau, C. M., & Richardson, G. A. (1993). The epidemiology of alcohol, marijuana, and cocaine use among women of childbearing age and pregnant women. *Clinical Obstetrics and Gynecology, 36*, 232–245.

Day, N. L., Jasperse, D., Richardson, G., Robles, N., Sambamoorthi, U., Scher, M., et al. (1989). Prenatal exposure to alcohol: Effect on infant growth and morphological characteristics. *Pediatrics, 84*, 536–541.

Day, N. L., Leech, G. A., Richardson, M. D, Cornelius, N., Robles, N., & Larkby, C. (2002). Prenatal alcohol exposure predicts continued deficits in offspring size at 14 years of age. *Alcoholism: Clinical and Experimental Research, 26*, 1584–1591.

Day, N. L., & Richardson G. A. (1991). Prenatal alcohol exposures: A continuum of effects. *Seminars in Perinatology, 15*(4), 271–279.

Day, N. L., Richardson, G. A., Geva, D., & Robles, N. (1994). Alcohol, marijuana, and tobacco: Effects of prenatal exposure on offspring growth and morphology at age six. *Alcoholism: Clinical and Experimental Research, 18*, 786–794.

Day, N. L., Robles, N., Richardson, G., Geva, D., Taylor, P., Scher, M., et al. (1991). The effects of prenatal alcohol use on the growth of children at three years of age. *Alcohol: Clinical and Experimental Research, 15*, 67–71.

Dorris-Robert, T., & Lindley-Doyle, F. (1968). Personality correlates and antecedents of drinking patterns in adult males. *Journal of Consulting and Clinical Psychology, 32*(1), 2–12.

Dotson, J. A. W., Henderson, D., & Magraw, M. (2003). A public health program for preventing fetal alcohol syndrome among women at risk in Montana. *Neurotoxicology and Teratolology, 25*, 757–761.

Dowdell, P. M. (1981, October). Alcohol and pregnancy: A review of the literature, 1968–1980. *Nursing Times*, 1825–1831.

Drews, C. D., Coles, C. D., Floyd, R. L., & Falek, A. (2003). Prevalence of prenatal drinking assessed at an urban public hospital and a suburban private hospital. *Journal of Maternal-Fetal and Neonatal Medicine, 13*(2), 85–93.

Dunnagan, T., Haynes, G., Christopher, S., & Leonardson, G. (2003). Formative evaluation of a multisite alcohol consumption intervention in pregnant women. *Neurotoxicology Teratolology, 25*, 745–755.

Ebrahim, S. H., Luman, E. T., Floyd, R. L., Murphy, C. C., Bennett, E. M., & Boyle, C. A. (1998). Alcohol consumption by pregnant women in the United States during 1988–1995. *Obstetrics and Gynecology, 92*(2), 187–199.

Ernhart, C. B., Marrow-Tlucack, M., Sokol, R. J., & Martier, S. (1988). Under-reporting of alcohol use in pregnancy. *Alcoholism: Clinical and Experimental Research, 12*, 506–511.

Ernhart, C. B., Sokol, R. J., Martier, S., Moron, P., Nadler, D., Ager, J. W., & Wolf, A. (1987). Alcohol teratogenicity in the human: A detailed assessment of specificity, critical period, and threshold. *American Journal of Obstetrics and Gynecology, 156*(1), 33–39.

Eustace, L. W., Kang, D. H., & Coombs, D. (2003). Fetal alcohol syndrome: A growing concern for health care professionals. *Journal of Obstetric Gynecologic and Neonatal Nursing, 32*(2), 215–221.

Ewing, J. A. (1984). Detecting alcoholism: The CAGE questionnaire. *Journal of the American Medical Association, 252,* 1905–1907.

Fleming, M. F., Barry, K. L., Manwell, L. B., Johnson, K., & London, R. (1997). Brief physician advice for problem and alcohol drinkers: A randomized controlled trial in community-based primary care practices. *JAMA, 277*(13), 1039–1045.

Fleming, M., & Manwell, L. B. (1999). Brief intervention in primary care settings. *Alcohol Research and Health, 23,* 128–137.

Floyd, R. L., & Sidhu, J. S. (2004). Monitoring prenatal alcohol exposure. *American Journal of Medical Genetics Part C (Seminars in Medical Genetics), 127C,* 3–9.

Fogel, C. I., & Melyea, M. (2001). Psychological risk factors in pregnant inmates: A challenge for nursing. *Maternal-Child Nursing, 26,* 10–16.

Gladstone, J., Levy, M., Nulman, I., & Koren, G. (1997). Characteristics of pregnant women who engage in binge alcohol consumption. *Canadian Medical Association Journal, 156,* 789–794.

Gladstone, J., Nulman, I., & Koren, G. (1996). Reproductive risks of binge drinking during pregnancy. *Reproductive Toxicology, 10,* 3–13.

Graham, J. M., Hanson, J. W., Darby, B. L., Barr, H. M., & Streissguth, A. P. (1988). Independent dysmorphology evaluations at birth and 4 years of age for children exposed to varying amounts of alcohol in utero. *Pediatrics, 81,* 772–778.

Grant, T., Ernst, C. C., Pagalilauan, G., & Streissguth, A. (2003). Postpartum follow-up effects of paraprofessional intervention with high risk women who abused alcohol and drugs during pregnancy. *Journal of Community Psychology, 31,* 211–222.

Handmaker, N. S., Miller, W. R., & Manicke, M. (1999). Findings of a pilot study of motivational interviewing with pregnant drinkers. *Journal of Studies on Alcohol, 60,* 285–287.

Handmaker, N. S., & Wilbourne, P. (2001). Motivational interventions in prenatal clinics. *Alcohol Research and Health, 25,* 219–229.

Hankin, J., &, Sokol, R. (2003). Brief postpartum intervention protects previously born children from alcohol-related developmental delay. *American Journal of Obstetrics and Gynecology, 189*(Suppl.), S148–S156.

Hannigan, J. H., & Armant, D. R. (2000). Alcohol in pregnancy and neonatal outcomes. *Seminars in Neonatology, 5,* 243–254.

Hayes, M. J., Brown, E., Hofmaster, P. A., Davare, A. A., Parker, K. G., & Raczek, J. A. (2002). Prenatal alcohol intake in a rural, Caucasian clinic. *Family Medicine, 34,* 120–125.

Hazelett, S. E., Liebelt, R. A., Brown, W. J., Androulakakis, V., Jarjoura, D., & Truitt, E. B. (1998). Evaluation of acetaldehyde-modified hemoglobin and other markers of chronic heavy alcohol use: Effects of gender and hemoglobin concentration. *Alcoholism: Clinical and Experimental Research, 22,* 1813–1819.

Henshaw, S. K. (1998). Unintended pregnancy in the United States. *Family Planning Perspectives, 30*(1), 24–29, 46.

Hindemarch, I., Kerr, J. S., & Sherwood, N. (1991). The effects of alcohol and other drugs on psychomotor performance and cognitive function. *Alcohol and Alcoholism, 26*(1), 71–79.

Ingersoll, K., Floyd, L., Sobell, M., & Velasquez, M. M. (2003). Project CHOICES Intervention Research Group: Reducing the risk of alcohol-exposed pregnancies—a study of a motivational intervention in community settings. *Pediatrics, 111*(5, Part 2), 1131–1135.

Iosub, S. M., Fuchs, M., Bingol, N., Rich, H., Stone, D. S., Gromisch, D. S., et al. (1985). Familial fetal alcohol syndrome: Incidence in blacks and Hispanics. *Alcoholism: Clinical and Experimental Research, 9,* 185–189.

Ismail, M. A., & Moawad, A. (1984). Drugs and teratogenic agents. In C. C. Lin, & M. I. Evans (Eds.), *Intrauterine growth retardation* (pp. 125–142). New York: McGraw-Hill.

Iyasu, S., Randall, L. L., Welty, T. K., Hsai, J., Kinney, H. C., & Mandell, F. (2002). Risk factors for sudden infant death syndrome among Northern Plains Indians. *Journal of the American Medical Association, 288,* 2717–2713.

Jacobs, E. A., Cooperman, S. M., Jeffe, A., & Kulig, J. (2000). Fetal alcohol syndrome and alcohol related neurodevelopmental disorders. *Pediatrics, 106,* 358–361.

Jacobson, J. L., Jacobson, S. W., Sokol, R. J., Martier, S. S., Ager, J. W., & Kaplan-Estrin, M. G. (1993). Teratogenic effects of alcohol on infant development. *Alcohol: Clinical and Experimental Research, 17,* 174–183.

Jacobson, S. W., Chiodo, L. M., Sokol, R. J., & Jacobson, J. L. (2002). Validity of maternal report of prenatal alcohol, cocaine, and smoking in relation to neurobehavioral outcome. *Pediatrics, 109,* 815–825.

Jessup, M. (1988). Fetal alcohol syndrome: Prevention and intervention for the nurse. *California Nurse, 84*(1), 12–13.

Jones, K. L., & Chambers, C. (1998). Biomarkers of fetal exposure to alcohol: Identification of at-risk pregnancies. *Journal of Pediatrics, 133*(3), 316–318.

Jones, K. L., & Smith, D. W. (1973). Recognition of the fetal alcohol syndrome in early infancy. *Lancet, 2*(7836), 999–1001.

Kaminski, M., Rumeau, C., & Schwartz, D. (1978). Alcohol consumption in pregnant women and the outcome of pregnancy. *Alcoholism: Clinical and Experimental Research, 2,,* 155–163.

Kesmodel, U., Wisborg, K., Olsen, S. F., Henriksen, T. B., & Secher, N. J. (2002). Moderate alcohol intake during pregnancy and the risk of stillbirth and death in the first year of life. *American Journal of Epidemiology, 155,* 305–312.

Larsson, G., Bohlin, A. B., & Tunell, R. (1985). Prospective study of children exposed to variable amounts of alcohol in utero. *Archives of the Diseases of Children, 60,* 315–321.

Lemoine, P., Harousseau, H., Borteyru, J. P., & Menuet, J. C. (1968). Les enfants de parents alcooliques: anomalies observees, a propos de 127 cas (Children of alcoholic parents: Anomalies observed in 127 cases). *Oest Medical, 21*(6), 476–482.

Livy, D. J., Miller, K., Maier, S. E., & West, J. R. (2003). Fetal alcohol exposure and temporal vulnerability: Effects of binge-like alcohol exposure on the developing rat hippocampus. *Neurotoxicology Teratology, 25,* 447–458.

Lundsberg, L. S., Bracken, M. B., & Staftlas, A. F. (1997). Low-to-moderate gestational alcohol use and intrauterine growth retardation, low birthweight, and premature delivery. *Annals of Epidemiology, 7,* 498–508.

Manwell, L. B., Fleming, M. F., Mundt, M. P., Stauffacher, E. A., & Barry, K. L. (2000). Treatment of problem alcohol use in women of childbearing age: Results of a brief intervention trial. *Alcoholism Clinical and Experimental Research, 24*, 1517–1524.

Marbury, M. C., Linn, S., Monson, R., Schoenbaum, S., Stubblefield, P. G., & Ryan, K. J. (1983). The association of alcohol consumption with outcome of pregnancy. *American Journal of Public Health, 73*, 1165–1168.

Martinez-Frias, M. L., Bermejo, E., Rodriguez-Pinilla, & Frias, J. L. (2004). Risk for congenital anomalies associated with different sporadic and daily doses of alcohol consumption during pregnancy: A case-control study. *Birth Defects Research, 70*(Part A), 194–200.

May, P. A. (1996). Research issues in the prevention of fetal alcohol syndrome and alcohol-related birth defects. In J. M. Howard, S. E. Martin, P. D. Mail, M. E. Hilton, E. D. Taylor, & M. E. Hilton (Eds.), *Women and alcohol: Issues for prevention research* (pp. 351–360). Bethesda, MD: National Institutes of Health, National Institute on Alcohol Abuse and Alcoholism.

May, P. A., Hymbaugh, K. J., Aase, J. M., & Samet, J. M. (1983). Epidemiology of fetal alcohol syndrome among American Indians of the Southwest. *Social Biology, 30*, 374–387.

Miller, W. R. (2000). Rediscovering fire: Small interventions, large effects. *Psychology of Addictive Behavior, 14*(1), 6–18.

Miller, W. R., & Rollnick, S. (2002). *Motivational interviewing: Preparing people for change* (2nd ed.). New York: Guilford Press.

Mirsky, A. F. (1987). Behavioral and psychophysiological markers of disordered attention. *Environmental Health Perspective, 74*, 191–199.

Morse, B. A., & Hutchins, E. (2000). Reducing complications from alcohol use during pregnancy through screening. *Journal of the American Women's Association, 55*(4), 225–228.

Moore, C., Jones, J., Lewis, D., & Buchi, K. (2003). Prevalence of fatty acid ethyl esters in meconium specimens. *Clinical Chemistry, 49*, 133–136.

Moore, C., Lewis, D., & Leikin, J. (1995). False-positive and false-negative rates in meconium drug testing. *Clinical Chemistry, 41*, 1614–1616.

Naimi, T. S., Lipscomb, L. E., Brewer, R. D., & Gilbert, B. C. (2003). Binge drinking in the preconception period and the risk of unintended pregnancy: Implications for women and their children. *Pediatrics, 111*, 1136–1141.

National Institute on Drug Abuse (NDA). (1996). National Pregnancy and Health Survey: Drug Use Among Women Delivering Livebirths: 1992. Rockville, MD: National Institutes of Health (NIH Publication No. 96-3819).

Phares, T. M., Morrow, B., Lansky, A., Barfield, W. D., Prince, C. B., Marchi, K. S., et al. (2004). Surveillance for disparities in maternal health-related behaviors—selected states, Pregnancy Risk Assessment Monitoring System (PRAMS), 2000–2001. *Morbidity and Mortality Weekly Review, 53*(SS04), 1–13.

Polygenis, D., Wharton, S., Malmberg, C., Sherman, N., Kennedy, D., Koren, G., & Einarson, T. R. (1998). Moderate alcohol consumption during pregnancy and the incidence of fetal malformations: A meta-analysis. *Neurotoxicology and Teratology, 20*, 61–67.

Rasch, V. (2003). Cigarette, alcohol and caffeine consumption: Risk factors for spontaneous abortion. *Acta Obstetrica Gynecologica Scandinavica, 82*(2), 182–188.

Rosett, H. L., Weiner, L., Zuckerman, B., McKinlay, S., & Edelin, K. C. (1980). Reduction of alcohol consumption during pregnancy with benefits to the newborn. *Alcoholism: Clinical and Experimental Research, 4*, 178–184.

Rouquette, J. (1957). *Influence de l'intoxicacion alocoolique parentele sur le développement physique et psychique des jeunes enfants.* Unpublished master's thesis, University of Paris, Paris, France.

Rowe, J. (1989). Nursing assessment of children of alcoholics. *Journal of Pediatric Nursing: Nursing Care of Children and Families, 4*(4), 248–255.

Russell, M. (1994). New assessment tools for risk drinking during pregnancy: T-ACE, TWEAK and others. *Alcohol Health and Research World, 18*(1), 55–61.

Russell, M., Martier, S. S., Sokol, R. J., Mudar, P., Jacobson, S., & Jacobson, J. (1996). Detecting risk drinking during pregnancy: A comparison of four screening questionnaires. *American Journal of Public Health, 56*, 1435–1439.

Sampson, P. D., Streissguth, A. P., & Bookstein, F. L. (1997). Incidence of fetal alcohol syndrome and prevalence of alcohol-related neurodevelopmental disorder. *Teratology, 56*, 317–326.

Savage, C., Wray, J., Ritchey, P. N., Sommers, M., Dyehouse, J., & Fulmer, M. (2003). Current screening instruments related to alcohol consumption in pregnancy and a proposed alternative method. *Journal of Obstetric Gynecologic and Neonatal Nursing, 32*, 437–446.

Selzer, M. L. (1971). The Michigan Alcoholism Screening Test: The quest for a new diagnostic instrument. *American Journal of Psychiatry, 127*, 1653–1658.

Serdula, M. K., Mokdad, A. H., Byers, T., & Siegel, P. Z. (1999). Assessing alcohol consumption: Beverage-specific versus grouped-beverage questions. *Journal of Studies on Alcohol, 60*, 99–102.

Shu, X. O., Hatch, M. C., Mills, J., Clemens, J., & Susser, M. (1995). Maternal smoking, alcohol drinking, caffeine consumption and fetal growth: Results from a prospective study. *Epidemiology, 6*(2), 115–120.

Simmons, R. W., Wass, T., Thomas, J. D., & Riley, E. P. (2002). Fractionated simple and choice reaction time in children with prenatal exposure to alcohol. *Alcoholism Clinical and Experimental Research, 26*, 1412–1419.

Sobel, L. C., Brown, J., Leo, G. I., & Sobell, M. B. (1996). The reliability of the Alcohol Timeline Followback when administered by telephone and by computer. *Drug and Alcohol Dependence, 42*, 49–54.

Soderberg, B. L., Sicinska, E. T., Blodget, E., Cluette-Brown, J. E., Suter, P. M., Schuppisser, T., et al. (1999). Preanalytical variables affecting the quantification of fatty acid ethyl esters in plasma and serum samples. *Clinical Chemistry, 45*(12), 2183–2190.

Sokol, R. J. (1981). Alcohol and abnormal outcomes of pregnancy. *Canadian Medical Association Journal, 125*, 143–148.

Sokol, R. J., Ager, J., Martier, S., Debanne, S., Ernhart, C., Kuzma, J., & Miller, S. I. (1986). Significant determinants of susceptibility to alcohol teratogenicity. *Annals of the New York Academy of Sciences, 477*, 87–102.

Sokol, R. J., & Clarren, S. K. (1989). Guidelines for use of terminology describing the impact of prenatal alcohol on the offspring. *Alcohol: Clinical and Experimental Research, 13*, 597–598.

Sokol, R. J., Delancey-Black, V., & Nordstrom, B. (2003). Fetal alcohol spectrum disorder. *Journal of the American Medical Association, 290*(22), 2996–2999.

Sokol, R. J., Martier, S. S., & Ager, J. W. (1989). The T-ACE questions: Practical prenatal detection of risk drinking. *American Journal of Obstetrics and Gynecology*, 160, 663–670.

Sommers, M. S., Savage, C., Wray, J., & Dyehouse, J. M. (2003). Laboratory measures of alcohol (ethanol) consumption: Strategies to assess drinking patterns with biochemical measures. *Biological Research in Nursing*, 4(3), 203–217.

Stoler, J. M., Huntington, K. S., Peterson, C. M., Peterson, K. P., Daniel, P., Aboagye, K. K., et al. (1998). The prenatal detection of significant alcohol exposure with maternal blood markers. *Journal of Pediatrics*, 133, 346–352.

Stoler, J. M., Ryan, L. M., & Holmes, L. B. (2002). Alcohol dehydrogenase 2 genotypes, maternal alcohol use and infant outcome. *Pediatrics*, 141, 780–785.

Stratton, K., Howe, C., & Battaglia, F. (1996). *Fetal alcohol syndrome: Diagnosis, epidemiology, prevention and treatment*. Washington, DC: National Academy Press.

Streissguth, A. P., Barr, H. M., Kogan, J., & Bookstein, F. L. (1996). Understanding the occurrence of secondary disabilities in clients with fetal alcohol syndrome (FAS) and fetal alcohol effects (FAE): Final report to the Centers for Disease Control and Prevention (CDC) (Tech. Rep. No. 96-06). Seattle: University of Washington, Fetal Alcohol and Drug Unit.

Streissguth, A. P., Bookstein, F. L., Barr, H. M., Press, S., Sampson, P. D., et al. (1998). Fetal alcohol behavior scale. *Alcoholism: Clinical and Experimental Research*, 22(2), 325–333.

Streissguth, A. P., Bookstein, F. L., Sampson, P. D., & Barr, H. M. (1989). Neurobehavioral effects of prenatal alcohol: Part 3. PLS analysis of neuropsychologic tests. *Neurotoxicology and Teratology*, 11, 493–507.

Struck, J. (2003). Four-state FAS consortium: Model for program implementation and data collection. *Neurotoxicology Teratology*, 25, 643–649.

Substance Abuse and Mental Health Services Administration (SAMHSA). (2002). *Results from the 2001 National Household Survey on Drug Abuse: Summary of national findings* (Vol. 1, NHSDA Series H-17, DHHS Pub. No. SMA 02-3758). Rockville, MD: Department of Health and Human Services, Office of Applied Studies. Retrieved September 4, 2004, from http://www.oas.samhsa.gov/NHSDA/2k1NHSDA/vol1/Chapter3.htm

————. (2003a). *Results from the 2002 National Survey on Drug Use and Health: National Findings* (NHSDA Series H-22, DHHS Pub. No. SMA 03-3836). Rockville, MD: Department of Health and Human Services, Office of Applied Studies. Retrieved September 4, 2004, from http://www.oas.samhsa.gov/nhsda/2k2nsduh/Results/2k2Results.htm#highlights

————. (2003b). *The National Survey on Drug Use and Health (NSDUH)*. Retrieved September 7, 2004, from http://www.oas.samhsa.gov/2k3/NSDUH/nsduh.htm

————. (2004). *Substance use among pregnant women during 1999 and 2000*. Retrieved September 7, 2004, from http://www.oas.samhsa.gov/2k3/pregnancy/pregnancy.pdf

Sullivan, W. C. (1899). A note on the influence of maternal inebriety on offspring. *Journal of Mental Science*, 45, 489–507.

Thornberry, J., Bhaskar, B., Krulewitch, C. J., Wesley, B., Hubbard, M. L., Das, D., et al., (2002). Audio computerized self-report interview use in prenatal clinics. *Computers, Informatics, Nursing*, 20(2), 46–52.

U.S. Department of Health and Human Services. (2000a, November). *Healthy People 2010: Understanding and Improving Health and Objectives for Improving Health* (2nd ed.). Washington, DC: U.S. Government Printing Office.

————. (2000b, June). *10th special report to the U.S. Congress on alcohol and health.* Bethesda, MD: National Institutes of Health.

U.S. Department of Health and Human Services, Substance Abuse and Mental Health, Office of Applied Studies. (2004). *SAMHSA data archive.* Retrieved September 7, 2004, from http://www.oas.samhsa.gov/samhda.htm

U.S. Department of Health and Human Welfare. (1979). *Healthy people: The Surgeon General's report on health promotion and disease prevention.* Washington, DC: Author.

U.S. Department of Treasury, U.S. Department of Health and Human Services. (1980, November). *Report to the President and Congress on health hazards associated with alcohol and methods to inform the general public of these hazards.* Washington, DC: U.S. Government Printing Office.

Ulleland, C. N. (1972). The offspring of alcoholic mothers. *Annals of the New York Academy of Science, 197,* 167–169.

Weber, M. K., Floyd, R. L., Riley, E. P., & Snider, D. E. (2002). National Task Force on Fetal Alcohol Syndrome and Fetal Alcohol Effect: Defining the national agenda for fetal alcohol syndrome and other prenatal alcohol-related effects. *Morbidity and Mortality Weekly Review, 51*(RR14), 9–12.

Wekselman, K., Spiering, K., Hetteberg, C., Kenner, C., & Flandermeyer, A. (1995). Fetal alcohol syndrome from infancy through childhood: A review of the literature. *Journal of Pediatric Nursing, 10,* 296–303.

West, J. R., & Goodlett, C. R. (1990). Teratogenic effects of alcohol on brain development. *Annals of Medicine, 22,* 319–325.

Whiteside-Mansell, L., Crone, C. C., & Conners, N. A. (1999).The development and evaluation of an alcohol and drug prevention and treatment program for women and children: The AC-CARES Program. *Journal of Substance Abuse Treatment, 16,* 265–275.

Whitty, J. E., & Sokol, R. J. (1996). Alcohol teratogenicity in humans: Critical period, thresholds, specificity and vulnerability. In H. L. Spohr & H. C. Steinhausen (Eds.), *Alcohol, pregnancy and the developing child* (pp. 3–13). New York: Cambridge University Press.

Wilford, J. A., Richardson, G. A., Leech, S. L., & Day, N. L. (2004). Verbal and visuospatial learning and memory function in children with moderate prenatal alcohol exposure. *Alcoholism: Clinical and Experimental Research, 28,* 497–507.

Williams, L. M., Morrow, B., Lansky, A., Beck, L. F., Barfield, W., Helms, K., et al. (2003). Surveillance for selected maternal behaviors and experiences before, during, and after pregnancy: Pregnancy Risk Assessment Monitoring System (PRAMS), 2000. *Morbidity and Mortality Weekly Report, 52*(SS-11), 1–15.

Windham, G. C., Fenster, L., Hopkins, B., & Swan, S. H. (1995). The association of moderate maternal and paternal alcohol consumption with birthweight and gestational age. *Epidemiology, 6,* 591–597.

Wolfgan, L. (1997). Charting recent progress: Advances in alcohol research. *Alcohol and Health Research World, 21,* 227–286.

Yang, Q., Witkiewicz, B. B., Olney, R. S., Liu, Y., Davis, M., Khoury, M. J., et al. (2001). A case-control study of maternal alcohol consumption and intrauterine growth retardation. *Annals of Epidemiology, 11,* 497–503.

Chapter 5

Alcohol, Children, and Adolescents

Carol J. Loveland-Cherry

ABSTRACT

Alcohol use in children and adolescents continues to be a major health concern. There is a rich literature on correlates and antecedents of alcohol use in children and adolescents, and concerted efforts have been made to develop, implement, and evaluate intervention strategies. This chapter provides a review of the intervention studies to prevent alcohol use in these groups. The interventions are categorized by their primary focus: school, family, and community. The studies were limited to those with either an experimental or a quasi-experimental design and published results.

Keywords: alcohol and children, alcohol and adolescents, alcohol and schools, school-based interventions, family-based interventions

Alcohol continues to be a widely used drug among adolescents (Johnston, O'Malley, Bachman, & Schulenberg, 2004). Since 1975, the Monitoring the Future (MTF) Project has provided annual data on substance use in a representative sample of adolescents in private and public schools. The original survey was of adolescents in grade 12, and it was extended to grades 8 and 10 in 1991 (Johnston et al., 2004). Estimates of use vary depending on the specified time period, gender, geographic location, age/grade, and race/ethnicity. Based on data from the MTF national annual survey (Johnston et al., 2004), 44% of 8th graders, 66% of 10th graders, and 77% of 12th graders report ever trying alcohol. Further, 20% of 8th-grade, 35% of 10th-grade, and 48% of 12th-grade students report alcohol use in the last 30 days. Approximately 43% of adolescents ages 12 to 17 report having ever used alcohol, 33.9% reported use in the past year, and more than 17.3% report use in the past month (Substance Abuse and Mental Health Services Administration [SAMHSA], 2001). Occasions of heavy drinking, defined as five or more drinks in a row during the prior 2-week interval (Johnston et al., 2004), were reported by 12%, 22%, and 28% of the respondents (8th, 10th, and 12th grade, respectively). MTF data show that trends in alcohol use parallel those of illicit drugs.

African American and Asian adolescents consistently report initiating alcohol use later and in lesser quantities than do their White counterparts. Males initiate drinking earlier and with patterns of heavier use (including heavy, episodic binge drinking) than do females. Drinking increases with age and peaks at age 21, when 67.5% report alcohol use (SAMHSA, 2001).

Although a relatively small percentage of adolescents who report consuming alcohol develop addiction, alcohol use has significant impact on adolescent morbidity and mortality. Further, there is evidence that early drinking is linked to alcohol dependence at later ages (Foxcroft, Ireland, Lister-Sharp, Lowe, & Breen, 2002; Grant, 1997).

DEFINITIONS, METHODS, AND RATIONALE
FOR NURSING SCIENCE

For the purpose of this review, the child and adolescent population was limited to individuals who are school age (5–18 years). Another chapter in this volume addresses the age group of young people over the age of 18. Data for children younger than 11 are extremely rare, but an attempt was made to locate any reports for this age group. Adolescence has been divided into periods, or phases. Although there is some variation in the definition of the phases, the use of early (11–14 years of age), middle (15–16 years of age), and late (17–19 year of age) adolescence is generally accepted. The focus was on children and adolescents in the United States, but relevant studies from the rest of the world published in English were considered.

A comprehensive search online using the Medline, Cumulative Index of Nursing and Allied Health Literature (CINAHL) databases and the Cochrane library was conducted for studies published from 1990 to 2003. Search keywords that were used included *children, adolescents, substance abuse, substance use, alco-*

hol, drugs, and *prevention.* Inclusion criteria comprised studies (1) published in refereed journals, (2) published in English, (3) reporting the results of research, (4) with a stated focus on prevention of substance use or misuse in children and adolescents, and (5) published between January 1990 and December 2003.

A total of 269 articles was identified with this search mechanism. The next step in defining the articles to be reviewed was to limit the references to those that reported results from a study that evaluated the efficacy of an intervention to prevent alcohol use in children ages 5 to 18 years using either an experimental or quasi-experimental design. Using this next level of screening, 67 articles were identified. These sources constituted the basis for this review. In addition to the studies that met these criteria, six major reviews of programs to decrease alcohol use in children and adolescents, and the literature that describes the epidemiology of the problem, were used.

The authors of these studies are from a variety of disciplines, including psychology, education, public health, medicine, sociology, and nursing. The number of studies from nurse-scientists is very limited, but this is not surprising. Overall, few published intervention studies are evident from nurse-researchers, and even fewer still in the area of alcohol research. The reasons for this are numerous, but it is useful to speculate on some contributing factors. Nurses have had limited exposure to information on substance use; until recently, content on substance use, especially in children and adolescents, was limited in nursing curricula. Further, the emphasis in nursing practice was on inpatient care with primarily infants, young children, and adults, or well-child care with young children. Adolescents were not often seen in primary care or in inpatient settings. The dearth of studies was so evident that Shalala (1996) commented on the often-neglected health needs of adolescents.

As nursing care moved into the community and a growing focus on the health risks of adolescents was highlighted, nurses began to focus on the health needs of this population, from both a practice and a research perspective. As the need for multidisciplinary approaches for this population became evident, nurse-scholars began to address the gaps in science. However, the number of nurse-researchers in this area of study remains limited. A focus on health promotion and prevention with adolescents around major risk behaviors, such as alcohol use, is consistent with nursing's commitment to and focus on prevention. Further, nurse-scientists have much to contribute to work in this area because their ecological perspective and knowledge of growth and development, health, and important social units.

THEORETICAL APPROACHES FOR UNDERSTANDING ADOLESCENT ALCOHOL USE

A variety of theoretical approaches have been used to understand adolescent alcohol use and risk behaviors. They include social cognitive theory (Bandura,

1977), problem behaviors (Jessor & Jessor, 1977), the theory of reasoned action/ theory of planned behavior (Ajzen, 1991; Ajzen & Fishbein, 1980), and ecological models. The most effective approaches are viewed as being multilevel and addressing components of the environment conceptualized by an ecological perspective. These approaches provide the basis for identifying factors that are correlates and antecedents of alcohol use in youth. Byrnes (2003) suggests a two-pronged approach to reducing these behaviors that is based on the assumption that "people are likely to take risks if both of the following conditions are true: (a) They are given the *opportunity* to take a risk, and (b) they have the *propensity* to take that risk when given the opportunity" (p. 17). Interventions, then, would focus on reducing the opportunities for youth to engage in risk behaviors and their propensity to do so.

Factors Influencing Adolescent Alcohol Use

There is a considerable literature that provides the empirical basis for interventions to prevent adolescent alcohol use. It is useful to classify the various factors related to adolescent alcohol use as protective or risk factors and whether they fall into the several important environments that have been identified as important for children and adolescents: family, schools, peers, and communities.

Family/Parents

Families continue to be a major social environment for children in which attitudes and behaviors develop (Kumpfer, 1998; Loveland-Cherry, Ross, & Kaufman, 1999). Further, parents and siblings are powerful role models for children and adolescents. Protective factors related to the family include family support (Barnes & Windle, 1987; Brook, Whiteman, Balka, & Hamburg, 1992; Loveland-Cherry, Leech, Laetz, & Dielman, 1996), sibling and parent attitudes toward drinking, authoritative parenting style, norm setting, monitoring, and nurturance (Biglan, Duncan, Ary, & Smolkowski, 1995; Dishion, Patterson, Stoolmiller, & Skinner, 1991; Steinberg, Fletcher, & Darling, 1994). Risk factors include sibling and parent, especially mother's, drinking behaviors (Hawkins, Catalano, & Miller, 1992), attitudes supportive of alcohol use, and parental permissiveness (Brook et al., 1992; Dielman, Butchart, & Shope, 1993; Johnson & Pandina, 1991). Family factors are more influential in younger children and in early adolescence, are replaced by peer factors during middle adolescence, then regain importance with peer factors in later adolescence.

School

As children move through adolescence, schools constitute an increasingly important component of the context for the development of risk behaviors (Abrams & Clayton, 2001). Dealing with transitions is a major characteristic of moving through the educational process. These transitions require changes in relationships and achievement, and often are accompanied by reevaluation of attitudes, beliefs, and behaviors. Schools become a major environment where peer interactions occur. Indicators of successful achievement such as school attachment and receiving good grades are associated with less adolescent alcohol use (Abbey, Pilgrim, Hendrickson, & Buresh, 2000). In contrast, absenteeism and poor grades are associated with initiation and level of alcohol use. Interactions with teachers and peers, and the context of the school, can be either a protective or a risk factor, depending on their nature.

Peers

As adolescence progresses, peer relationships become increasingly important in terms of behaviors. Peer alcohol use, peer pressure to use alcohol, and peer tolerance or approval of alcohol use have all been supported as risk factors for alcohol use in children and adolescents. The influence of peer risk factors appears to peak during middle adolescence (Huba, Wingard, & Bentler, 1980).

Communities

Social environmental norms, social support, and opportunities for nonuse of alcohol are protective factors for children and adolescents (Resnick et al., 1997). Communities provide an important context related to availability of alcohol and access to opportunities for participation in activities that strengthen social bonds and provide alternatives to risk-related activities (Wagenaar & Perry, 1995).

Given the multiple sources of protective and risk factors, interventions to prevent or delay the onset of alcohol use have focused on one or more of these critical environments. Multilevel studies that include two or more critical social environmental systems are less common but have been proposed as being the most desirable. The results from the review of literature for prevention of alcohol use in children and adolescents are organized by the focal location for the interventions.

SCHOOL-BASED INTERVENTIONS

Given the concentration of children and adolescents in schools, it is not surprising that the majority of the interventions to decrease alcohol use in this population were conducted in schools. Support for school-based programs increased with the influx of federal funds in the late 1980s (Gorman, 1998). School-based alcohol prevention programs generally are universal interventions that focus on prevention of alcohol use in early adolescence and reduction of overall prevalence (Hansen, 1993). Approaches vary and include knowledge only, affective only, a combination of knowledge and affective, peer programs that include refusal skills and/or social and life skills, and alternatives, including alternative activities and building personal competence (Tobler, 1986). Knowledge only programs use a single approach—presentation of legal, biological, and psychological effects of drug abuse by a teacher with minimum discussion; the intent is to scare adolescents. Affective only programs also use a single approach but focus on self-esteem building, self-awareness, feelings, values clarification, experiential, and humanistic psychology. Knowledge and affective components can be combined in programs that focus on problem solving and decision making. Peer programs build on positive peer influence and incorporate peer teaching, counseling, helping, and facilitating, and peer participation. Refusal skills programs focus on interpersonal enhancement, resistance skills, "saying no" techniques, surveys, showing "everybody isn't doing it," peer role models, assertiveness skills, and intervention techniques around drinking and driving. Social and life skills programs focus on developing both interpersonal (communication skills, modeling, feedback with social reinforcement, assertiveness) and intrapersonal skills (affective education—self-esteem building, feelings, self-awareness, values clarification, anxiety reduction, and coping skills). Alternative programs include positive activities that are more appealing than drug use and/or competence building activities (Tobler, 1986, p. 541).

In the current review, 35 publications contained reports of school-based interventions outcomes (see Table 5.1). They represent 21 different intervention programs. Eight of the programs were designed and implemented with elementary school populations (Catalano et al., 2003; Clayton, Cattarello, & Johnstone, 1996; Hanson & Graham, 1991; Hawkins, Catalano, Kosterman, Abbott, & Hill, 1999; Lynam et al., 1999; Prinz, Dumas, Smith, & Laughlin, 2000; Ringwalt, Ennett, & Holt, 1991; Rosenbaum, Flewelling, Bailey, Ringwalt, & Wilkinson, 1994; Schinke & Tepavac, 1995; Schinke, Tepavac, & Cole, 2000; Shope, Dielman, Butchart, Campanelli, & Kloska, 1992). Eleven interventions focused on middle school students (Allison, Silverman, & Dignam, 1990; Bagnall, 1990; Botvin, Baker, Dusenbury, Botvin, & Diaz, 1995; Botvin, Baker, Dusenbury, Tortu, & Botvin, 1990; Botvin, Griffin, Diaz, & Ifill-Williams, 2001; Caplan et al., 1992; Ellickson & Bell, 1990, 1992; Ellickson, Bell, & Harrison, 1993; Ellickson, Bell, & McGuigan, 1993; Gilason, Yngvadottir, & Benediktsdottir, 1995; Mathias, 2003; Newman, Anderson, & Farrell, 1992; Ross, Richard, & Potvin, 1998; Werch, 1997; Werch et al., 2000; Werch, Anzalone, et al., 1996; Werch, Carlson, Pappas, & DiClemente, 1996; Werch, Pappas, Carlson, & DiClemente, 1999; Wilhelmsen, Laberg, & Klepp, 1994). The remaining eight studies described interventions implemented with high school samples (Brem-

TABLE 5.1   School-based Intervention: Significant Alcohol Effects

Authors	Setting, population, and design	Conceptual approach	Intervention description	Change in alcohol measures
Bagnall (1990)	1,560 12- and 13-year-old students from England, Wales, and Scotland		Pupil participation through small group work and role play; focus on media messages, parental attitudes, peer group pressure; 4 hours of classroom time over four or five social education slots	10 months—fewer reports of alcohol consumed in last 7 days, $F(1,4) = 4.32, p < .1$, and fewer reports of consuming more than 3 drinks, $F(1,4) = 10.47; p < .05$
Botvin, Griffin, Diaz, & Ifill-Williams (2001)	5,222 seventh graders from 29 New York City schools, 61% African American, 22% Hispanic, 6% Asian, 6% White, and 5% mixed/other backgrounds	Cognitive-behavioral approach	Life Skills Training—drug resistance skills, antidrug norms, and development of important personal and social skills; 15 sessions in grades 7 and 10 booster sessions in grade 8	3 month—lower drunkenness; 1 year—less frequency, $F(1,3,530) = 14.7, p < .0001$, less drunkenness, $F(1,3,504) = 7.1, p < .0040$, lower quantity $F(1,3,503) = 11.6, p < .0007$

(continued)

TABLE 5.1 *(continued)*

Authors	Setting, population, and design	Conceptual approach	Intervention description	Change in alcohol measures
Botvin, Baker, Dusenbury, Botvin, & Diaz (1995)	3,597 12th graders from 56 schools; 91% White Attrition 40%		Life Skills Training—15 class periods in grade 7, 10 sessions in grade 8, 5 sessions in grade 9; information and skills for resisting social influences to use drugs, personal and social skills	6 years—full sample, lower problem drinking, 0.34 (0.20) vs. 0.33 (0.03) vs. 0.40 (0.02), $p < .01$ (intervention workshop training, intervention videotape training, control, respectively); high-fidelity sample (2,752 students from 50 schools who received 60% of intervention), lower weekly drinking, 0.24 (0.02) vs. 0.20 (0.02) vs. 0.29 (0.02) $p < .01$; heavy drinking, 0.53 (0.03) vs. 0.52 (0.02) vs. 0.59 (0.02), $p < .01$ (intervention workshop training, intervention videotape training, control, respectively)

TABLE 5.1 *(continued)*

Authors	Setting, population, and design	Conceptual approach	Intervention description	Change in alcohol measures
Botvin, Baker, Dusenbury, Tortu, & Botvin (1990)	4,466 of 5,954 seventh graders from 56 schools in New York state; 91% White, 2% Black, 2% Hispanic, 1% Native American		Life Skills Training—15 class periods in grade 7, 10 sessions in grade 8, 5 sessions in grade 9; information and skills for resisting social influences to use drugs, personal and social skills; three groups compared—two prevention groups; teachers trained in 1-day workshop vs. 2-hour videotape; control	3 years—NS for drinking frequency and quantity; lower frequency of getting drunk for videotape teacher training group vs. control $F(2,3,678) = 3.25$, $p = .0391$
Caplan, Weissberg, Grober, Sivo, Grady, & Jacoby (1992)	282 sixth and seventh graders—206 from inner-city schools (90% Black, 8% Hispanic, 2% mixed origins) and 76 from suburban schools (99% White and 1% Hispanic) in Connecticut		Positive Youth Development Program—20-session curriculum with six units (stress management, self-esteem, problem solving, substances and health, assertiveness, social networks) in two 50-minute class periods per week over 15 weeks	Increase in intention to use beer, $F(1,218) = 3.75$, $p < .05$, and hard liquor, $F(1,218) = 5.22$, $p < .05$; frequency of 3 or more drinks at one time, $F(1,213) = 3.65$, $p < .05$; having too much to drink, $F(1,213) = 3.68$, $p < .05$; and quantity, $F(1,213) = 5.65$, $p < .05$, control students

(continued)

TABLE 5.1   *(continued)*

Authors	Setting, population, and design	Conceptual approach	Intervention description	Change in alcohol measures
Cuijpers, Jonkers, deWeerdt, & deJong (2002)	1,405 of 1,930 students from 12 schools Attrition: 27%	Theory of planned behavior, social cognitive theory, model of behavioral change	The Healthy School and Drugs—5 components implement over a 3-year period, coordinating committee, series of educational lessons; school regulations on drug use, system of early detection of students with drug problems and interventions; parental involvement through manuals, brochures	1, 2, and 3 years—less alcohol use (proportion users 0.328 vs. 0.428 $p = .05$ in year 1, 0.566 vs. 0.654 $p < .01$ in year 2, 0.738 vs. 0.805 $p < .01$ in year 3; frequency 0.442 vs. 0.569, $p < .01$ in year 3; quantity $M = 4,06$, $SD = 7.20$; $M = 5.27$, $SD = 7.57$, $p < .01$, in year 3, drinks per session $M = 4,79$, $SD = 4.30$; $M = 5.82$, $SD = 5.78$, $p < .001$, in year

TABLE 5.1   *(continued)*

Authors	Setting, population, and design	Conceptual approach	Intervention description	Change in alcohol measures
Ellickson & Bell (1990); Ellickson, Bell, & McGuigan (1993); Ellickson, Bell, & Harrison (1993)	Seventh graders from 30 schools in California and Oregon Attrition: 53%–57%	Health belief model and self-efficacy theory	Project ALERT—8 lessons during grade 7 and 3 booster lessons in grade 8; designed to build motivation and skills to resist substance use; team vs. adult leader	6 years—early small reductions in grade 7 were NS by grade 8; 3, 12, and 15 months—modest (28%, $p = .04$) reductions in drinking for nonusers (44%, $p = .07$) experimenters, and ($p = .06$) users; effects were largely associated with the teen leader intervention groups and disappeared by grade 8
Goldberg, MacKinnon, Elliot, Moe, Clarke, & Cheong (2000)	3,207 athletes from 31 high school football teams in 3 cohorts Attrition: 31.3%		Adolescents Training and Learning to Avoid Steroids (ATLAS) Interactive classroom and exercise training sessions by peer educators and facilitated by coaches and strength trainers	1 year—new occurrences of drinking and driving lower in experimental group (% change in *SD* units: 10.7 vs. 12.1, $p = .004$); index of alcohol and other drug use lower in experimental group (% change in *SD* units: 3.9 vs. 8.4, $p < .05$)

(continued)

TABLE 5.1   *(continued)*

Authors	Setting, population, and design	Conceptual approach	Intervention description	Change in alcohol measures
Hansen & Graham (1991); Hansen, Graham, Wolkenstien, & Rohrbach (1991)	2,416 of 3,011 students in 12 junior high schools in Los Angeles and Orange counties in California; two cohorts— fifth grade and seventh grade; 52% White, 29% Latino, 10% Asian, 4% Black, 5% other Attrition: 19.8%		Adolescent Alcohol Prevention Trial Information; normative training; combined	1 year—less alcohol use in normative training group, 11.24 vs. 0.60 for resistance and 0;21 for combined, $p <$ .01; delay in onset of ever being drunk for normative training, 25.19 vs. 0.03 for resistance, and 2.24 for combined, $p < .0001$
Komro, Perry, Murray, Veblen-Mortenson, Williams, & Anstien (1996)	24 school districts and communities in northeastern Minnesota; 20 intervention and comparison schools	Perry and Jesser's model of health promotion and prevention of adolescent drug abuse	Project Northlands—Peer Participation Program component: planners took part in planning and promoting alcohol-free social activities for their peers; attenders attended events only; nonparticipants	1 year— planners: less alcohol use in past year than attenders, $F(2,26) = 2.73$, $p = .04$; less alcohol use in last month than attenders and nonparticipants, $F(2,26) = 6.96$, $p < .01$; planners less likely to intend to use alcohol when age 21 and in next year than attenders, $F(2,2) = 2.17$, $p = .05$

TABLE 5.1 *(continued)*

Authors	Setting, population, and design	Conceptual approach	Intervention description	Change in alcohol measures
Newman, Anderson, & Farrell (1992)	Two cohorts— 3,500 students in 87 classes and 3,500 students in 84 classes in 9 junior high schools in 2 sequential years	Problem behavior theory, social cognitive theory, role theory, educational immunization	Resisting Pressures to Drink and Drive— videotaped examples of refusal skills, role playing, frequency and quantity of alcohol use, riding with a drinking driver	One year—NS for use, smaller increase in times riding with drinking driver, $F(2,170) = 24.95$, $p < .05$
Schinke & Tepavac (1995)	2,475 third to sixth graders from 11 suburban Midwestern elementary schools	Social learning theory, problem-behavior theory	Million Dollar Machine (MDM)— introduced in interactive, live assembly conducted by a robot; learning objectives emphasized in classroom for 8 weeks	6 months— fourth graders less actual and potential drinking, $F(2,24) = 3.63$, $p < .05$
Schinke, Tepavac, & Cole (2000)	1,396 Native American students in grades 3 to 5 from 27 elementary students on 10 reservations in 5 states Attrition: 14.11%	Life skills training, culturally tailored	Resistance skills, problem solving, personal coping, interpersonal communication; community involvement component added to one group	30 and 42 months—lower alcohol use, $F(2,1,182) = 4.75$, $p < .01$; $F(2,1,171) = 6.03$, $p < .001$

(continued)

TABLE 5.1   *(continued)*

Authors	Setting, population, and design	Conceptual approach	Intervention description	Change in alcohol measures
Shope, Copeland, Maharg, & Dielman (1996)	1,041 students who completed grade 12 posttest of 2,031 grade 10 pretested	Social learning theory	Alcohol Misuse Prevention Study (AMPS)—5 45-minute sessions on consecutive days; awareness of short-term effects of alcohol, risks of alcohol misuse, situation and social pressures to misuse alcohol; development of refusal skills— focus on grade 10 intervention	2 years—less alcohol misuse, $F(2,1,910) = 4.06, p < .017$
Shope, Dielman, Butchart, Campanelli, & Kloska (1992)	Over 5,000 fifth and sixth graders from 49 schools	Same	Same	26 months— less misuse in previous drinkers, $F(2,1,302) = 4.2, p < .02$
Shope, Elliott, Raghunathan, & Waller (2001)	4,635 of 6,081 10th graders in southeastern Michigan in original study who obtained a driver's license by June 1997; 83% White, 17% non-White	Same	Same	7 years—fewer serious offenses in first year of driving (80% risk of serious offense, $p = .056$), especially for those in the low-drinking, nondisapproving-parents group; NS after first year

TABLE 5.1 *(continued)*

Authors	Setting, population, and design	Conceptual approach	Intervention description	Change in alcohol measures
Wynn, Scfhulenberg, Maggs, & Zucker (2000)	232 to 361 sixth to tenth grades Attrition: 36%	Same	Same	Cross-sectional at each grade—no effects on overindulgence in grades 6 and 7; norms-mediated effects on overindulgence (indirect effect = -0.09, $p < .05$); intervention exerted an indirect effect on 10th-grade alcohol overindulgence through 8th-grade norms and through alcohol overindulgence (indirect effect = -0.06, $p < .01$)
Sussman, Dent, Stacy, & Craig (1998)	21 continuation high schools with 1,074 of 2,001 high-risk students in southern California; 46% Latino, 37% White, 4% Asian American, 8% African American, 3% Native American, 2% other Attrition: 33%		Toward No Drug Abuse (TND)—9 sessions with three 50-minute sessions per week for 3 consecutive weeks; health motivation, social skills, decision making; school-as-community	1 year—lower use high pretest users ($t = 7/42$, $p < .01$)

TABLE 5.1 *(continued)*

Authors	Setting, population, and design	Conceptual approach	Intervention description	Change in alcohol measures
Werch, Pappas, Carlson, Edgemon, Sinder, & DiClemente (2000)	650 grade 6 students from 2 middle school in economically disadvantaged inner-city Jacksonville, FL; 85% African American, 12% Caucasian, 3% other Attrition: 52% to 53%	Multi-Component Motivational Stages (McMOS); health belief model, social learning theory, behavioral self-control theory	STARS (Start Taking Alcohol Risks Seriously)—2-phase, brief nurse consultation and six focused weekly follow-up consultations	Fewer intervention students in more advanced stages, $X^2 = 10.20$, 4 df, $p = .03$; fewer drank alcohol any length of time, $X^2 = 6.12$, 2 df, $p = .04$; fewer drank heavily in last 30 days, $X^2 = 3.89$, 1 df, $p = .04$; greater motivation to avoid alcohol, $F(1,315) = 8.15$, $p = .005$; less total alcohol risk, $F(1,315) = 4.31$, $p = .03$; less frequency of alcohol use, $F(1,314) = 8.51$, $p = .004$; and lower intention to use, $F(1,314) = 6.48$, $p = .01$ for magnet schools

TABLE 5.1 *(continued)*

Authors	Setting, population, and design	Conceptual approach	Intervention description	Change in alcohol measures
Werch, Pappas, Carlson, & DiClemente (1999)	138 sixth to eighth graders in innercity Florida schools; 84% African American, 13% Caucasian	Same	Same	At 3-month posttest—decrease in heavy use (t = –2.33, df = 120, p = .02)
Werch, Anzalone, Brokiewicz, Felker, Carlson, & Castellon-Vogel (1996)	104 sixth to eighth graders in innercity schools; 88% African American, 10% Caucasian	Same; resistance, self-efficacy	STARS—3-phase, self-instructional module with audiotape, brief nurse or physician consultation, follow-up consultations	At 10-week posttest—less use, 30-day quantity, F = 5.92, p = .01)
Wilhelmsen, Laberg, & Klepp (1994)	909 of 915 seventh graders from 12 schools in Bergen (Norway) school district Attrition: 4.8%	Theory of reasoned action	Elected peer leaders in three conditions: highly role-specified, less role-specified, and comparison; social norms, managing drinking pressure, attitudes toward alcohol use; 10 sessions over a 2-month period	1 month—significant effect for norms, $F(1,485)$ = 5.91, p < .05, alcohol use, $F(1,485)$ = 4.11, p < .05; effects for the highly role-specified condition (students more involved)

NS = Not Significant

berg & Arborelius, 1994; Collins & Cellucci, 1991; Cuijpers, Jonkers, de-Weerdt, & deJong, 2002; Goldberg, Halpern-Felsher, & Millstein, 2002; Scott, Surface, Friedli, & Barlow, 1999; Sheehan et al., 1996; Shope et al., 2000; Shope, Copeland, Maharg, & Dielman, 1996; Sussman, Dent, Stacy, & Craig, 1998; Wynn, Schulenberg, Maggs, & Zucker, 2000; Wynn, Schulenberg, Kloska, & Laetz, 1997).

Originally, the school-focused programs were not scientifically based and showed limited outcomes, but this situation changed over the past two decades (Hansen, 1993). Investigators became informed about risk factors, theoretical formulations, and more effective approaches. The factors related to alcohol use include normative beliefs, personal commitment, values, consequence beliefs, resistance skills, alternative, goal-setting skills, decision-making skills, self-esteem, stress skills, assistance skills, and life skills, in descending order of magnitude of the correlations.

Another change in the last decade is focusing programs on prevention in elementary grades, or "upstream" interventions designed for implementation prior to the onset of problems. Earlier programs targeted middle school and high school grades—that is, the years of greatest initiation of drinking. Recently, the rationale for building protective factors and decreasing risk factors prior to the highest initiation age has gained strength. Results of previous reviews (Greenberg et al., 2003; Tobler & Stratton, 1997) indicate that high-intensity, interactive programs are most effective in alcohol prevention. Trends have shifted from programs based on a "scare" approach to more scientifically based interventions delivered at earlier grade levels and for longer duration.

The critical question is, over the past decade, how have school interventions fared? Data on both short- and long-term effects are available from a number of programs. The programs will be examined by the major conceptual approach and variables that provided the focus of the intervention.

In light of the correlations between the various approaches and alcohol use, it is surprising to see that development of resistance skills was the most common emphasis for school interventions and was evident in 8 of the interventions, 4 as a singular component (Botvin et al., 1990, 1995, 2001; Caplan et al., 1992; Clayton et al., 1996; Ellickson & Bell, 1990; Ellickson, Bell, & Harrison, 1993; Ellickson, Bell, & McGuigan, 1993; Griffin et al., 2003; Lynam et al., 1999; Ringwalt et al., 1991; Rosenbaum et al., 1994) and 10 as a major focus in combination with other approaches (Cuijpers et al., 2002; Goldberg et al., 2000; Hansen & Graham, 1991; Newman et al., 1992; Ross et al., 1998; Schinke et al., 2000; Sheehan et al., 1996; Shope et al., 1996; Shope, Elliott, Raghunathan, & Waller, 2001; Sussman et al., 1998; Werch, Anzalone, et al., 1996; Werch, 1997; Werch, Carlson, et al., 1996; Werch et al., 2000; Werch et al., 1999; Wilhelmsen et al., 1994; Wynn et al., 1997, 2000). A resistance skills approach was most often combined with a knowledge component and often with a component that clarified peer norms.

The majority of the studies examined alcohol outcomes, including initiation of alcohol use, frequency and quantity of drinking alcohol, problems resulting from alcohol misuse, and the effects on mediating variables. A limitation of the studies was the short periods of follow-up for evaluation of outcomes. When looked at 3 months or less postintervention, decreases in heavy use (Bagnall, 1990; Botvin et al., 2001; Werch et al., 1996), use on a 30-day quantity measure (Werch et al., 1996), actual use (Bagnall, 1990; Ellickson & Bell, 1990), and potential drinking (Caplan et al., 1992; Schinke & Tepavac, 1995; Wilhelmsen et al., 1994) were reported. At 1 year posttest, findings included less frequency and quantity, less drunkenness (Botvin et al., 2001; Cuijpers et al., 2002), lower use in high pretest users (Sussman et al., 1998), and less alcohol use (Hansen & Graham, 1991).

Several studies included longer term evaluations. Schinke and colleagues (2000) found lower alcohol use at 3.5 years posttest from a culturally tailored life skills program with Native American students implemented in grades 3 to 5. Four studies that evaluated the efficacy of the Drug Abuse Resistance Education (DARE) program, one of the most widely implemented interventions, found no effects on alcohol use (Clayton et al., 1996; Lynam et al., 1999; Ringwalt et al., 1991; Rosenbaum et al., 1994), and thus the main objective of DARE failed. Several studies (Gilason et al., 1995; Sheehan et al., 1996; Wynn et al., 2000) found no significant effects, short or long term, for other interventions. Outcomes of the Alcohol Misuse Prevention Study (AMPS) included less alcohol misuse at 2 years (Shope et al., 1992, 1996) and fewer serious offenses in the first year of driving (Shope et al., 2001). Ellickson and colleagues (1993) found that early effects of Project ALERT disappeared at longer term follow-up.

Botvin and colleagues published the longest follow-up of effects (with the exception of Lynam et al., 1999). The Life Skills Training program developed by Botvin was implemented in grades 7, 8, and 9. At 3 years posttest, they found that less drunkenness persisted, but not less frequency and quantity. At 6 years posttest, the finding of less drunkenness/problem drinking continued to be evident in the full sample. Outcomes were also examined in a "high-fidelity sample" that consisted of 2,752 students who received 60% of the intervention. In this group, less weekly drinking, heavy drinking, and problem drinking were noted.

Besides alcohol use and misuse outcomes, researchers often reported changes in the mediating factors that represented the dynamic of the intervention. An increase in knowledge about alcohol and drinking was reported in several studies (Botvin et al., 1990, 2001; Collins & Cellucci, 1991; Cuijpers et al., 2002; Hansen & Graham, 1991; Newman et al., 1992; Shope et al., 1992, 1996; Wynn et al., 2000). Researchers also reported changes in response to peer pressure, stress management, conflict resolution, impulse control social and emotional adjustment, problem-solving self-efficacy (Caplan et al., 1992), perceptions of peer and adult alcohol use (Botvin et al., 2001; Ellickson et al., 1993; Werch et al., 1996), self-respect (Schinke & Tepavac, 1995), and self-efficacy (Cuijpers et al., 2002; Ellickson et al., 1993; Hansen & Graham, 1991). However, changes in mediating factors did not necessarily match up with changes in alcohol use or misuse.

The programs were implemented with a variety of populations that included both high- and low-risk youth in urban, suburban, and rural settings in a variety of geographic settings throughout the United States, as well as in Iceland (Gilason, Yngvadottir, & Benediktsdottir, 1995), Canada (Ross et al., 1998), Norway (Wilhelmsen et al., 1994), Scotland (Bagnall, 1990), Sweden (Bremberg & Arborelius, 1994), and the Netherlands (Cuijpers et al., 2002). The majority of the studies were conducted with urban middle school populations. The diversity of the samples is a strength of this group of studies; a number of the researchers recruited samples that allowed for examination of the effects of school-based interventions with White and African American (see, e.g., Caplan et al., 1992; Werch et al., 1996), Latino (see, e.g., Botvin et al., 2001; Hansen & Graham, 1991; Sussman et al., 1998), and Native American (Schinke et al., 2000) adolescents. However, not all of the school-based interventions were evaluated across diverse populations, and conclusions about generalizibility of any of the programs would be premature.

The programs varied in length from a brief intervention to multiple sessions (5–15) with boosters at subsequent years. The programs with more sessions delivered over a longer period of time demonstrated stronger effects. Health professionals, teachers, research staff, and peers implemented interventions. One study (Ellickson, Bell, & McGuigan, 1993) compared the impact of adolescent peer and adult educator teams with adult educator only. The researchers found that the former were more effective in achieving positive changes about cognitive risk factors such as estimates of peer alcohol use and peer pressure to use alcohol. Ellickson et al.'s findings reinforced Tobler's (1992) meta-analysis findings that peer programs were most effective when delivered by mental health professionals/ counselors, followed by peer leaders and teachers. The combination of peer and health educators appears to have a synergistic effect.

Reviews of school-based programs synthesized the findings and clarified efficacy (see, e.g., Flay, 2000; Gorman, 1998; Hansen, 1992, 1993; Tobler, 1986, 1992; Wagner & Waldron, 2001). Although schools have been a common locus for alcohol prevention programs, little evaluation of these programs was evident until the 1980s (Gorman, 1998). Evaluation of the early programs was discouraging; effect sizes were small and inconsistent. Based on a meta-analysis of 143 prevention programs, Tobler (1986) concluded that "knowledge only" and "affective only" programs were not efficacious in reducing alcohol use and should be discontinued. In contrast, peer programs that combine positive peer influence with specific skill training were low intensity, cost effective, and decreased alcohol use. Alternative programs, though intensive and costly, were effective for special high-risk populations.

A more recent review (Flay, 2000) supported Tobler's conclusions. First-generation programs with information only often increased substance use. Affective approaches (second-generation programs) were equally ineffective, and third-generation approaches (personal and skills training) showed small but consistent effects. More recent studies, Flay (2000) concluded, indicate that changing normative beliefs "may be more important than skills development" (p. 862). Finally, Flay observed that program effects tended to decay over time, but they could be sustained with the use of booster sessions.

Summary

Although school-based interventions were the most prevalent in the literature, the effects were inconsistent, relatively small, and short-lived. These conclusions are similar to those of Foxcroft and colleagues (2004) in the *Cochrane Review of Primary Prevention for Alcohol Misuse in Young People*. There is little consistency in the analytic approaches to the data or even to the definition of outcomes. In some instances, the data are broken down and analyzed on three or more levels. The results of these analyses make it difficult to obtain a coherent picture of the efficacy of the intervention. Few studies have demonstrated long-term results that would lead to practice recommendations. The investigators did not address program replicability, cost effectiveness, or sustainability, so these programs had limited payoff. The most effective programs implemented the intervention over a substantial period of time (i.e., 15 sessions) and included booster sessions. Moving the science forward about school-based interventions is a challenging goal. Perhaps the most productive approach would be a radical one: hold a consensus conference; commission review and meta-analysis papers; invite the major scientists working in this area; and conduct a frank appraisal of critical correlates, approaches, and analytic strategies; then draw conclusions about the critical questions still to be addressed and develop a strategic plan for progress.

FAMILY-BASED INTERVENTIONS

In light of the modest success of school-based programs, together with the large literature on family correlates of adolescent alcohol use, researchers moved to development and evaluation of parent- or family-based interventions. Until recently, there were a limited number of family interventions. They are more complex and costly to design and deliver. There are limited systematic evaluations of family-based interventions evident in the literature, but in the decade from 1990 to 2000, family interventions increased as an option for investigators (Hogue & Liddle, 1999). The National Institute on Alcohol Abuse and Alcoholism (NIAAA) funded a number of intervention trials that evaluated the efficacy of either standalone family interventions or multitiered interventions with a family component. Results of these studies are beginning to appear in the literature.

Family interventions can be standalone interventions or part of broader, multifactorial intervention (Loveland-Cherry, 2000). Of the family studies (see Table 5.2) included in this review, eight were part of either community-based (Perry et al., 1993, 1996; Rohrbach et al., 1995; St. Pierre, Mark, Kaltreider, & Aiken, 1997; Williams, Perry, Farbakhsh, & Veblen-Mortenson, 1999) or school-based interventions (Dishion et al., 1998; Dishion & Kavanagh, 2000; Tolan & McKay, 1996; Werch, 1997; Werch et al., 1991, 1999, 2000). The remaining family-based interventions were designed and implemented as standalone programs: Iowa Strengthening Families Program (ISFP) (Kumpfer, 1998; Kumpfer, Molgaard, & Spoth, 1996; Spoth, Redmond, & Lepper, 1999; Spoth, Redmond, & Shin, 1998, 2001; Spoth, Redmond, Trudeau, & Shin, 2002; Spoth, Reyes, Redmond, & Shin, 1999), Family Matters (Bauman et al., 2001), Families in Action (Abbey et al., 2000; Bogenschneider & Stone, 1997), Child and Parent Relations (CAPR) (Loveland-Cherry et al., 1999), Preparing for the Drug-Free Years (PDFY) (Catalano, Kosterman, Hagerty, Hawkins, & Spoth, 1998; Spoth, Redmond, Haggert, & Ward, 1995), the Shadow Project (Boyd-Hall, 2003), Family Effectiveness Training (Szapocznik, Santisteban, Rio, Perez-Vidal, Santisteban, & Kurines, 1989), Michigan State Multiple Risk Child Outreach Programs (Maguin, Zucker, & Fitzgerald, 1994; Nye, Zucker, & Fitzgerald, 1999), Parent-based Intervention Strategies to Reduce Adolescent Alcohol-Impaired Driving (Jaccard & Turrisi, 1999), and SUPER STARS (Emshoff, Avery, Raduka, Anderson, & Calvert, 1996).

The samples for family-based interventions were not as diverse as those for school-based interventions. Although some studies (Hawkins et al., 1999; Loveland-Cherry & Looman, 2003; Rohrbach et al., 1995; St. Pierre et al., 1997; Werch et al., 1999, 2000) had samples that included sufficient numbers in subgroups to do meaningful analyses, most of the studies had samples that were largely or totally Caucasian. Thus, the knowledge culled from this research is limited to certain segments of the population. As the diversity of the population increases and alcohol use becomes an issue in these segments, it will be important to understand if the interventions developed and evaluated with majority populations can be generalized to other groups.

All of the family interventions were conceptually based, and the theoretical approaches were characterized by an ecological perspective that allowed for multilevel interventions. Adolescents, parents, families, schools, and communities were targeted for intervention. As with school-based projects, adolescents' initiation of alcohol use, frequency and quantity of use, and heavy use were the outcomes. Intervention dynamics focused on changing adolescents' intentions,

TABLE 5.2   Family-based Interventions: Significant Alcohol Effects

Authors	Setting, population, and design	Conceptual approach	Intervention description	Change in alcohol measures
Dishion, Andrews, Kavanagh, & Soberman (2001); Dishion & Kavanagh (2000)	158 families— 119 intervention and 59 quasi-control; 1,200 adolescents Attrition: 34%	Social interactional framework with multiple gating model	Adolescent Transitions Program (ATP)—3 levels: universal, The Family Resource Room; selected, The Family Check-up; indicated, A Menu of Services; 12 group sessions	1 year—reduced alcohol use
Hawkins, Catalano, Kosterman, Abbott, & Hill (1999)	598 18-year-olds who entered study in grade 5; 44% White, 26% African American, 22% Asian American, 5% Native American, 3% other Attrition: 7%	Social development model	Parent training: behavior management skills; in grade 2: "Catch 'Em Being Good"; grades 2–4: session "How to Help Your Child Succeed in School"; grades 5 and 6: "Preparing for the Drug (Free) Years" plus teacher training	8 years—less heavy alcohol use, 15.4% intervention vs. 25% controls ($p = .04$)
Loveland-Cherry, Ross, & Kaufman (1999)	892 students in grade 4 from 3 Midwestern school districts; 86% European American Attrition: 19%	Social cognitive theory, problem behavior theory, family systems theory	Child and Parent Relations—3 hour-long in-home sessions, family meetings, and follow-up telephone calls between in-home sessions; intervention in grade 4 and booster in grade 7	4 years— decreased alcohol use in nonprior drinking intervention students; higher rate of increase for use and misuse for prior drinkers

(continued)

TABLE 5.2   *(continued)*

Authors	Setting, population, and design	Conceptual approach	Intervention description	Change in alcohol measures
Perry et al. (1993, 1996); Williams et al. (1999)	2,351 adolescents from 24 school districts in rural and small towns in Minnesota	Comprehensive ecological model	Project Northlands, 3 themes—Slick Tracy Home Team Program, Amazing Alternatives!, and power Lines; parent–child activities, newsletter, events at schools, facilitators for local teen groups, and membership on community task forces	Delayed onset and prevalence of alcohol use
Williams, Perry, Farbakhsh, & Veblen-Mortenson (1999)	2,191 of 2,351 students from 24 school districts in northeastern Minnesota; 945 White, 5.5% Native American Attrition: 19%		Project Northlands, comprehensive program; 2 phases—Phase I, grades 6–8; parent involvement emphasis in first 2 years—4 weeks of parent–child activities, Northland Notes for Parents, plays, members of community task forces, facilitators for local TEENS groups	3 years—NS lower rates

TABLE 5.2 *(continued)*

Authors	Setting, population, and design	Conceptual approach	Intervention description	Change in alcohol measures
Chou et al. (1998); Rohrback et al. (1995)	22,500 students for grades 6 or 7 in 15 communities in Kansas City (Kansas City, KS, and Kansas City, MO) metropolitan area and 3 cohorts of students from 57 middle or junior high schools in Indianapolis area; 70% White	Comprehensive ecological model	Midwestern Prevention Project—10-session youth education program and 10 homework sessions—STAR (Students Taught Awareness and Resistance)	1 year—decreased alcohol use; 3 years—NS
Spoth, Redmond, Trudeau, & Shin (2002)	Grade 7 students from 36 schools in Midwestern state; 96% Caucasian		Compared two intervention groups, SFP 10–14 (revised ISFP) and Life Skills Training (LST), LST only and control; boosters in grade 8	1 year—reduced rates of alcohol initiation: 30% reduction for SFP 10–14
Spoth, Redmond, & Shin (2001)	667 sixth graders and their parents from 33 public schools in a Midwestern state; 99% Caucasian Attrition: 33%	PDFY—social development model; ISFP—biopsychosocial model	Compared two interventions, 5-session PDFY and 7-session ISFP and control	4 years—lower proportion of new use of alcohol and greater relative reduction in being drunk for ISFP; lower rate of use for PDFY and ISFP

(continued)

TABLE 5.2 *(continued)*

Authors	Setting, population, and design	Conceptual approach	Intervention description	Change in alcohol measures
Spoth, Redmond, & Lepper (1999); Spoth, Reyes, Redmond, & Shin (1998); Spoth, Redmond, & Shin (1999)	446 families (317 at posttest year 1 and 294 at posttest year 2)	Same	ISFP—2-hour sessions, once a week for 7 weeks, separate parent and child sessions followed by a family session	1 and 2 years— lower rates of alcohol initiation; effect size 0.26 and 0.39; relative reduction 29.3–60.5 2 years—PDFY and ISFP students more likely to remain in 1-year non-use status at 2-year posttest
Werch, Carlson, Pappas, & DiClemente (1999); Werch et al. (2000)	650 sixth graders in inner-city Jacksonville, FL; 85% African American, 12% Caucasian, 3% other Attrition: 25%	Multi-Component Motivational States (McMOS) model	STARS for Families Program—series of 10 mailed physician-endorsed prevention postcards with a key fact to emphasize with child; same risk factors found in student STARS consultation	6 months— decreased alcohol use for magnet school students who received the intervention $(F(1,314) = 8.51, p = .004)$

ISFP = Iowa Strengthening Families Program; PDFY = Preparing for the Drug-Free Years; NS = Not Significant; TEENS = The Exciting and Entertaining Northland Students

beliefs, knowledge, school attachment, family problems, school problems, self-esteem, self-efficacy, and perceptions of peer/family alcohol use. Further, modifications occurred in family/parent protective and risk factors such as knowledge and beliefs about adolescent development and alcohol use, communication, monitoring, values and attitudes, parental responsiveness, family cohesion, parent–child relationships, and parenting skills.

Family interventions that were incorporated into school- or community-based interventions employed homework assignments or newsletters sent home with the child and requiring focused parent–child interactions. For example, the Midwestern Prevention Project had 10 homework sessions involving active interviews and role plays with parents and family members to complement media coverage and the educational program. In contrast, the Metropolitan Area Child Study and the Adolescent Transitions Program (ATP) involved families in a variety of activities within the school setting itself. The standalone interventions required more family interaction and involved families either individually or in groups in homes, schools, and churches in rural or urban communities. The intensity of the interventions varied from homework activities to 28 sessions over 10 months.

Outcomes of family-based studies included either adolescent alcohol use/misuse or mediating factors. Three studies reported outcomes for mediating variables, such as parents' communication to avoid drugs, perceptions of peer alcohol use, susceptibility to peer pressure (Werch et al., 1991), parental monitoring (Bogenschneider & Stone, 1997), and family cohesion, family fighting, school attachment, self-esteem, and anti–alcohol use beliefs (Abbey et al., 2000). The others reported outcomes of adolescent alcohol use/misuse, including initiation of alcohol use covering periods from less than 6 months to eight years post intervention.

Two of these showed no significant effects at 11 months (Boyd-Hall, 2003) or at 1 year (Bauman et al., 2001); one reported less alcohol use at 1 year (Rohrbach et al., 1995) but not at 3 years (Chou et al., 1998). Short-term effects were demonstrated for two interventions; the STARS for Families Program (Werch et al., 1999, 2000) and ATP (Dishion et al., 1998; Dishion & Kavanagh, 2001). Several investigators demonstrated longer term effects. Loveland-Cherry and colleagues (1999) found decreased alcohol use and misuse in non–prior drinking students at 4 years postintervention. Interestingly, they also found a higher rate of increase for use and misuse for prior drinkers after an initial decrease. Hawkins and colleagues (1999) reported the most resilient effects at 8 years; adolescents in this intervention reported less heavy alcohol use. A project in progress by Spoth and colleagues in Iowa is comparing several family interventions. To date, they have demonstrated consistent efficacy at 1, 2, and 4 years (Spoth et al., 1999, 2001, 2002; Spoth, Redmond, & Shin, 2001; Spoth, Redmond, & Lepper, 1999). Limited effects were found for the PDFY aspect of the program, but outcomes in both cases were decreasing use and delaying initiation of use.

The three studies that investigated mediating variables (Werch, Pappas, Carlson, & DiClemente, 1999; Werch, Pappas, Carlson, Edgemon, Sinder, & DiClemente, 2000; Werch, Young, et al., 1991) found significant intervention effects. Werch and colleagues (1991) found significant effects for the Keep a Clear Mind intervention at 2 weeks posttest. Parents in the experimental condition reported more recent and greater frequency of communication to avoid drugs, and students reported less perception of peer use of alcohol and less susceptibility to peer pressure.

Summary

Taken as a whole, family interventions may produce at least short-term effects for intention to delay alcohol use and to decrease use and heavy use of alcohol. However, with few exceptions, the effect size is small and does not hold up over time. Foxcroft and colleagues (2004) identified the Strengthening Families Program as having the most potential to be an effective family intervention, but it needs to be validated in larger and more diverse samples.

COMMUNITY-BASED INTERVENTIONS

Community-based interventions (see Table 5.3) comprised the smallest number of studies, with a total of 8 programs described in 11 reports. There was a variety of intervention approaches, including some with special populations. The approaches included culturally specific interventions for African American adolescents (Belgrave, 2002) and for Native American adolescents (Cheadle et al., 1995), an intervention on sales of alcohol (Grube, 1997), brief interventions in an emergency room (ER) (Monti et al., 1999), an intervention with adolescents in residential facilities (Morehouse & Tobler, 2000), an intervention with pregnant and parenting female adolescents (Palinkas, Atkins, Miller, & Ferreira, 1996), two community trials (Perry et al., 1996, 2000; Stevens, Mott, & Youells, 1996), and one intervention in primary care pediatric practices (Stevens, Olson, Gaffney, & Tosteson, 2002). This variety of subpopulations and intervention approaches makes it difficult to summarize or generalize across the community-based interventions.

Five of the studies identified the use of a conceptual model. Belgrave (2002) used relation theory and Africentric theory for the Project Naja and social cognitive theory for the Cultural Enhancement Program. A social influence model, derived from social learning/cognitive theory, provided the conceptual framework for the Shifting Gears Program (Klepp, Kelder, & Perry, 1995). Project PALS was developed within problem behavior theory (Palinkas et al., 1996). Project Northlands (Perry et al., 1996, 2000) was framed within social cognitive theory, with an emphasis on environmental and personal factors. The predominant use of social cognitive theory is not surprising because these interventions focused strongly on the person–environment interaction.

The samples for this group of studies were diverse, with the smaller studies reaching specific populations, either specific ethnic groups or socially specific groups such as adolescents in residential facilties or pregnant adolescents. The samples for the two larger community trials were composed primarily of White adolescents.

Only four of eight programs reported significant intervention effects. A community-based approach to prevent underage sales of alcohol (Grube, 1997)

TABLE 5.3 Community-based Interventions

Authors	Setting, population, and design	Conceptual approach	Intervention description	Change in alcohol measures
Klepp, Kelder, & Perry (1995)	2 of 6 communities, matched on population size (~100,000 each) in Minnesota; primarily Caucasian, middle-class; grade 6 cohorts Attrition: 45% in the intervention community and 69% in the reference community	Social influence model, derived from social learning theory	Shifting Gears—school-based peer-led program to delay or prevent tobacco, marijuana, and alcohol use; building social skills enabling students to resist pressure to use drugs; 6 sessions; component of Minnesota Heart Health program	6 years—at year 3, intervention community participants had fewer drinking occasions, 1.9 vs. 2.2, $p = $ .019, and fewer occasions of problem drinking (20% vs. 30%, $p = $ .028), than reference community peers; differences became smaller each year and were not significant in subsequent years; at year 3, intervention participants reported few drinking and driving occasions in last 3 months than those in the reference community; results did not persist over time

(continued)

TABLE 5.3   *(continued)*

Authors	Setting, population, and design	Conceptual approach	Intervention description	Change in alcohol measures
Monti et al. (1999)	94 (of 141) alcohol-positive adolescents presenting in an ER		Randomized to 35–40 minutes of brief motivational interview (MI) or 5 minutes of standard care (SC)	3 and 6 months—no significant group differences for alcohol consumption; drinking and driving—SC nearly 4 times more likely to report drinking and driving (85%) than MI (662%), $X^2(1, N = 73) = 5.82$, $p < .05$; moving violations—MI less likely to have moving violations (3%) than SC (23%), $X^2(1, N = 62) = 5.17$, $p < .05$; alcohol-related injuries—MI (21%) have fewer injuries than SC (50%), $X^2(1, N = 82) = 7.72$, $p < .01$; alcohol-related problems—MI have fewer problems $(M = 0.89, SD = 1.18)$ than SC $(M = 1.44, SD = 1.43)$, $F(1.78) = 45/10$, $p < .05$, effect size $= 0.23$

TABLE 5.3 *(continued)*

Authors	Setting, population, and design	Conceptual approach	Intervention description	Change in alcohol measures
Morehouse & Tobler (2000)	132 intervention and 201 comparison group youth (primarily African American and Latino) ages 13–19 from six residential facilities for problem youth Attrition: 21%		RSAP—focus on wellness; student assistant counselors; training and consultation to residential child care, clinical, and teaching staff to increase awareness and skill in AOD prevention strategies; meet with all youth on entry, prevention education groups, with discussion and role play in 6–8 sessions, outreach activities; independent 45-minute group counseling for youths with alcohol or substance abusing parents; individual 45-minute counseling; referral to AOD treatment programs; facilitates involvement in 12-step programs; Adolescent Resident Task Force to change culture and norms of facility; conducted by Student Assistance Service Corp.	5 years—pretest/posttest comparison, frequency–quantity index ($t_{262} = 4.25, p = .000$), and number-of-drugs index ($t_{262} = 4.99, p = .000$), significantly lower at posttest for intervention and not for comparison group ($t_{453} = 0.43, p = .67$, and $t_{454} = 1.19, p = .06$, respectively); cross-sectional intervention vs. cross-sectional comparison—difference in quantity–frequency index—with lower scores for intervention ($t_{428} = 5.28, p = .000$), effect size = 0.51

(continued)

TABLE 5.3   *(continued)*

Authors	Setting, population, and design	Conceptual approach	Intervention description	Change in alcohol measures
Perry et al. (1996)	24 school districts and communities in northeastern Minnesota, 20 intervention and comparison schools	Social cognitive theory, emphasis on environmental factors and personal factors	Project Northlands, Phase I—Slick Tracy Home Team Program and community-wide task forces in grade 6, Amazing Alternatives peer participation program, four Home Program booklets with parents, Northland Notes for Parents, classroom curriculum and community-wide task forces in grade 7; PowerLines classroom curriculum, theater production, Northland Notes for Parents, and community-wide task forces in grade 8; community task forces included policy, discussions with local alcohol merchants, distribution of materials to support policies, sponsorship of alcohol-free activities for young teens	3 years—less alcohol use in intervention schools/communities (16% $\pm$ 1.7% vs. 17.5% $\pm$ 1.8%, $p < .05$); lower onset rates for baseline nonusers (5.3% $\pm$ 4.6% vs. 9.8% $\pm$ 4.6%, $p < .05$)

TABLE 5.3   *(continued)*

Authors	Setting, population, and design	Conceptual approach	Intervention description	Change in alcohol measures
Perry et al. (2000)	Same		Project Northlands, Phase II—5 intervention strategies: community organizing, parent education, youth development, media, school curriculum	1 year—intervention students reported drinking less, but NS difference; baseline nonusers in intervention reported marginally ($p <$ .07) less past week alcohol use

AOD = Alcohol and Other Drugs; ER = Emergency Room; NS = Not significant; RSAP = Residential Student Assistance Program

demonstrated significantly reduced sales to minors in two of three experimental communities. The intervention included three strategies: enforcement of underage sales laws, responsible beverage service training (RBS), and media advocacy. Results were based on intervention versus comparison communities and outlets that received training versus those that did not. Significant results were from the community comparisons but not for the training effects. The authors cautioned that the training effects may not have reached significance because of small numbers. Further, the authors pointed out that the results were for underage sales, relationships between availability of alcohol as reflected in sales, and perceived availability, whereas underage drinking behaviors were not determined.

Brief interventions delivered in the ER were effective in decreasing drinking/driving behaviors, moving violations, alcohol-related problems, and alcohol-related injuries, but not alcohol consumption (Monti et al., 1999). All of the adolescents, regardless of study condition, decreased their alcohol consumption, so this may be the result of experiencing an alcohol-related injury. Further, the intervention focused on decreasing sequelae of drinking and not drinking itself.

The Residential Student Assistance Program (RSAP) (Morehouse & Tobler, 2000) was effective in preventing and reducing alcohol use in high-risk adolescents who are in residential facilities. This "captive audience" of adolescents is not exposed to alcohol prevention interventions because they are not in school. In this project, only the adolescents received treatment because there was no family present. Reportedly, five of the six facilities continued the program postintervention.

The results from Project Northlands, a major community trial, were mixed. At 3-year follow-up of Phase I, which included parent and classroom approaches, interventions in schools and communities showed less alcohol use and lower onset rates of alcohol use for baseline nonusers. However, in Phase II no significant effects occurred at 1-year follow-up. The final results of the trial were not available at the time of the 2000 publication. Based on available information, the effects of the multilevel intervention appear to dissipate over time.

Summary

The eight community-based interventions were directed at special populations but showed mixed results. For the large community trials (e.g., Project Northlands), multilevel, creative strategies were developed, but only short-term effects were seen, and they were not sustained over time. The review of these studies was particularly disappointing as community-based interventions hold the greatest promise for success. Foxcroft and colleagues (2004) spoke against creating new interventions for each special group because this strategy is not cost effective; they recommended instead that efforts should be directed toward finding a single community intervention that works across diverse groups.

CONCLUSION

There have been significant investments of time, effort, and money in developing and evaluating interventions to prevent alcohol use and misuse in children and adolescents. Certainly, prevention interventions are logical strategies to decrease morbidity and mortality in these age groups. Another rationale, with some supporting evidence, is that delaying the initiation of alcohol use and preventing use and misuse will produce positive health consequences at later ages. Unfortunately, no efficacious interventions have been developed so far at the individual, family, school, or community level. At best, studies have demonstrated short-term effects that were not sustained over time.

Orleans and colleagues (1999) used McKinlay's population-based intervention model to evaluate population promotion on six behaviors. The model proposed intervention types: downstream, midstream, and upstream. Downstream interventions target individuals; they are designed for persons with a risk factor or risk-related disease/condition, and they emphasize changing (rather than preventing) health-damaging behaviors. Midstream interventions attempt to change and/or prevent health-damaging behaviors; they involve "mediation through important organizational channels or natural environments" (Orleans et al., 1999, p. 76). Upstream interventions are macro-level state and national public policy/environmental strategies "to strengthen social norms and supports for health behaviors and to redirect unhealthy societal and industry counter-forces" (Orleans et al., 1999, p. 76). An organized, systematic evaluation of existing alcohol interventions is warranted, followed by development and testing of innovative interventions for prevention of alcohol use in children and adolescents.

Concurrently, methodological issues must be addressed. One helpful strategy would be to define outcome measures that can be used consistently across studies. This recommendation is consistent with that of Foxcroft and colleagues (2004), who pointed out that such measures could determine important predictors of alcohol misuse, morbidity, and mortality at later life stages. Improvements in other aspects of design and analysis are warranted. Large-scale randomized con-trolled trials with evaluation of long-term effects are needed. The use of sophisti-cated analytic approaches, such as hierarchical linear modeling and mixed model approaches, would more appropriately analyze the multilevel, nested data that are collected. Finally, when promising interventions are identified, replication of these programs is in order, including examination of effectiveness, cost effec-tiveness, feasibility, and sustainability. Federal funding of such replication studies is needed.

Foxcroft and colleagues (2004) suggest using the *International Guide for Monitoring Alcohol Consumption and Relation Harm* (World Health Organization, 2000) as a framework for reviewing indicators of alcohol use and misuse. Further, they recommend the development of a classification system for interventions allowing for grading on a 4-point scale, from A to D. A indicates a safe, efficacious, and effective intervention recommended for use; B, that efficacy of the interven-tion has been established but further evaluation is needed to determine effective-ness and safety (B rating interventions could be used as part of a primary research program or a surveillance program); C, that safety and efficacy are not known (C rating interventions should be used only as part of a primary research program with appropriate methodology); and D, that safety and/or efficacy have been unsatisfactory and that the intervention should not be used.

A more systematic process for tracking alcohol prevention interventions for children and adolescents is needed to bring coherence to existing research. Such an approach would necessitate interdisciplinary participation, and nurse-scientists need to be ready to participate. Nurse-scientists have the broad perspec-tive that would benefit this research area. Funding sources, such as the National Institute on Drug Abuse and the National Institute on Alcohol Abuse and Alcoholism, have been open to funding nurse-researchers as principal investiga-tors, and the agencies view nurse-researchers as valuable members of interdisci-plinary teams.

ACKNOWLEDGMENTS

I would like to acknowledge the contributions of Wendy Looman, PhD, RN, who was a doctoral student in the University of Michigan School of Nursing and who provided invaluable assistance in conducting the literature searches that form the basis for this review. Dr. Looman currently is on the faculty of the University of Minnesota School of Nursing.

REFERENCES

Abbey, A., Pilgrim, C., Hendrickson, P., & Buresh, S. (2000). Evaluation of a family-based substance abuse prevention program targeted for the middle school years. *Journal of Drug Education, 30*(2), 213–228.

Abrams, D. B., & Clayton, R. R. (2001). Transdisciplinary research to improve brief interventions for addictive behaviors. In P. M. Moon, S. M. Colby, & T. A. O'Leary (Eds.), *Adolescents, alcohol, and substance abuse: Reaching teens through brief interventions*. New York: Guilford Press.

Allison, K. W., Crawford, I., Leone, P. E., Trickett, E., Perez-Febles, A., Burton, L. M., et al. (1999). Adolescent substance use: Preliminary examinations of school and neighborhood context. *American Journal of Community Psychology, 27*(2), 111–141.

Allison, K. R., Silverman, G., & Dignam, C. (1990). Effects on students of teacher training in use of a drug education curriculum. *Journal of Drug Education, 20*(1), 31–46.

Ajzen, I. (1991). The theory of planned behavior. *Organizational Behavior and Human Decision Processes, 50*, 179–211.

Ajzen, I., & Fishbein, M. (1980). *Understanding attitudes and predicting social behavior*. Englewood Cliffs, NJ: Prentice-Hall.

Bagnall, G. (1990). Alcohol education for 13 year olds—does it work? *British Journal of Addiction, 85*, 89–96.

Bandura, A. (1977). Self-efficacy: Toward a unifying theory of behavioral change. *Psychological Review, 84*, 191–215.

Barnes, G. M., & Windle, M. (1987). Family factors in adolescent alcohol and drug abuse. *Pediatrician, 14*, 13–18.

Bauman, K. E., Foshee, V. A., Ennett, S. T., Pemberton, M., Hicks, K. A., King, T. S., et al. (2001). Influence of a family program on adolescent tobacco and alcohol use. *American Journal of Public Health, 91*(4), 604–610.

Belgrave, F. Z. (2002). Relational theory and cultural enhancement interventions for African American adolescent girls. *Public Health Reports, 117*(1 Suppl.), 76–81.

Bell, N. J., Forthun, L. F., & Sun, S. W. (2000). Attachment, adolescent competencies, and substance use: Developmental considerations in the study of risk behaviors. *Substance Use and Misuse, 35*(9), 1177–1206.

Biglan, A., Duncan, T. E., Ary, D. V., & Smolkowski, K. (1995). Peer and parental influence on adolescent tobacco use. *Journal of Behavioral Medicine, 18*(4), 315–330.

Bogenschneider, K., & Stone, M. (1997). Delivering parent education to low and high risk parents of adolescent via age-paced newsletters. *Family Relations, 46*(2), 123–134.

Botvin, G. J., Baker, E., Dusenbury, L., Botvin, E. M., & Diaz, T. (1995). Long-term follow-up results of a randomized drug abuse prevention trial in a white middle-class population. *Journal of the American Medical Association, 273*(14), 1106–1112.

Botvin, G. J., Baker, E., Dusenbury, L., Tortu, S., & Botvin, E. M. (1990). Preventing adolescent drug abuse through a multimodal cognitive-behavioral approach: Results of a 3-year study. *Journal of Consulting and Clinical Psychology, 58*(4), 437–446.

Botvin, G. J., Griffin, K. W., Diaz, T., & Ifill-Williams, M. I. (2001). Drug abuse prevention among minority adolescents: Posttest and one-year follow-up of a school-based preventive intervention. *Prevention Research, 2*(1), I–B.

Botvin, G. J., Malgady, R. G., Griffin, K. W., Scheier, L. M., & Epstein, J. A. (1998). Alcohol and marijuana use among rural youth: Interaction of social and intrapersonal influences. *Addictive Behaviors, 23*(3), 379–387.

Boyd, G. M. (1999). Alcohol and the family: Opportunities for prevention. *Journal of Studies on Alcohol,* (Suppl. 13), 5–9.

Boyd-Ball, A. J. (2003). A culturally responsive, family-enhanced intervention model. *Alcoholism, Clinical and Experimental Research, 27*(8), 1356–1360.

Bremberg, S., & Arborelius, E. (1994). Effects on adolescent alcohol consumption of a school based student centered health counselling programme. *Scandinavian Journal of Social Medicine, 22*(2), 113–119.

Brook, J. S., Whiteman, M., Balka, E. B., & Hamburg, B. A. (1992). African American and Puerto Rican drug use: Personality, familial, and other environmental risk factors. *Genetic, Social, and General Psychology Monographs, 118*(4), 417–438.

Byrnes, J. P. (2003). Changing views on the nature and prevention of adolescent risk taking. In D. Romer (Ed.), *Reducing adolescent risk: Toward an integrated approach* (pp. 11–17). Thousand Oaks, CA: Sage.

Caplan, M., Weissberg, R. P., Grober, J. S., Sivo, P. J., Grady, K., & Jacoby, C. (1992). Social competence promotion with inner-city and suburban young adolescents: Effects on social adjustment and alcohol use. *Journal of Consulting and Clinical Psychology, 60*(1), 56–63.

Carlson, J. M., Moore, M. J., Pappas, D. M., Werch, C. E., Watts, G. F., & Edgemon, P. A. (2000). A pilot intervention to increase parent–child communication about alcohol avoidance. *Journal of Alcohol and Drug Education, 45*(2), 59–70.

Catalano, R. F., Gainey, R. R., Fleming, C. B., Haggerty, K. I. P., & Johnson, N. O. (1999). An experimental intervention with families of substance abusers: One-year follow-up of the focus on families project. *Addiction, 94*(2), 241–254.

Catalano, R., Mazza, J., Harachi, T., Abbott, R., Haggerty, K., & Fleming, C. (2003). Raising healthy children through enhancing social development in elementary school: Results after 1.5 years. *Journal of School Psychology, 41*(2), 143–164.

Cheadle, A., Pearson, D., Wagner, E., Psaty, B. M., Diehr, P. F., & Koepsell, T. (1995). A community-based approach to preventing alcohol use among adolescents on an American Indian reservation. *Public Health Reports, 110*(4), 439–447.

Chou, C., Montgomery, S., Pentz, M. A., Rohrbach, L. A., Johnson, A., Flay, B. R., et al. (1998). Effects of a community-based prevention program on decreasing drug use in high risk adolescents. *American Journal of Public Health, 88*(6), 944–948.

Clayton, R. R., Cattarello, A. M., & Johnstone, B. M. (1996). The effectiveness of drug abuse resistance education (Project DARE): 5-year follow-up results. *Preventive Medicine, 25,* 307–318.

Collins, D., & Cellucci, T. (1991). Effects of a school-based alcohol education program with a media prevention component. *Psychological Reports, 69*(1), 191–197.

Cuijpers, P., Jonkers, R., deWeerdt, I., & deJong, A. (2002). The effects of drug abuse prevention at school: The "Healthy School and Drugs" project. *Addiction, 97,* 167–173.

Dent, C. W., Sussman, S., & Stacy, A. W. (2001). Project Towards No Drug Abuse: Generalizability to a general high school sample. *Preventive Medicine, 32*(6), 514–520.

Dielman, T. E., Butchart, A. T., & Shope, J. T. (1993). Structural equation model tests of patterns of family interaction, peer alcohol use, and intrapersonal predictors of adolescent alcohol use and misuse. *Journal of Drug Education, 23,* 273–316.

Dishion, T. J., Andrews, D. W., Kavanagh, K., & Soberman, L. H. (2001). Preventive interventions for high-risk youth: The adolescent transitions program. In R. D. Peters & R. J. McMahon (Eds.), *Preventing childhood disorders, substance abuse, and delinquency.* Thousand Oaks, CA: Sage.

Dishion, T. L., & Kavanagh, K. (2000). A multilevel approach to family-centered prevention in schools: Process and outcome. *Addictive Behaviors, 25*(6), 899–911.

Dishion, T. J., & Kavanagh, K. (2001). An ecological approach to family intervention for adolescent substance use. In E. F. Wagner & H. B. Waldron (Eds.), *Innovations in adolescent substance abuse interventions* (pp. 127–142). New York: Pergamon.

Dishion, T. J., Patterson, G. R., Stoolmiller, M., & Skinner, M. L. (1991). Family, school, and behavioral antecedents to early adolescents' involvement with antisocial peers. *Developmental Psychology, 27,* 172–180.

Ellickson, P. L., & Bell, R. M. (1990). Drug prevention in junior high: A multi-site longitudinal test. *Science, 247*(16), 1299–1305.

Ellickson, P. L., Bell, R. M., & Harrison, E. R. (1993). Changing adolescent propensities to use drugs: Results from Project ALERT. *Health Education Quarterly, 20*(2), 227–242.

Ellickson, P. L., Bell, R. M., & McGuigan, K. (1993). Preventing adolescent drug use: Long-term results of a junior high program. *American Journal of Public Health, 83*(6), 856–861.

Ellickson, P. L., Tucker, J. S., Klein, D. J., & McGuigan, K. A. (2001). Prospective risk factors for alcohol misuse in late adolescence. *Journal of Studies on Alcohol, 62*(6), 773–782.

Emshoff, J., Avery, E., Raduka, G., Anderson, D. J., & Calvert, C. (1996). Findings from SUPER STARS: A health promotion program for families to enhance multiple protective factors. *Journal of Adolescent Research, 11*(1), 68–96.

Flay, B. R. (2000). Approaches to substance use prevention utilizing school curriculum plus social environmental change. *Addictive Behaviors, 25*(6), 861–885.

Foxcroft, D. R., Ireland, D., Lister-Sharp, D. J., Lowe, G., & Breen, R. (2002). Primary prevention for alcohol misuse in young people. *The Cochrane Database of Systematic Reviews* 2002, Issue 3. Art. No.: CD00 10-1002/14651858.CD003024.

Gilason, T., Yngvadottir, A., & Benediktsdottir, B. (1995). Alcohol consumption, smoking and drug abuse among Icelandic teenagers: A study into the effectiveness of the "Skills for Adolescence" programme. *Drugs: Education, Prevention and Policy, 2*(3), 243–258.

Goldberg, J. H., Halpem-Felsher, B. L., & Millstein, S. G. (2002). Beyond invulnerability: The importance of benefits in adolescents' decision to drink alcohol. *Health Psychology, 21*(5), 477–484.

Goldberg, L., MacKinnon, D. P., Elliot, D. L., Moe, E. L., Clarke, G., & Cheong, J. W. (2000). The adolescents training and learning to avoid steroids program. *Archives of Pediatric and Adolescent Medicine, 154,* 332–338.

Gorman, D. M. (1998). The irrelevance of evidence in the development of school-based drug prevention policy, 1986–1996. *Evaluation Review, 22*(1), 118–146.

Grant, B. F. (1997). Prevalence and correlates of alcohol use and DSM-IV alcohol dependence in the United States: Results of the National Longitudinal Alcohol Epidemiologic Survey. *Journal of Studies on Alcohol, 58,* 464–473.

Greenberg, M. T., Weissberg, R. P., O'Brien, M. U., Zins, J. E., Frederick, L., Resnik, H., et al. (2003). Enhancing school-based prevention and youth development through coordinated social, emotional, and academic learning. *American Psychologist, 58*(6–7), 466–474.

Griffin, K. W., Botvin, G. J., & Nichols, T. R. (2004). Long-term follow-up effects of a school-based drug abuse prevention program on adolescent risky driving. *Prevention Science, 5*(3), 207–212.

Grube, J. W. (1997). Preventing sales of alcohol to minors: Results from a community trial. *Addiction, 92*(Suppl. 2), 251–160.

Hansen, W. B. (1992). School-based substance abuse prevention: A review of the state of the art in curriculum, 1980–1990. *Health Education Research, 7,* 403–430.

———. (1993). School-based alcohol prevention programs. *Alcohol Health and Research World, 17*(1), 54–60.

Hansen, W. B., & Graham, J. W. (1991). Preventing alcohol, marijuana, and cigarette use among adolescents: Peer pressure resistance training versus establishing conservative norms. *Preventive Medicine, 20,* 414–430.

Hawkins, J. D., Catalano, R. F., Kosterman, R., Abbott, R., & Hill, K. (1999). Preventing adolescent health-risk behaviors by strengthening protection during childhood. *Archives of Pediatrics and Adolescent Medicine, 153*(3), 226–234.

Hawkins, J. D., Catalano, R. F., & Miller, J. Y. (1992). Risk and protective factors for alcohol and other drug problems in adolescence and early adulthood: Implications for substance abuse prevention. *Psychological Bulletin, 112*(1), 64–105.

Hogue, A., & Liddle, H. A. (1999). Family-based preventive intervention: An approach to preventing substance abuse and antisocial behavior. *American Journal of Orthopsychiatry, 69*(3), 278–293.

Huba, G. J., Wingard, J. A., & Bentler, P. M. (1980). Framework for an interactive theory of drug use. *NIDA Research Monograph, 30,* 95–101.

Jaccard, J., & Turrisi, R. (1999). Parent-based intervention strategies to reduce adolescent alcohol-impaired driving. *Journal of Studies on Alcohol* (Suppl. 13), 84–93.

Jessor, R., & Jessor, S. L. (1977). *Problem behavior and psychosocial development: A longitudinal study of youth.* New York: Academic.

Johnson, V., & Pandina, R. J. (1991). Effects of the family environment on adolescent substance use, delinquency, and coping styles. *American Journal of Drug and Alcohol Abuse, 17*(1), 71–88.

Johnston, L. D., O'Malley, P. M., Bachman, J. G., & Schulenberg, J. E. (2004). *Monitoring the future: National survey results on drug use, 1975–2003. 1: Secondary school students* (NIH Pub. No. 04-5507). Bethesda, MD: National Institute on Drug Abuse.

Klepp, K. I., Kelder, S. H., & Perry, C. L. (1995). Alcohol and marijuana use among adolescents: Long-term outcomes of the class of 1989 study. *Annals of Behavioral Medicine, 17*(1), 19–24.

Komro, K. A., Perry, C. L., Murray, D. M., Veblen-Mortenson, S., Williams, C. L., & Anstine, P. S. (1996). Peer-planned social activities for preventing alcohol use among young adolescents. *Journal of School Health, 66*(9), 328–334.

Komro, K. A., Perry, C. L., Williams, C. L., Stigler, M. H., Farbakhsh, K., & Veblen-Mortenson, S. (2001). How did Project Northland reduce alcohol use among young adolescents? Analysis of mediating variables. *Health Education Research, 16*(1), 59–70.

Kosterman, R., Hawkins, J. D., Haggerty, K. P., Spoth, R., & Redmond, C. (2001). Preparing for the drug free years: Session-specific effects of a universal parent-training intervention with rural families. *Journal of Drug Education, 31*(1), 47–68.

Kumpfer, K. L., Molgaard, V., & Spoth, R. (1996). The strengthening families program for the prevention of delinquency and drug use. In R. D. Peters & R. J. McMahon (Eds.), *Preventing childhood disorders, substance abuse, and delinquency* (pp. 241–267). Thousand Oaks, CA: Sage.

Kumpfer, K. (1998). Selective prevention interventions: The Strengthening Families program. *National Institute on Drug Abuse Research Monograph, 177*, 160–207.

Loveland-Cherry, C. J. (2000). Family interventions to prevent substance abuse: Children and adolescents. *Annual Review of Nursing Research, 18*, 195–218.

Loveland-Cherry, C. J., Leech, S. L., Laetz, V. B., & Dielman, T. E. (1996). Correlates of alcohol use and misuse in 4th grade children: Psychosocial, peer, parental and family factors. *Health Education Quarterly, 23*(4), 497–511.

Loveland-Cherry, C. J., & Looman, W. S. (2004). Parent, peer, and child risk factors for alcohol use in two cohorts of elementary school children. In J. E. Donovan, S. L. Leech, R. A. Zucker, C. J. Loveland-Cherry, J. M. Jester, H. E. Fitzgerald, et al. Really underage drinkers: Alcohol use among elementary students. *Alcoholism: Clinical and Experimental Research, 28*(2), 341–349.

Loveland-Cherry, C. J., Ross, L. T., & Kaufman, S. R. (1999). Effects of a home-based family intervention on adolescent alcohol use and misuse. *Journal of Studies on Alcohol* (Suppl. 13), 94–102.

Lynam, D. R., Milich, R., Zimmerman, R., Novak, S. P., Logan, T. K., Martin, C., et al. (1999). Project DARE: No effects at 10-year follow-up. *Journal of Consulting and Clinical Psychology, 67*(4), 590–593.

Maguin, E., Zucker, R. A., & Fitzgerald, H. E. (1994). The path to alcohol problems through conduct problems: A family-based approach to very early intervention with risk. *Journal of Research on Adolescence, 4*, 249–269.

Mathias, R. (2003). School prevention program effective with youths at high risk for substance use. *NIDA Notes, 18*(5), 1–3.

Monti, P. M., Colby, S. M., Barnett, N. P., Spirito, A., Rohsenow, D. L., Myers, M., et al. (1999). Brief intervention for harm reduction with alcohol-positive older adolescents in a hospital emergency department. *Journal of Consulting and Clinical Psychology, 67*(6), 989–994.

Morehouse, E., & Tobler, N. S. (2000). Preventing and reducing substance use among institutionalized adolescents. *Adolescence, 35*(137), 1–28.

Newman, I. M., Anderson, C. S., & Farrell, K. A. (1992). *Journal of Drug Education, 22*(1), 55–67.

Nye, C. L., Zucker, R. A., & Fitzgerald, H. E. (1999). Early family-based intervention in the path to alcohol problems: Rationale and relationship between treatment process characteristics and child and parenting outcomes. *Journal of Studies on Alcohol* (Suppl. 13), 10–21.

Orleans, C. T., Gruman, J., Ulmer, C., Emont, S. L., & Hollendonner, J. K. (1999). Rating our progress in population health promotion: Report card on six behaviors. *American Journal of Health Promotion, 14*(2), 75–82.

Palinkas, L. A., Atkins, C. J., Miller, C., & Ferreira, D. (1996). Social skills training for drug prevention in high-risk female adolescents. *Preventive Medicine, 25,* 692–701.

Perry, C. L., Williams, C. L., Komro, K. A., Veblen-Mortenson, S., Forster, L. L., Bernstein-Lachter, R., et al. (2000). Project Northland High School interventions: Community action to reduce adolescent alcohol use. *Health Education and Behavior, 27*(1), 29–49.

Perry, C. L., Williams, C. L., Forster, J. L., Wolfson, M., Wagenaar, A. C., Finnegan, J. R., et al. (1993). Background, conceptualization, and design of a community-wide research program on adolescent alcohol use: Project Northland. *Health Education Research, 8,* 125–136.

Perry, C. L., Williams, C. L., Veblen-Mortenson, S., Toomey, L., Komro, K. A., Anstine, P. S., et al. (1996). *American Journal of Public Health, 8*(7), 956–965.

Prinz, R. J., Dumas, J. E., Smith, E. P., & Laughlin, L. E. (2000). The EARLY ALLIANCE Prevention Trial: A dual design to test reduction of risk for conduct problems, substance abuse, and school failure in childhood. *Controlled Clinical Trials, 21,* 286–302.

Resnick, M. D., Bearman, P. S., Blum, R. W., Harris, K. M., Jones, J., et al. (1997). Protecting adolescents from harm. findings from the national longitudinal study on adolescent health. *JAMA, 278*(10), 823–832.

Ringwalt, C., Ennett, S. T., & Holt, K. D. (1991). An outcome evaluation of project DARE (Drug Abuse Resistance Education). *Health Education Research, 6*(3), 327–333.

Rohrbach, L. A., Hodgson, C. S., Broder, B. I., Montgomery, S. B., Flay, B. R., Hansen, W. B., et al. (1995). Parental participation in drug abuse prevention: Results from the Midwestern Prevention Project. In G. M. Boyd, J. Howard, & R. A. Zucker (Eds.), *Alcohol problems in prevention research* (pp. 173–195). Hillsdale, NJ: Erlbaum.

Rosenbaum, D. P., Flewelling, R. L., Bailey, S. L., Ringwalt, C. L., & Wilkinson, D. L. (1994). Cops in the classroom: A longitudinal evaluation of drug abuse resistance education (DARE). *Journal of Research in Crime and Delinquency, 31*(1), 3–31.

Ross, C., Richard, L., & Potvin, L. (1998). One year outcome evaluation of an alcohol and drug abuse prevention program in a Quebec high school. *Canadian Journal of Public Health, 89*(3), 166–170.

Schinke, S. P., & Tepavac, L. (1995). Substance abuse prevention among elementary school students. *Drugs and Society, 8*(3–4), 15–27.

Schinke, S. P., Tepavac, L., & Cole, K. C. (2000). Preventing substance use among Native American youth: Three year results. *Addictive Behaviors, 25*(3), 387–397.

Scott, D. M., Surface, J. L., Friedli, D., & Barlow, T. W. (1999). Effectiveness of student assistance programs in Nebraska schools. *Journal of Drug Education, 29*(2), 165–174.

Shalala, D. E. (1996, September). Keynote address. Presented at the National Conference on Drug Abuse Prevention Research, Washington, DC.

Sheehan, M., Schonfeld, C., Ballard, R., Schofield, F., Najman, J., & Siskind, V. (1996). A three-year outcome evaluation of a theory-based drink driving education program. *Journal of Drug Education, 26*(3), 295–312.

Shope, J. T., Copeland, L. A., Maharg, R., & Dielman, T. E. (1996). Effectiveness of a high school alcohol misuse program. *Alcoholism: Clinical and Experimental Research, 20*(5), 791–798.

Shope, J. T., Dielman, T. E., Butchart, A. T., Campanelli, P. C., & Kloska, D. D. (1992). *Journal of Studies on Alcohol, 53*(2), 106–121.

Shope, J. T., Elliott, M. R., Raghunathan, T. E., & Waller, P. F. (2001). Long-term follow-up of a high school alcohol misuse prevention program's effect on students' subsequent driving. *Alcoholism, Clinical, and Experimental Research, 25*(3), 403–410.

Spoth, R., Redmond, C., & Lepper, H. (1999). Alcohol initiation outcomes of universal family-focused preventive interventions: One- and two-year follow-ups of a controlled study. *Journal of Studies on Alcohol* (Suppl. 13), 103–111.

Spoth, R., Redmond, C., & Shin, C. (1998). Direct and indirect latent-variable parenting outcomes of two universal family-focused preventive interventions: Extending a public health-oriented research base. *Journal of Consulting and Clinical Psychology, 66*(2), 385–399.

———. (2001). Randomized trial of brief family interventions for general populations: Adolescent substance use outcomes 4 years following baseline. *Journal of Consulting and Clinical Psychology, 69*(4), 627–642.

Spoth, R., Reyes, M. L., Redmond, C., & Shin, C. (1999). Assessing a public health approach to delay onset and progression of adolescent substance use: Latent transition and log-linear analyses of longitudinal family preventive intervention outcomes. *Journal of Consulting and Clinical Psychology, 67*(5), 619–630.

Spoth, R. L., Redmond, C., Trudeau, L., & Shin, C. (2002). Longitudinal substance initiation outcomes for a universal preventive intervention combining family and school programs. *Psychology of Addictive Behaviors, 16*(2), 129–134.

Steinberg, L., Fletcher, A., & Darling, N. (1994). Parental monitoring and peer influences on adolescent substance use. *Pediatrics, 93*(6), 1060–1064.

Stevens, M. M., Mott, L. A., & Youells, F. (1996). Rural adolescent drinking behavior: Three-year follow-up in the New Hampshire substance abuse prevention study. *Adolescence, 13*(121), 159–166.

Stevens, M. M., Olson, A. L., Gaffney, C. A., & Tosteson, T. D. (2002). A pediatric, practice-based, randomized trial of drinking and smoking prevention and bicycle helmet, gun, and seatbelt safety promotion. *Pediatrics, 109*(3), 490–497.

St. Pierre, T. L., Mark, M. M., Kaltreider, D. L., & Aikin, K. J. (1997). Involving parents of high-risk youth in drug prevention: A three-year longitudinal study in boys and girls clubs. *Journal of Early Adolescence, 17*(1), 21–50.

Substance Abuse and Mental Health Services Administration. (2002). *Results from the 2001 National Household Survey on Drug Abuse: Volume 1. Summary of National Findings* (Office of Applied Studies, NHSDA Series H-17, DHHS Pub. No. SMA 02-3758). Rockville, MD.

Sussman, S., Dent, C. W., Stacy, A. W., & Craig, S. (1998). One-year outcomes of Project Towards No Drug Abuse. *Preventive Medicine, 27*, 632–642.

Szapocznik, J., Santisteban, D., Rio, A., Perez-Vidal, A., & Kurtines, W. M. (1989). Family effectiveness training: An intervention to prevent drug abuse and problem behaviors in Hispanic adolescents. *Hispanic Journal of Behavioral Sciences, 11*(1), 4–27.

Tobler, N. S. (1986). Meta-analysis of 143 adolescent drug prevention programs: Quantitative outcome results of program participants compared to a control or comparison group. *Journal of Drug Issues, 16*(4), 37–567.

————. (1992). Drug prevention programs can work: Research findings. *Journal of Addictive Diseases, 11*(3), 1–27.

Tobler, N. S., & Stratton, H. H. (1997). Effectiveness of school-based drug prevention programs: A meta-analysis of the research. *Journal of Primary Prevention, 18*(1), 71–128.

Tolan, P. H., & McKay, M. M. (1996). Preventing serious antisocial behavior in inner-city children: An empirically based family intervention program. *Family Relations, 45*, 148–155.

Wagenaar, A. C., & Perry, C. L. (1995). Community strategies for the reduction of youth drinking: Theory and application. In G. M. Boyd, J. Howard, & R. A. Zucker (Eds.), *Alcohol problems among adolescents: Current directions in prevention research* (pp. 197–223). Hillsdale, NJ: Erlbaum.

Wagner, E. F., Dinklage, S. C., Cudworth, C., & Vyse, J. (1999). A preliminary evaluation of the effectiveness of a standardized student assistance program. *Substance Use and Misuse, 34*(11), 1571–1584.

Wagner & Waldon

Werch (1997)

Werch, C. E., Anzalone, D. M., Brokiewicz, L. M., Felker, J., Carlson, J. M., & Castellon-Vogel, E. A. (1996). An intervention for preventing alcohol use among inner-city middle school students. *Archives of Family Medicine, 5*, 146–152.

Werch, C. E., Carlson, J. M., Pappas, D. M., & DiClemente, C. C. (1996). Brief nurse consultations for preventing alcohol use among urban school youth. *Journal of School Health, 66*(9), 335–338.

Werch, C. E., Pappas, D. M., Carlson, J. M., & DiClemente, C. C. (1999). Six-month outcomes of an alcohol prevention program for inner-city youth. *American Journal of Health Promotion, 13*(4), 237–240.

Werch, C. E., Pappas, D. M., Carlson, J. M., Edgemon, P., Sinder, J. A., & DiClemente, C. C. (2000). Evaluation of a brief alcohol prevention program for urban school youth. *American Journal of Health Behavior, 24*(2), 120–131.

Werch, C. E., Young, M., Clark, M., Garrett, C., Hooks, S., & Kersten, C. (1991). Effects of a take-home drug prevention program on drug-related communication and beliefs of parents and children. *Journal of School Health, 61*(8), 346–350.

Wilhelmsen, B., Laberg, J., & Klepp, K. (1994). Evaluation of two student and teacher involved alcohol prevention programmes. *Addiction, 89*, 1157–1165.

Williams, C. L., Perry, C. L., Farbakhsh, K., & Veblen-Mortenson, S. (1999). Project Northland: Comprehensive alcohol use prevention for young adolescents, their parents, schools, peers and communities. *Journal of Studies on Alcohol* (Suppl. 13), 112–124.

World Health Organization. (2000). *International guide for monitoring alcohol consumption and related harm.* Department of Mental Health and Substance Dependence, Noncommunicable Diseases and Mental Health Cluster, World Health Organization.

Wynn, S. R., Schulenberg, J., Kloska, D. D., & Laetz, V. B. (1997). The mediating influence of refusal skills in preventing adolescent alcohol misuse. *Journal of School Health, 67*(9), 390–395.

Wynn, S. R., Schulenberg, J., Maggs, J. L., & Zucker, R. A. (2000). Preventing alcohol misuse: The impact of refusal skills and norms. *Psychology of Addictive Behaviors, 14*(1), 36–47.

Chapter 6

College Students' Alcohol Use: A Critical Review

Carol J. Boyd, Sean Esteban McCabe, and Michele Morales

ABSTRACT

This integrative review of college students' alcohol use covers research papers as well as review and theoretical papers published between 1990 and 2004. To conduct this review, abstracts were identified by searching Medline (PubMed), Ingenta, ERIC, PsycInfo, and Health Reference Center Academic using the following words: alcohol and college drinking, binge drinking, college students and undergraduates and the years 1990 to 2004. From an initial list of over 400 abstracts, 203 papers were identified and considered for this review. A developmental perspective of college drinking was assumed, and the chapter is organized within five domains: biology, identity, cognition, affiliation, and achievement. In addition, research pertaining to the harmful consequences of college drinking and the assessment of risky drinking is reviewed and discussed. The chapter concludes with the identification of gaps in knowledge and implications for future research.

Keywords: underage drinking, binge drinking, college, alcohol

Binge drinking and its concomitants are considered the greatest public health problem on American college campuses; indeed, binge drinking (also referred to as heavy episodic drinking) is the leading cause of injury and death among college students and young adults (Hingson, Heeren, Zakocs, Kopstein, & Wechsler, 2002; Wechsler, Dowdall, Davenport, & Castillo, 1995). Over the past decade, the public's awareness of binge drinking and other forms of alcohol misuse by college students has increased; few health topics have been more studied and publicly discussed.

To address the serious consequences of alcohol use and abuse by college students, the National Advisory Council to the National Institute on Alcohol Abuse and Alcoholism (NIAAA) established a task force in 2001 to examine college students' alcohol use, drinking that is usually illegal because students are underage. By all accounts the composition of the task force was unique; college presidents and leading researchers worked together to create a series of reports that would be both scientific and useful to a wide audience. Their review papers appeared as 18 articles in the *Journal of Studies on Alcohol* (see Supplement 14, March 2002), and the task force report was placed on the Web (www.college drinkingprevention.gov). The terminology recommended in the National Advisory Council's report (pp. 6–7) will also be used throughout this chapter (see Table 6.1).

Toward the goal of providing a synthesis that will be useful to nurse-researchers, a developmental perspective was chosen, and the literature was discussed as it pertains to this perspective. This integrative review covers studies that were published between 1990 and 2004, although some earlier studies also are cited. The discussion is limited to research with samples drawn from 2- and 4-year colleges and universities within the United States and theoretical or review papers specific to college populations. Given the extensive number of studies on this topic, concentration centered on national and multiinstitutional studies (e.g., several university student bodies included in the sample) that use random and representative samples. In addition, studies using international or convenience samples and/or samples drawn from one campus are reviewed when such studies provide new and interesting insights.

METHOD

Medline (PubMed), Ingenta, ERIC, PsycInfo, and Health Reference Center Academic were searched using the following words: *alcohol and college drinking, binge drinking, college students*, and *undergraduates*. Only abstracts published after 1990 were considered. In addition, the authors' own research provided a literature base, as did relevant government reports (e.g., from the NIAAA) released within the previous 10 years. Once the initial search was completed, all of the abstracts that included U.S. samples of undergraduate students and dealt with the topic of college alcohol consumption were printed and reviewed by the authors. From

TABLE 6.1   Terms and Definitions

Term	Other terms	Operational definitions
Alcohol consumption	Drinking	Use of any alcoholic beverage
Alcohol-free housing		Residence halls that require students to commit to not bringing or consuming alcohol within the housing unit (Finn, 1996)
Binge drinking	Heavy episodic drinking	Where 4 or 5 drinks were consumed in a row, at least once, in a previous 2-week period (Wechsler et al., 1995)
College student(s)	Undergraduate, student	College students are considered part or full time, enrolled in community college, technical schools, or 4-year traditional colleges or universities
College/university	Institution of higher learning	Two- or 4-year institution that provides postsecondary education
Frequent binge drinking		Where 4 or 5 drinks were consumed in a row on three or more occasions in a 2-week period (Wechsler et al., 1995)
High-risk drinking	Risky drinking, heavy drinking	Modified from the NIAAA definition to include 57 Drinks in a 28-day period for men, 29 drinks in a 28-day period for women. Alternatively, four or more binge episodes in a 28-day period for both men and women (Kokotailo et al., 2004)
Developmental transitions	Life changes, developmental trajectories	"Paths that connect us to transformed physical, mental and social selves" (Schulenberg et al., 1997, p 1)
Non-binge drinking	Non-problem drinking	Less alcohol consumption (than binge drinking) and is considered a more moderate form of drinking behavior (Wechsler et al., 1994)
Primary adverse consequences	Primary consequences from heavy drinking	Consumption by itself is not a major social issue; rather, it is a problem only if it generates consequences. Primary adverse consequences are usually described in terms of social, legal, educational, and medical consequences experienced by the drinker (Wechsler, Davenport, Dowdall, Moeykens, & Castillo, 1994)
	Social consequences	Physical or verbal aggression, marital difficulties, loss of important social relationships
	Legal consequences	Arrests for driving while intoxicated, minor in possession, public inebriation, open container, etc.

(continued)

TABLE 6.1   *(continued)*

Term	Other terms	Operational definitions
	Educational/vocational consequences	Academic difficulties, termination of employment, etc.
	Medical consequences/physical problems	Acute and chronic medical problems associated with drinking, such as physical injury, liver disease, or alcohol poisoning
Residence halls	Dormitories	University-sponsored housing
Secondary adverse consequences	Secondhand effects or secondary consequences of heavy drinking	Students' alcohol-related consequences that affect students who were not binge drinkers, such as sleep disturbances, vandalism, and physical attacks (Wechsler, Davenport, Dowdall, Moeykens, & Castillo, 1994)
Substance-free housing		Residence halls that require students to commit to not consuming alcohol, drugs, or tobacco products within the housing unit (Finn, 1996)
Unrestricted housing		University/college-sponsored housing that does not specifically stipulate rules regarding alcohol and tobacco (Finn, 1996)

NIAAA = National Institute on Alcohol Abuse and Alcoholism

the initial list of over 400 abstracts, the authors began choosing the articles to be reviewed.

Abstracts were given highest priority for a formal review if the sample contained college students, had national, representative, and random samples, used valid and reliable measures, and included multivariate analytic techniques. Further, abstracts were given priority if the topic was specific to college populations and, thus, specifically contributed to our understanding of college students' alcohol use. Priority was also given to articles published in what are considered the top-tier substance abuse journals and/or conducted by researchers known for their work in the alcohol field, regardless of sample or research design.

Generally, the best designed studies used either random or very large national samples and/or longitudinal or panel designs. Thus, the descriptive insights provided by qualitative research were dwarfed by the shear volume of large, random sample studies. Even so, when qualitative or exploratory studies offered new insights or promising perspectives, these studies were included in the review. From the abstract review, 203 articles were selected for this review. Approximately 33% of the articles were derived from one of three large national studies (discussed later). Twenty-three of the abstracts were review articles.

HISTORICAL OVERVIEW

Institutions of higher education historically have had trouble with alcohol misuse. During the Middle Ages, student drunkenness was prevalent among European universities; following the drunken feast day of St. Scholastica at Oxford University in 1354, for example, a bloody fight broke out between students and local townspeople, and 63 students died (Hastings, 1936). In the mid-17th century, a group of 50 students attending Harvard University formed a drinking society that consumed over 270 barrels of beer during an academic year (Morison, 1936). Over the past two centuries, there have been several instances of alcohol-related disturbances by college students that have strained many "town and gown" relationships.

It is estimated that more than 1,400 U.S. college students ages 18 to 24 and enrolled in 2- and 4-year colleges and universities died from alcohol-related unintentional injuries in 1998 (Hingson et al., 2002). The serious consequences continue to this day; each year, alcohol-related deaths involving college students are reported by the press. Alcohol-related tragedies involving college students also impact the mortality and morbidity of individuals not attending colleges or universities. Tragically, a University of Colorado student, for example, was convicted of vehicular homicide when he killed a music teacher while driving under the influence (see U.S. Department of Education, 2002).

Although drinking has long been a part of the collegiate experience, empirical research examining collegiate alcohol use was not initiated until the late 1940s. In 1949, the first known nationwide study surveyed 15,000 college students and showed that at least 79% of the men and 65% of the women consumed alcohol (Straus & Bacon, 1953). Blane and Hewitt (1977) later reviewed 68 studies to determine the extent of drinking among college students. The studies were divided into three distinct time periods: (1) pre-1966, (2) 1966–1970, and (3) 1971–1975. Blane and Hewitt (1977) found an increase in the prevalence of drinking between the first and second time periods and a decline between the second and third time periods.

A new wave of longitudinal and national studies were launched in the late 1970s and the early 1980s as a result of the societal concern about alcohol and other drug use among youth (e.g., Jessor & Jessor, 1977; Johnston, O'Malley, & Eveland, 1978; Kandel, 1975). These studies later revealed that the use of alcohol and binge-drinking behavior among college students peaked in the early 1980s, declined slightly during the mid-1980s, but has generally remained unchanged in the early 2000s (Hanson & Engs, 1992; Johnston, O'Malley, & Bachman, 2003; Wechsler, Lee, Kuo, Seibring, et al., 2002), although women's drinking behaviors may be changing (Wechsler, Lee, Kuo, Seibring, et al., 2002). Over the last 20 years, even with numerous interventions aimed at reducing underage drinking, studies consistently show that more than 90% of college students have consumed alcohol upon entering college and overall, approximately 40% to 45% engage in binge drinking while in college (Johnston et al., 2003; O'Malley & Johnston, 2002; Wechsler, Lee, Kuo, & Lee, 2000). There is increasing evidence that the amount consumed and the number of episodes per 2-week period (e.g., frequent binge drinking) are escalating among college students (Wechsler, Lee, Kuo, & Lee, 2000), particularly among women (Wechsler, Lee, Kuo, Seibring, et al., 2002). However, these increases are seen not only among college students, but also in young adults within the general population (Naimi et al., 2003).

There are three large national studies that are the most often cited when discussing prevalence, trends, and consequences associated with alcohol and other drug use among U.S. college students. These studies—College Alcohol Study (CAS) (e.g., Wechsler, Lee, Kuo, Seibring, et al., 2002); the CORE Survey (e.g., Presley, Meilman, & Cashin, 1996); and Monitoring the Future (MTF) study (e.g., Johnston, O'Malley, & Bachman, 1986–2002)—are considered state-of-the-art surveys, each with different strengths and weaknesses, but all providing similar estimates. Because each study includes somewhat different measurement and sampling techniques, taken in combination, the three studies provide a breadth of published data that is singular. However, although the breadth of data makes an outstanding contribution to the substance abuse field, there is a liability to consider. These large epidemiological studies of college students' drinking behaviors have never been theory-based, and, generally, the current theories (e.g., developmental perspective) have been developed after analyzing the epidemiological data. Thus, three large national studies, each with a unique set of strengths but with several shared weaknesses, are predominantly driving the theory development in this area.

The MTF, CORE, and CAS studies generally have produced remarkably stable data that reveal a high degree of behavioral continuity in collegiate binge drinking over the past 20 years. Of note, all three databases revealed that the binge-drinking rate among college students has remained substantially higher than the national rates for other young adults; approximately 40% of undergraduates engaged in binge drinking compared with approximately 35% in the noncollege populations of the same age (Johnston et al., 2003). During high school, those students who planned on going to college were less likely to binge drink; however, once in college, the proportion of full-time traditional-age college students who binge drink increased by 12%, whereas their noncollege peers decreased by 3% (Bachman, Wadsworth, O'Malley, Johnston, & Schulenberg, 1997). This shift was even more prominent for female students as compared with male students; female undergraduates appear to be increasingly heavy drinkers. Using CAS data, in 1993, only 17% of women undergraduates were frequent binge drinkers, but by 2001, 21% of the nation's undergraduate women were frequent binge drinkers. Men's frequent binging also increased during this period, from 22% to 25%. Although Wechsler, Lee, Hall, Wagenaar, and Lee's (2002) most recent findings indicated that approximately 41% of women undergraduates were binge drinkers compared with 49% of men, MTF data from 2002 indicated rates of 33% and 51%, respectively. However, MTF samples were limited to 19- to 22-year-old students, included students attending 2-year colleges and universities, and used a slightly different measure of binge drinking (five or more drinks in a row in the past 2 weeks for both men and women) and thus cannot necessarily be generalized to the 4-year undergraduate population used in the CAS.

The CAS was funded by the Robert Wood Johnson Foundation to collect data on alcohol use/abuse by full-time undergraduate students enrolled at 4-year colleges and universities (Wechsler, Lee, Kuo, Seibring, et al., 2002). Half of the sampled schools were larger than 10,000 students; almost one fifth had student bodies between 5,001 and 10,000, and one third had student bodies smaller than 5,000 students. Women's and historically Black colleges were oversampled. In 1993, the CAS study began with 140 schools; since that time, samples of students have been collected in 1997, 1999, and 2001, so that cross-sectional trends can be determined. Unfortunately, the overall response rate decreased over time from 70% in 1993 to 52% in 2001 (Wechsler, Lee, Kuo, Seibring, et al., 2002). There are several advantages of the CAS study: The sample is large so that subgroups of students can be analyzed, schools can be grouped by college characteristics, and the CAS study includes several individual and contextual variables that are especially relevant to the collegiate environment. In addition, there is considerable attention paid to instrument reliability and validity. Limitations of the CAS include small samples from individual institutions. Further, the sample does not include non-college-bound individuals or individuals attending institutions other than 4-year colleges and universities, which limits the generalizability of all studies using CAS data. To date, the CAS database has produced well over 50 published studies on college student drinking, each study reflecting the design strengths and weaknesses of the CAS (see http://www.hsph.harvard.edu/cas/ and Dowdall & Wechsler, 2002; Gassman, Demone, & Wechsler, 2002; Harford, Wechsler, & Muthen, 2002; Hingson et al., 2002; Knight et al., 2002; Wechsler, Lee, Hall, et al., 2002; Wechsler, Lee, Kuo, Seibring, et al., 2002; Wechsler, Lee, Nelson, & Kuo, 2002; Wechsler & Nelson, 2001; Williams, Chaloupka, & Wechsler, 2002).

The CORE was funded by the Drug Prevention in Higher Education Program of the Fund for the Improvement of Postsecondary Education (FIPSE). The first national, cross-sectional CORE study of college students was conducted in 1989. Like the CAS, the CORE study was specifically designed for use with college students; unlike the CAS, institutions participated on a voluntary basis, so the self-selected sample was not nationally representative. The CORE study annually surveys over 58,000 students from 56 4-year and 22 2-year institutions of higher education (Presley et al., 1996). Dissimilar to the CAS, the CORE study surveys full- and part-time undergraduate and graduate college students regarding prevalence and consequences of alcohol and other drug use. The CORE study, different from the CAS, defined binge drinking as consuming five or more drinks in a row for both men and women and has consistently shown an overall binge-drinking rate of approximately 40% among undergraduate college students. The CORE study shares many of the advantages of the CAS but also includes 2-year colleges and universities, as well as the more traditional 4-year schools. However, the voluntary nature of the sampling plan and the noninclusion of individuals not attending college limit inferences made to the general population of college students. In addition, response rates remain low from some of the schools included in the CORE, and, like the CAS, the data are cross-sectional. The CORE database (e.g., http://www.siu.edu/departments/coreinst/public_html/index.html) has produced well over 20 published studies, and although these published studies suffer from similar design limitations, the research produces data similar to the CAS, thereby providing some confidence in its validity (e.g., Cashin, Presley, & Meilman, 1998; Delk & Meilman, 1996; Leichliter, Meilman, Presley, & Cashin, 1998; Meilman, 1993; Meilman et al., 1993; Meilman, Cashin, McKillip, & Presley, 1998; Meilman, Leichliter, & Presley, 1998, 1999; Meilman, Presley, & Cashin, 1995; Meilman, Presley, & Lyerla, 1994; Presley, Meilman, & Cashin, 1997; Perkins, Meilman, Leichliter, Cashin, & Presley, 1999; Presley, Meilman, & Lyerla, 1994; Presley, Meilman, Lyerla, & Karmos, 1995).

The third national study, MTF, represents the only random sample and longitudinal research project among the three national studies (Johnston et al., 1986–2002). The MTF Study has examined alcohol and other drug use among students enrolled in both secondary and postsecondary schools since 1976. In 1976, the MTF study surveyed 17,000 high school seniors, and in 1977, these investigators began their biennial mail follow-up surveys of representative subsamples of high school seniors. Unlike the CAS and the CORE, the MTF surveys undergraduates enrolled part- and full-time in 2- and 4-year institutions of higher education. For over 2 decades, the MTF study has consistently shown that approximately 40% of college students have reported binge drinking while in college (Johnston et al., 1986–2002; O'Malley & Johnston, 2002). Like the CAS and CORE, the MTF study has shown gender differences with respect to drinking behaviors.

The advantages to the MTF are similar to the CAS and CORE but also include available data since 1976. Further, the study is ongoing, longitudinal, and includes non-college students for comparison (O'Malley & Johnston, 2002). The main limitations of the MTF study include the relatively small sample of college students each year that are tracked in the longitudinal panel study. The MTF database has produced numerous monographs, reports, and published studies focusing on college students (see http://www.monitoringthefuture.org/ and Johnston et al., 1986–2002, 2003; O'Malley & Johnston, 2002; Schulenberg et al.,

2001; Schulenberg, Bachman, O'Malley, & Johnston, 1994; Schulenberg & Maggs, 2002).

To date, these three epidemiological surveys using national databases represent some of the most comprehensive attempts at assessing drinking behavior among college students; in some cases, subsamples and regional differences have been examined. Although using somewhat different measures in establishing prevalence, these studies collectively established several important findings. First, male collegians generally engage in heavy drinking more often than their female classmates, although there is evidence that the differences between males and females are decreasing (O'Malley & Johnston, 2002; Wechsler, Lee, Kuo, Seibring, et al., 2002). Second, collegians are more likely to engage in binge drinking than their same-age peers not attending college (Johnston et al., 2003; Schulenburg & Maggs, 2002). Third, White collegians engage in heavy episodic drinking more often than their non-White classmates (e.g., O'Malley & Johnston, 2002; Presley et al., 1996; Wechsler, Lee, Kuo, Seibring, et al., 2002). Finally, students who engage in binge drinking have significantly higher rates of alcohol-related consequences than students who are non-binge drinkers or non-drinking students (Wechsler, Davenport, Dowdall, Moeykens, & Castillo, 1994). Unfortunately, the MTF, CAS, and CORE data have failed to produce studies that adequately examine collegiate drug use (in combination with alcohol), although there is research showing that college alcohol misuse is a multidimensional problem that involves drugs (Boyd, McCabe, & d'Arcy, 2003). More generally, the studies aimed at explaining drinking patterns have most often focused on selected risk groups such as athletes and fraternity and sorority members and not on more marginalized high-risk groups, such as students who identify as lesbian, gay, or bisexual (e.g., Abbey, 2002; McCabe, Boyd, Hughes, & d'Arcy, 2003; Perkins, 2002).

A DEVELOPMENTAL PERSPECTIVE: BIOLOGY, IDENTITY, COGNITION, AFFILIATION, AND ACHIEVEMENT

The time between high school and college is a period of major developmental transition. Students move away from their parents' homes to start college, and the campus environment presents opportunities for independence, new social networks, and different living arrangements (Cantor, Norem, Niedenthal, Langston, & Brower, 1987; Pascarella & Terenzini, 1991; Schulenberg & Maggs, 2002). The college years mark a time of personal growth, albeit with added vulnerability. It is in this developmental transition that alcohol use usually increases and binge drinking occurs.

Drawing on the MTF's longitudinal panel of young adults, Schulenberg and colleagues (Schulenberg et al., 2001; Schulenberg, O'Malley, Bachman,

Wadsworth, & Johnston, 1996; Schulenberg, Wadsworth, et al., 1996) used these data to guide the development of a theoretical perspective that includes the concept of developmental trajectories. Likewise, Maggs (Maggs, 1997; Schulenberg et al., 2001; Schulenberg, O'Malley, et al., 1996; Schulenberg, Wadsworth, et al., 1996), drawing on data from the University Life Transitions Project Telephone Diary Study, now advocates using a multidimensional developmental perspective that recognizes several pathways toward adulthood. Both Schulenberg and Maggs studies situate college drinking (and its consequences) in the context of normative developmental tasks and transitions, acknowledging that precollege drinking behaviors can be associated with college as demonstrated by CAS, CORE, and MTF, as well as other research (Bachman et al., 1997; Barnes, Welte, & Dintcheff, 1992; Hingson, Heeren, Zakocs, Winter, & Wechsler, 2003; Presley et al., 1996; Schulenberg et al., 1996; Wechsler et al., 1995; Wechsler, Dowdall, Maenner, Gledhill-Hoyt, & Lee, 1998; Wechsler, Lee, Hall, et al., 2000; Yu & Shacket, 2001).

Schulenberg and colleagues (Schulenberg, O'Malley, et al., 1996), in a four-wave study of MTF data, documented six trajectories of binge drinking that applied to 90% of their sample of young adults between the ages of 18 and 24. The six trajectories included chronic (two or more binge episodes in the previous 2 weeks across all four waves); decreased (started as frequent binge drinker in high school at wave 1, then decreased to no frequent binge drinking by wave 4); increased (no frequent binge drinking in high school at wave 1 but increased to frequent binge drinking by wave 4); fling (no frequent binge drinking in high school at wave 1 or 4, but some frequent binge drinking at wave 2 and/or 3); rare (some binge drinking during one of the four waves but no frequent binge drinking across any of the waves); and never (no binge drinking across the four waves). The data revealed that the trajectories varied depending on whether a high school student goes to college and on the gender and ethnicity of the adolescent; women were underrepresented in the chronic and increased groups and overrepresented in the never groups. White youths were generally overrepresented in all binge drinking trajectories except the never group. Finally, college students were overrepresented in the increase and fling trajectories and underrepresented in the decrease trajectory relative to their same-age peers not attending college (Schulenberg & Maggs, 2002; Schulenberg, O'Malley, et al., 1996).

Labouvie's (1996) longitudinal data suggested that drinking behavior outcomes differed little for men and women; both genders tend toward lower levels of overall drinking as they leave college and the age of first alcohol use neither predicted alcohol use by age 20 nor the consequences from alcohol abuse by age 30 (Labouvie, Bates, & Pandina, 1997). Schulenberg and Maggs (2002) in their review of the extant literature on secondary and college drinking noted that it is more normative to drink during adolescence than to not drink; in fact, MTF data consistently reveals that approximately 60% of 10th graders in the U.S.

consumed alcohol in the previous year. For this reason, Maggs surmises that despite its illegality and potential risks, drinking appears to serve important social functions for many college students; however, while it may help achieve valuable social goals (e.g., making friends) these same behaviors threaten short-term health and safety (Maggs, 1997). Schulenberg and Maggs (2002) suggest that to understand the risks, as well as the normative aspects of college drinking one must consider several domains. These domains can be conceptually organized around five areas: biology, identity, cognition, affiliation, and achievement (see Schulenberg, Wadsworth, et al., 1996, and Schulenberg & Maggs, 2002, for reviews).

Biology and Background

Several biological models of substance abuse have focused on independent genetic risk factors apart from family environment, although both genetics and environment are predictors of alcohol abuse or dependence among college students (Baer, 2002). During the transition to adulthood, biology and background converge to create both risk and protection.

Although many biological models have focused on the genetic links to alcohol dependency, there are fewer links for binge drinking by college students (Glantz & Pickens, 1992). There is some research to show that college students with an altered aldehyde dehydrogenase (ALDH) enzyme are less likely to binge drink. The gene for this enzyme is altered in a majority of Asians, which results in an enzyme that does not efficiently metabolize acetaldehyde, leading to an alcohol-flush reaction (Luczak, Wall, Shea, Byun, & Carr, 2001). This aversive consequence may be protective against alcohol abuse and is similar to the reaction produced by disulfiram.

A genetic factor that may place some students at higher risk for alcohol abuse involves a particular variant of the serotonin transporter gene. Herman, Philbeck, Vasilopoulos, and Paolo (2003), using a convenience subsample of 204 ($N = 268$) Caucasian college students, found that the presence of the short variant (S) of the serotonin transporter polymorphism (5-HTTLPR) was associated with differences in drinking behaviors. Although most of the population is heterozygous for the gene, about 30% of Caucasians are homozygous (i.e., carry duplicates of the long or short gene). Students who were homozygous for the short version of 5-HTT were more likely to engage in binge-drinking behavior, including a greater number of drinks per occasion. The authors concluded that 5-HTTLPR influences alcohol consumption in late pubescence (Herman et al., 2003), although they were unable to determine whether students with two short versions of 5-HTT are at greater risk for developing alcohol dependency in later adulthood.

There have been some attempts to link anxiety sensitivity to alcohol use, particularly heavy use (Lawyer, Karg, Murphy, & McGlynn, 2002). Lawyer and colleagues (2002), using a convenience sample of 245 university students, had students complete two anonymous questionnaires for an undergraduate psychology course. Negatively reinforced drinking was operationalized as high scores on scales that included drinking because of conflict with others, unpleasant emotions, and physical discomfort. Lawyer et al. found that anxiety sensitivity (i.e., fear of cognitive dyscontrol, observable anxiety symptoms, fear of respiratory and/or cardiac symptoms) was a factor in negatively reinforced drinking for both men and women, but particularly for men. These authors noted that because anxiety sensitivity appears to be associated with heavy drinking by college students in negatively reinforcing situations, the relevance of anxiety sensitivity should be considered in prevention programs for college students.

There is some empirical evidence that family drinking history may play a role in the etiology of alcohol-related problems among college students, although, to date, the research is scant and tends to use samples from clinical populations (Baer, 2002; Perkins & Berkowitz, 1991). In a survey of 860 college students, Perkins and Berkowitz (1991) examined the children of alcohol-dependent parents and the students' collegiate drinking experiences. They found that students, regardless of sex, were more likely to have a drinking problem if they had a parent or grandparent diagnosed or treated for alcohol dependency. They also found that students who had their homes disrupted by parental alcohol use/abuse (without a diagnosis of alcoholism) were more likely to have problems as well. However, Engs (1990) reported rates of drinking that were indistinguishable when comparing college students with and without parents who had drinking problems, an indication that further research is needed in this area.

At this time, and given the inconsistency in the data, it appears that the biological models may be more effective in describing associations and less about the possible causes of alcohol abuse among college students. Clearly, it is difficult to separate the family environmental factors from the biological factors when examining drinking among college students. Nonetheless, genetic predisposition, as well as family characteristics, may mediate the relationship between a developmental transition and alcohol use.

Identity: Self-Definition and Psychological Well-being

According to Schulenberg and Maggs (2002), college students experience changes in self-definition as they move from high school to college; in fact, college students often question previous beliefs and develop new behaviors and identities. Identity formation, however, occurs within a paradoxical set of perceptions—unstable self-definition and a stable sense of well-being. This instability is thought to lead to experimentation and risk taking, which in turn leads to a more stable, adult identity. Accordingly, drinking may function as a means to explore personal identities; some of these identities (e.g., athlete, sorority sister) function as risk factors for college drinking, although they are time-limited (Schulenberg & Maggs, 2002).

Racial and ethnic identities represent factors that are strongly associated with heavy episodic drinking behavior. In 2002, using the CAS database, Wechsler and colleagues (Wechsler, Lee, Kuo, Seibring, et al., 2002) reported on trends among several ethnic/racial groups; the prevalence of African American college students who engaged in binge drinking increased from 17% in 1993 to 22% in 2001, although this increase was not statistically significant. Hispanic and Native American students significantly decreased binge drinking during the same time period, with Hispanic and Native American students reporting a 6% decline. Generally, White and Hispanic students tend to drink more than other ethnic or racial groups, and Asian and African American college students tend to report less alcohol use and binge drinking (Hanson & Engs, 1992; Keefe & Newcomb, 1996; O'Malley & Johnston, 2002; Presley et al., 1996; Wechsler, Lee, Hall, et al., 2000; Wechsler, Lee, Kuo, Seibring, et al., 2002). These racial patterns of alcohol consumption have remained fairly consistent over the past 20 years, as evidenced by the CAS and MTF studies (Johnston et al., 2003, O'Malley & Johnston, 2002; Wechsler, Lee, Kuo, Seibring, et al., 2002). Although there have been descriptive attempts to consider race or ethnicity in some of these national studies, the literature shows a notable lack of attention to the important influences of acculturation or differences within racial subgroups.

Gender identity is a risk factor that is often associated with heavy episodic drinking and alcohol abuse. On average, women do not drink as much as their male counterparts; however, women who abuse alcohol are often more likely to suffer negative consequences (O'Malley & Johnston, 2002), including health and social consequences such as sexual assault (Abbey, 2002). Wechsler and colleagues (Wechsler, Lee, Kuo, Seibring, et al., 2002) in the 2001 CAS survey found an increase in drinking among students attending all-women's colleges. In fact, there is preliminary evidence from both the CAS and CORE datasets that some female undergraduates are increasing their quantity and frequency of drinking; however, at this time, it is unclear what factors are driving this increase, and more research is needed. Nonetheless, although college women's alcohol use may be increasing, prevalence rates for binge drinking remain below men's, as documented by a wide range of studies using the CAS, CORE, and MTF databases (see Bachman et al., 1997; Baer, Kivlahan, & Marlatt, 1995; Davis & Hunnicut, 1991; Gfroerer, Greenblatt, & Wright, 1997; Johnston et al, 2003; Presley et al., 1996; Wechsler et al., 1995, 1998; Wechsler, Lee, Hall, et al., 2000; Wechsler, Lee, Kuo, Seibring, et al., 2002).

The association among sexual identities and alcohol use among college students has been limited by the fact that national college-based studies have lacked questions about sexual identity (Johnston et al., 2003; Presley et al., 1996; Wechsler, Lee, Kuo, Seibring, et al., 2002). Existing data from single institutional studies provide some support for the relationship between sexual identity and alcohol use among college students (Debord, Wood, Sher, & Good, 1998; McCabe et al., 2003), and this support is further demonstrated in the general literature on alcohol use among lesbian, gay, and bisexual (LGB) populations. For example, DeBord and colleagues (1998) surveyed a small random sample of students at one college over 4 years and found heavier alcohol use among self-identified LGB college students than among a matched control group of heterosexual college peers. McCabe and colleagues (2003) furthered the study of sexual identity and alcohol use when they found important gender differences in the association between drinking behavior and sexual identity. Although there were no differences in drinking behaviors between college women who identified as lesbian and bisexual as compared with heterosexuals, gay and bisexual men were significantly less likely to report binge drinking than heterosexual men. The authors concluded that more research on the relationship between sexual identity and alcohol use was needed using national samples of college students. There has been at least one study that has examined the association between sexual behavior and alcohol use based on a national sample (Eisenberg & Wechsler, 2003). However, there have been no such national attempts to examine sexual identity, and there is growing recognition that more research is needed that examines the relationship between sexual orientation and alcohol use and consequences among college students (e.g., Abbey, 2002; McCabe et al., 2003; Perkins, 2002).

Cognitive Factors: Why, With Whom, and How Much?

The relationship between age and drinking experience is unclear, because age is inevitably confounded with alcohol experience and consumption, and thus, with increasing age, there should be increasing consumption (Lundahl, Davis, Adesso, & Lukas, 1997). However, this age-related increase in consumption is only true through the college years; after college, age and levels of consumption are not necessarily related.

Schulenberg and Maggs (2002) note that for many older adolescents bound for college, alcohol consumption is a given—college choices focus on with whom and how much, not on if. To be sure, many studies have linked alcohol expectancies and motivations to college drinking (e.g., Baer, 2002; Carey & Correia, 1997; Evans & Dunn, 1995; Goldstein, Wall, McKee, & Hinson, 2004; Perkins et al., 1999; Schulenberg, Wadsworth, et al., 1996).

One documented motivation to drink is to alleviate negative mood (e.g., Abbey, Smith, & Scott, 1993). Using an experimental design with a convenience sample of 302 undergraduates in Canada, Goldstein and colleagues (2004) examined whether mood induction influenced alcohol expectancies. They found that drinking motives did not moderate the relationship between alcohol expectancies and mood; however, mood primed types of alcohol expectancies. The priming was different for men and women. Physical expectancies, such as getting drunk, feeling dizzy and falling asleep, were more likely for women, and social-situational enhancements, such as enjoying friends, meeting people, and having a good time, were more likely for men. Likewise, Johnston and O'Malley (1986) reported on scales that measured motivations for using alcohol, although these scales may have failed to account adequately for the motivations of college women (Billingham, Parrillo, & Gross, 1993). Notwithstanding this possible gender bias, two scales were particularly useful for differentiating frequent and heavy alcohol users from infrequent drinkers: (1) Reduce Negative Affect scale and (2) To Get Drunk scale.

In a study of 371 college women, Perry, Miles, and Svikis (2004) found that approximately 40% of the sample drank in order to feel disinhibited. However, in a convenience sample of 284 college students Eggleston, Woolaway-Bickel, and Schmidt (2004) reported somewhat different results. They found that social anxiety (social evaluation) was related to decreased drinking by both men and women but was also associated with both positive and negative alcohol expectancies, particularly social facilitation expectancies.

Lundahl and colleagues (1997) examined the effects of gender, age, and family history of alcoholism on alcohol expectancies in a sample of 627 college students. Multivariate analyses indicated significant family history, gender, and age interactions; women over 20 years of age reported significantly lower alcohol expectancies of global positive effects than men. However, for college women under 20 years of age, global positive effects were higher than for women over 20, but this age pattern was not true for men. In addition, women reported greater alcohol expectancies related to power and aggression than did males, a finding that has been supported. Thombs's data (1993) suggesting that problem-drinking women differed from non-problem-drinking women on power and aggression expectancy scales. Lundahl and colleagues concluded that identifying the alcohol expectancies held by men and women at various ages would represent a first step in the development of age- and gender-specific prevention programs targeted at changing the cognitive expectancies that contribute to problem drinking by college students.

There is evidence that motivational factors (e.g., desire to get drunk or facilitate interactions) are related to drinking behaviors during the college years (Schulenberg, Wadsworth, et al., 1996); however, motivational factors have rarely been incorporated into college prevention models. Many cognitive-behavioral prevention models emphasize changing individuals' expectancies and other cognitions regarding alcohol in an effort to change individual behaviors. However, given the developmental perspective of Schulenberg and Maggs (2002) and the research on motivations to drink, one might anticipate that college-age drinkers are gaining far too many benefits (and experiencing relatively few consequences) to make this type of cognitive-educational approach useful for this age group.

College students do appear to practice some protective strategies in an effort to mitigate the harmful consequences of heavy episodic drinking. Benton et al. (2004) explored the relationships among gender, alcohol use, protective strategies, and harmful drinking consequences in a sample of 3,851 college students who were administered the CAS. They found that although women drank less than men, women were also more likely to practice protective strategies that limited intoxication levels (e.g., stopping drinks at least 1–2 hours before going home, alternating nonalcoholic beverages, making one's own drinks, and drinking in safe environments). For both men and women whose drinking exceeded the median average number of drinks (six drinks), there was a negative relationship between protective strategies and negative consequences (Benton et al., 2004), and, in general, as all students increased their drinking, they were less likely to use protective strategies and more likely to experience negative consequences.

Affiliations: Peers and Places

It is a truism that new affiliations occur in college. Because alcohol consumption is linked to peer relationships, these new affiliations may serve as a risk factor for increased alcohol use. For instance, the uncertainty of the new environment may reinforce the need for certain stable social milieus (e.g., fraternity living) and some alcohol expectancies (social facilitation). Several investigators have found that students who engaged in heavier alcohol use before college are more likely to join social fraternities or sororities (e.g., Baer et al., 1995; Lo & Globetti, 1995; Wechsler, et al., 1994), and these living arrangements become an independent risk factor for heavy, episodic drinking during the college years (Wechsler, Lee, Kuo, Seibring, et al., 2002).

Living arrangements are strongly associated with drinking among college students (Bachman et al., 1997; Boyd, McCabe, & d'Arcy, 2004; Weitzman, Nelson, & Wechsler, 2003). Bachman and colleagues (1997), in their national, longitudinal study, compared living in a residence hall with other living arrangements and found that residence hall life was a significant independent predictor of drinking behavior. Residence hall living provides distinct opportunities, such as parties and drinking games (Johnson, 2002), that could lead to increased alcohol use and binge drinking (Bachman et al., 1997; Maggs, 1997; Wechsler et al., 1995). Fraternity and sorority houses show similar associations with binge drinking (for a review, see Baer, 1994; Borsan & Carey, 1999; Lo & Globetti, 1995; Wechsler, Kuh, & Davenport, 1996). Undeniably, the highest rates of binge drinking occur among students living in fraternities and sororities (Cashin et al., 1998; Presley et al., 1996; Wechsler & Isaac, 1992; Wechsler, Lee, Hall, et al., 2000; Wechsler, Lee, Kuo, Seibring, et al., 2002). However, the relationship between these living arrangements and drinking pattern is not necessarily causal (Boyd et al., 2004). It is likely that there is a "selection" process that contributes to this association: First-year students who identify with the behaviors of fraternity/ sorority life are more likely to pledge into these organizations. Reciprocally, fraternities and sororities select new pledges that best represent their culture, in part by considering pledges' behaviors with alcohol. Lo and Globetti (1995) found that members of fraternities and sororities were significantly more likely to increase the frequency of their drinking over time relative to nonmembers.

Of course, not all undergraduate students live in unrestricted (traditional) residence halls, fraternities, or sororities houses, and many campuses now offer substance-free residence halls (Finn, 1996; Wechsler, Lee, Nelson, & Lee, 2001). Drawing on data from the 1999 CAS national sample, Wechsler and colleagues (2001) examined alcohol use, associated behaviors, and the secondary consequences of others' drinking among students living in unrestricted housing, substance-free housing, and alcohol-free housing. They found that residents in substance-free housing drank less than students in alcohol-free or nonrestricted housing. Precollege drinking was strongly associated with living arrangement; students who drank less in high school were more likely to select substance-free housing. Students in substance-free housing also were less likely to binge drink or suffer the negative consequences of others' heavy drinking (Wechsler et al., 2001). Like Wechsler and colleagues' findings, Boyd et al. (2004) conducted a cross-sectional, Web-based survey using a random sample of 2,041 undergraduate students attending a large public university in the Midwest recruited via email. Even when precollege drinking behavior was statistically controlled, for both men and women, living arrangements remained highly predictive of binge drinking; not surprisingly, substance-free housing conferred protective effects for both negative consequences and preventative behaviors. In addition, several researchers reported that living at home with family or parents—*not with peers*—was associated with less binge drinking among college students in both cross-sectional (Gfroerer et al., 1997; Wechsler et al., 1995) and national longitudinal studies (Bachman et al., 1997).

Achievement: Academics and Beyond

The association between academic performance and college drinking is mixed. Maney (1990) showed in a single institutional study that poor academic performance, measured by grade point averages, was associated with greater binge drinking, although McCabe, Boyd, Couper, Crawford, and d'Arcy (2002) did not find this same relationship between binge drinking and poor academic performance, for either men or women. Aergeerts and Buntinx (2002) found that alcohol abuse was not associated with poor academic performance, although alcohol dependence was associated with a 25% excess risk of failing grades (when compared with non-alcohol-dependent students). Boyd et al. (2004) reported on data from 739 students who had consumed alcohol in the previous year and were living in group housing; 20% of those living in a fraternity/sorority reported performing poorly on a test the previous year because of drinking, and 9% of students living in residence halls reported poor test performance. Further evidence for a relationship between heavy drinking and poor academic performance came from several national cross-sectional studies (Presley et al., 1996; Wechsler et al., 1995), but there was much weaker evidence in studies with longitudinal designs (Schulenberg et al., 1994; Wood, Sher, Erickson, & DeBord, 1997). For instance, Wood and colleagues (1997) used a longitudinal design at a single institution and showed that binge drinking was not predictive of poor academic performance over time, even though there was a cross-sectional association between binge drinking and poor academic performance. These equivocal findings regarding academic performance and alcohol consumption among college students corroborate MTF's longitudinal data and Schulenberg and colleagues' conclusions drawn from those data. In general, most college students who drink, even those who binge drink, leave their drinking and concomitant consequences behind and go on to successful lives. In fact, for college graduates, the transition to work is associated with declines in alcohol abuse (Bachman et al., 1997), a decline that is not as evident for adolescents going directly from high school to full-time employment (Schulenberg & Maggs, 2002). Additionally, data indicated that the successful transitions from college to work, and work to marriage, are associated with decreases in all forms of substance use (Bachman et al., 1997; Schulenberg, Wadsworth, et al., 1996).

ASSESSMENT OF ALCOHOL USE AMONG COLLEGE STUDENTS

Precollege drinking behavior has been associated with alcohol-related consequences while in college, as demonstrated by CAS, CORE, and MTF, as well as other research (Bachman et al., 1997; Barnes et al., 1992; Hingson et al., 2003; Presley et al., 1996; Schulenberg, O'Malley, et al., 1996; Wechsler et al., 1995, 1998; Wechsler, Lee, Kuo, & Lee, 2000; Yu & Shacket, 2001), and a proportion of the high-risk drinkers in college will go on to become alcohol dependent. Based on CAS data, it was estimated that 31% of U.S. college students attending 119 4-year colleges met the criteria of the *Diagnostic and Statistical Manual of Mental Disorders* (4th ed., *DSM-IV*) for alcohol abuse, and 6% met the criteria for alcohol dependence (Knight et al., 2002).

Although some experts argue that adolescent college drinking is normative, there are many problems associated with high-risk drinking; the longer adolescents continue heavy episodic drinking, the more likely they are to suffer social, physical, and legal consequences. College administrators irrefutably struggle with the best way to identify the minority of college drinkers at risk for developing severe health and social problems.

Myerholtz and Rosenberg (1998) conducted a survey of 100 randomly selected directors of collegiate alcohol programs. They found that directors most often reported using one of the following brief screening instruments when trying to identify problem drinkers among undergraduates: the Michigan Alcoholism Screening Test (MAST), the Substance Abuse Subtle Screening Inventory 2, the CAGE, or the MacAndrew Scale of the Minnesota Multiphasic Personality Inventory (MMPI). One of these instruments, the four-item CAGE (which sets its acronym from questions about cutting down, annoyance from others, guilt about drinking, and the need for a drink in the morning or eye opener), is often viewed as the most practical because of its brevity and ease of administration (Allen, Maisto, & Connors, 1995; Maisto, Connors, & Allen, 1995); however, the CAGE was designed to screen for lifetime alcohol dependency (Mayfield, McLeod, & Hall, 1974), and college students, for the most part, have not had the amount of drinking experiences needed to endorse one item on the CAGE (O'Hare & Tran, 1997). Notwithstanding its wide use in college settings, the CAGE does not provide information on quantity/frequency or on past versus present use. The CAGE generally has been less reliable in assessing both adult women and men when compared with the five/six-item TWEAK (Cherpitel, 1999).

The TWEAK, specifically designed for adult prenatal populations, has never been systematically studied with college populations. (TWEAK is an acronym for Tolerance [T1, number of drinks to feel high; T2], number of drinks one can hold], Worry about drinking, Eye-openers, Amnesia [blackouts], and Cut down on drinking [K/C]; Chan, Pristach, Welte, & Russel, 1993.) The relatively few college-based studies addressing questionnaires used as screening assessments (e.g., CAGE) raise disquieting issues of sensitivity and specificity with younger (Bisson, Nadeau, & Demmers, 1999) and university populations (Boyd et al., 2003; O'Hare & Tran, 1997); in fact, because so few college students are alcohol dependent, it is unlikely that either the CAGE or the TWEAK is adequate for assessing this population.

The fact that additional items may either enhance the CAGE or even function with greater specificity is supported by an earlier study by Heck and Williams (1995a). They suggested that the CAGE may be ineffective in screening college students for alcohol problems because it detects only more severe patterns of problem drinking, and typically, college students have not been drinking long enough to develop these problems. To develop a more useful screening questionnaire, Heck and Williams suggested using the CAGE, plus additional items to assess quantity and frequency. They found several elements significantly discriminated between problem drinkers and normal drinkers: (1) endorsing the "cut down" and "annoyed" questions on the CAGE, (2) never or rarely choosing nonalcoholic beverages at social events, (3) driving under the influence at least 6 times in the past year, and (4) having started regular alcohol use before college.

The Alcohol Use Disorders Identification Test (AUDIT) was developed by the World Health Organization as a brief written screening method to identify problem alcohol consumption in primary care settings (Kokotailo et al., 2004). Unlike the CAGE or the TWEAK, the AUDIT was specifically developed to identify high-risk drinking, not alcohol dependence. With this in mind, Kokotailo and colleagues studied 302 (185 female), predominantly White (90%) college students attending a college health clinic in order to determine the validity of the AUDIT for college populations. They used the revised third edition of the DSM (*DSM-III-R*) abuse and dependence criteria and 28-day alcohol use as criterion standards. They concluded that the AUDIT was a somewhat valid assessment with college students when using the traditional cutoff score of 8; in this case, the AUDIT had 82% sensitivity and 78% specificity in the detection of high-risk drinkers. However, the AUDIT was more valid if a cutoff score of 6 was used; thus, specificity increased to 91%, and sensitivity was 60%. Unfortunately, because the sample was small, subgroup analyses by gender and/or race were not possible, so it is unclear whether the AUDIT is equally valid for college subpopulations.

Aertgeerts and colleagues (2000) used a sample of 3,564 (54% female) consecutive college first-year students with a mean age of 18 years, from one university in Belgium. In their cross-sectional study, they examined the sensitivity, specificity, and positive and negative predictive value of the CAGE and AUDIT. Using the *DSM-IV* criteria, 18% of the male students met the criteria for alcohol abuse, and 6% were alcohol dependent, in contrast to 4% and 2% of the female students who met the criteria for alcohol abuse and dependence, respectively. When using the *DSM-IV* criteria, Aertgeerts and colleagues found that a cutoff score of 1 on the CAGE was generally associated with a sensitivity of 42% and a specificity of 87%, and a score of 6 or more on the AUDIT gave a sensitivity of 80% and a specificity of 78%. However, for women, sensitivity and positive predictive value of both the CAGE and the AUDIT were lower than men. These researchers concluded that in their current forms neither the CAGE nor the AUDIT should be used in screening college students. However, they did find that by replacing one of the CAGE questions (Annoyed) with a question about driving Under the influence (CUGE), the sensitivity for the CUGE was 94%, and specificity was 89%. Of note, there was a dramatic decline in sensitivity from the CUGE with a cutoff of 2 or more. When the cutoff was 2, sensitivity was reduced to 38%, an indication that, like the CAGE, the CUGE is most dependent on a positive answer to only one question.

Although a variety of short, alcohol-screening instruments for identifying problem drinkers are available, these screening instruments are not necessarily valid for assessing the heavy episodic drinking that occurs within college populations. Indeed, research indicates that if either the CAGE or the AUDIT is used, it should be modified with additional questions or changes in scoring. The few validity studies that have used college-based populations revealed that these instruments often perform erratically—a major concern—because reliable, valid, and practical screening instruments are critical for obtaining accurate assessments of problem drinking among college students (Aergeerts et al., 2000; Heck & Williams, 1995a,b; O'Hare & Tran, 1997). Summaries of problem drinking assessment instruments can be found in the NIAAA's treatment handbook *Assessing Alcohol Problems: A Guide for Clinicians and Researchers* (Allen & Columbus, 1995).

HARMFUL CONSEQUENCES OF COLLEGE DRINKING

Although a normative developmental perspective has guided the discussions within this chapter, a host of harmful outcomes result from college students' drinking, particularly high-risk or binge drinking. It is these harmful outcomes that are the focus of most primary prevention and intervention programs for college students.

Perkins (2002), in his review of the present research dealing with consequences of alcohol misuse in college populations, noted some empirical support for the following consequences to the college drinker: academic impairment, memory loss (blackouts), physical illnesses, unintended and unprotected sexual activity, suicide, sexual coercion/acquaintance rape, impaired driving, legal problems, and impaired athletic performance.

Students who misuse alcohol have higher rates of injury according to the CORE and CAS data (Presley et al., 1996; Wechsler et al., 1994, 1998; Wechsler, Lee, Kuo, & Lee, 2000). Wechsler, Lee, Gledhill-Hoyt, and Nelson (2000) reported that data from the CAS revealed that 10% of nonbinge drinkers, 27% of binge drinkers, and 54% of frequent binge drinkers had at least one episode of memory loss (blackout) in the past year. Presley and colleagues (1996), using CORE data, also documented high rates of memory loss among college drinkers; in addition, injuries and alcohol poisonings posed notable threats to the health of students. Because heavy drinking by college students usually does not continue after graduation, most people believe that the health consequences from heavy drinking are short term and easily resolved (e.g., hangovers and sleep deprivation).

Data from the CAS and CORE studies document the ubiquitous nature of these secondary consequences on college campuses. Wechsler, Lee, Kuo, and

Lee (2002) reported that 61% of nonbingeing students living on college campuses reported sleep loss and interrupted study because other students were drinking. It was estimated that approximately one in three students who drank in the previous 12 months also drove (while under the influence), and about half of all fatal car crashes among this age group involved alcohol. On average, more than three college students in the United States die from alcohol-related car crashes every day, and alcohol-related driving behavior is the greatest single cause of death and injury among traditional-age undergraduate students in the United States (Hingson et al., 2002; Perkins, 2002; Wechsler, Lee, Nelson, & Kuo, 2002).

Alcohol related sexual assaults are common on campuses, although there is some variation in estimates, depending on the sample and definition of assault (Abbey, 2002; Mohler-Kuo, Lee, & Wechsler, 2003; Wechsler et al., 1994, 1998). Heavy drinking was also associated with high-risk sexual behavior and physical and sexual aggression. Sexual assaults on campus are most frequent among acquaintances and in the context of a date or party. Of course, the fact that alcohol misuse and sexual assault often co-occur on college campuses does not mean that alcohol causes assault; however, alcohol does play a role (Abbey, 2002). The association between alcohol and sexual assault proved to be complex, with multiple pathways linking these factors (for reviews, see Abbey, 2002; Abbey, Zawacki, Buck, Clinton, & McAuslan, 2001). College men's alcohol expectancies are associated with perceptions about increased sexuality and more willing sexual partners, including sexual assault perpetration (Abbey, Ross, McDuffie, & McAuslan 1996).

Use of other drugs may be another consequence of heavy drinking (Bachman et al., 1997; Johnston, O'Malley, & Bachman, 1999; Presley et al., 1996; Wechsler et al., 1995), although alcohol remains the primary psychoactive drug of choice among college students. After alcohol, cigarettes, marijuana, and prescription drugs are the most abused substances (Johnston et al., 2003; McCabe, Teter, & Boyd, 2005; Mohler-Kuo et al., 2003; O'Malley & Johnston, 2002). In their review of data from large, representative national datasets, O'Malley and Johnston (2002) noted that between 1995 and 1999, about 20% of college students smoked marijuana, and the majority of students (66%) who used marijuana also engaged in binge drinking. Another smaller group used cocaine, and most cocaine users (77%) engaged in binge drinking (Bachman et al., 1997).

Ecstasy use among college students began rising between 1997 and 2001; however, use has now leveled off. Using the CAS databases, Strote and colleagues (2002) examined the prevalence and changing patterns of Ecstasy use among college students in 1999. These researchers found that annual Ecstasy use rose from 2.8% to 4.7% between 1997 and 1999, a statistically significant increase; however, this was not universal. Data revealed that Ecstasy users were more likely to engage in several risky behaviors, such as binge drinking, sexual activity, and marijuana and cigarette smoking. There were, however, several limitations to the study. Most notably, these authors did not report the influence of other factors that have been shown to be correlated with drinking and drug use (e.g., high school drug use).

In two studies using large, random samples from one institution, researchers examined two forms of illicit drug use in their college population (Boyd et al., 2003; Teter, McCabe, Boyd, & Guthrie, 2003). Boyd and colleagues (2003) found that 10% of students reported lifetime Ecstasy use, and 3% reported past-month use. Among the 15 illegal substances listed, only alcohol and marijuana were more widely used. Men and women were equally likely to have ever used Ecstasy, and White students were more likely to report lifetime Ecstasy use than African American or Asian students. Class year was strongly associated with time of initiation. Teter and colleagues (2003) sampled 2,250 undergraduates and found that 3% of college students reported past-year use of methylphenidate (Ritalin) and that these illicit users were significantly more likely to use alcohol, Ecstasy, and cigarettes and to report adverse alcohol- and drug-related consequences compared with prescription stimulant users or nonusers.

Recently, the relationship between the nonmedical use of prescription stimulants and alcohol use was examined in a nationally representative sample of 10,904 college students attending 4-year colleges in the United States (McCabe, Knight, Teter, & Wechsler, 2005). Approximately 7% of college students reported lifetime nonmedical use of prescription stimulants, and 4% reported such use in the past year. Past-year nonmedical users of prescription stimulants were significantly more likely than nonusers of prescription stimulants to use alcohol, binge drink, and experience alcohol-related consequences. In particular, past-year nonmedical prescription stimulant users were over 10 times more likely than nonusers to report frequent binge drinking.

At this time, the college studies reporting illicit drug abuse in combination with alcohol abuse are limited by several factors, including sample and measurement issues. Many of these studies are derived from single institutions, and thus, generalizabiltiy is limited. Further, the studies from MTF, CAS, and CORE do not ask students about their medically prescribed use of prescription drugs, and thus, it is impossible to ascertain the extent to which students are also using prescription drugs legally. Finally, the motivations for the illegal use of prescription drugs by college students are not well documented—is it self-treatment or for purposes of intoxication?—and further study is needed in this area.

GAPS IN KNOWLEDGE AND IMPLICATIONS FOR RESEARCH

One shortcoming in assuming a developmental perspective, as described by both Schulenberg and Maggs, is that the perspective presupposes that drinking is normal; thus, college students' alcohol abuse and dependence problems tend to get less attention. There is, arguably, a dearth of research in areas related to college students' alcohol-related health problems (e.g., dependence), and clearly, more research is needed to characterize the relationships among alcohol consumption and acute and chronic problems among college students. There is a striking paucity of studies on brief screening for subgroups of students who meet the diagnostic criteria for alcohol dependence. Relative to the number of students who report symptoms that meet the diagnosis for alcohol abuse or dependence, very few of these students ever seek any treatment while in college (Knight et al., 2002). Data are needed to determine age-appropriate criteria for diagnosing college-student alcohol problems, including alcohol abuse and dependency.

More information is needed on the efficacy of brief interventions for young people between the ages of 16 and 25 years (Saunders, Kypri, Scott, Laforge, & Larimer, 2004). Fager and Melnyk (2004) provide an integrative review of 15 intervention studies that aimed to decrease alcohol use by college students. They reported that two major behavioral outcomes were used in their evaluation: reduced quantity, frequency, and intensity of alcohol use and decreased negative and primary consequences of alcohol use. Half of the studies reviewed tested brief motivational interventions, and four of the studies used an expectance approach (e.g., Does alcohol make you relax?). The research designs of the 15 studies limited confidence in the conclusions; many of the studies used unreliable measures of alcohol consumption and included small convenience samples with relatively short-term follow-up of 1 year or less (see Fager & Melnyk, 2004). Although some studies support the efficacy of brief interventions in reducing high-risk drinking, there is a question whether brief interventions are effective and appropriate for late adolescent populations, and there is little consensus as to what constitutes a "brief intervention" for college populations (see Saunders et al., 2004). Kypri, Saunders, and Gallagher (2003) examined the acceptability of several brief interventions and found that undergraduates expressed a reluctance to discuss their risky drinking with health professionals; however, they expressed interest in electronic assessment and feedback. In their study of 1,564 undergraduates, they found that electronic screening with brief intervention was one of the most popular interventions. Because younger college students are almost universally Internet literate, future applications of computer assessment and feedback are likely, and nurses should consider the Internet as an efficacious venue for brief interventions.

Minority populations remain underrepresented in studies of college students, and further research is needed that highlights the mechanisms behind the apparent protective factors of being African American or a woman and the apparent risk factors associated with being lesbian or gay. Moreover, there are several groups who are virtually invisible in prevention literature on college drinking, including students who choose not to drink for health, cultural, or religious reasons and students who are in recovery (therefore abstinent). We know little about how students within these subpopulations cope with their environments and seek out nondrinking peers and/or forge their identities.

Far greater research attention should be paid to the role high-risk drinking plays in the self-selection into certain living arrangements as well as how alcohol use interferes with social and emotional development (e.g., intimate relationships). Finally, although many studies support taking a developmental perspective, and certainly the Task Force of the National Advisory Council on Alcohol Abuse and Alcoholism appears to embrace the perspective, far more longitudinal research is needed to determine the factors that contribute to a college student's moving from one drinking pattern (heavy episodic) to another (lower consumption).

Over 1,400 U.S. college students ages 18 to 24 died in 1998 from alcohol-related unintentional injuries (Hingson et al., 2002). One unfortunate consequence of considering college drinking normative or developmental is that, until relatively recently, little attention focused on preventing college students' heavy episodic drinking. Drinking, including drinking games and songs, was assumed to be part of college culture (Johnson, 2002). However, even if college students' alcohol use is characterized as normative, prevention strategies that target reducing harm are badly needed.

In 2002 the Task Force of the National Advisory Council on Alcohol Abuse and Alcoholism issued a series of recommendations to researchers interested in addressing gaps in prevention knowledge that were based on their extensive review of extant prevention research (see www.collegedrinkingprevention.gov). The task force recommended that researchers focus their collective attention on the effects of the following in reducing the negative consequences of high-risk drinking: parental notification, disciplinary policies, academic environments (e.g., increased academic requirements), living environments (e.g., substance-free housing), and environmental characteristics (e.g., location of bars).

To date, little is known about the long-term effectiveness of community prevention approaches, such as the enactment of laws that affect consumption (e.g., minimum drinking age), the use of media approaches (e.g., advertising bans), and the deployment of social norms approaches (campus-wide campaigns to negate overestimations of alcohol and other drug use). Too often, researchers have used small convenience samples that do not necessarily focus on college students or case studies that are limited in their scope. Virtually all of the studies on community-based interventions suffer from inadequate control of covariates, sample limitations, and relatively short-term follow-up. Thus, the gap in our knowledge regarding effective prevention is waiting to be filled.

Although social norm approaches recently have been criticized as being ineffective (e.g., Wechsler et al., 2003), these programs have been embraced by a great many institutions because they represent a broad-based, universal approach (see Perkins, 2002). Social norm activities target the misperceptions many students hold about their peers and are meant to clarify the drinking misperceptions held by the general student body, specifically, those held by students at highest risk (Perkins, 2002; Perkins et al., 1999). What is surprising is how many institutions have embraced social norm campaigns and how few data are available supporting their efficacy. Far greater study is needed before these programs should be assumed to be universally effective.

CONCLUSION

Nurse-researchers are poised to advance knowledge in areas related to the assessment and prevention of high-risk drinking by college students. However, like all complex problems, high-risk drinking will never be understood through the findings of a single discipline; college students' drinking behaviors are far too complex to be claimed by one discipline. Nonetheless, the consequences of college students' binge drinking beg further attention, and nurse-scientists are in an excellent position to contribute to our understanding of this developmentally mediated but highly consequential adolescent behavior.

REFERENCES

Abbey, A. (2002). Alcohol-related sexual assault: A common problem among college students. *Journal of Studies on Alcohol* (Suppl. 14), 118–128.

Abbey, A., Ross, L. T., McDuffie, D., & McAuslan, P. (1996). Alcohol, misperception and sexual assault: How and why they are linked. In D. M. Buss & N. Malamuth (Eds.), *Sex, power, conflict: Evolutionary and feminist perspectives* (pp. 138–161). New York: Oxford University Press.

Abbey, A., Smith, M. J., & Scott, R. O. (1993). The relationship between reasons for drinking alcohol and alcohol consumption: An interactional approach. *Addictive Behaviors*, 18, 659–670.

Abbey, A., Zawacki, T., Buck, P. O., Clinton, A. M., & McAuslan, P. (2001). Alcohol and sexual assault. *Alcohol Research and Health*, 25(1), 43–51.

Aergeerts, B., & Buntinx, F. (2002). The relationship between alcohol abuse or dependence and academic performance in first-year college students. *Journal of Adolescent Health*, 31, 223–225.

Aergeerts, B., Buntinx, F., Bande-Knops, J., Vandermeulen, C., Roelants, M., Ansoms, S., et al. (2000). The value of CAGE, CUGE, AUDIT in screening for alcohol abuse and dependence among college freshman. *Alcoholism: Clinical and Experimental Research*, 24, 53–57.

Allen, J. P., & Columbus, M. (Eds.). (1995). *Assessing alcohol problems: A guide for clinicians and researchers*. Bethesda, MD: U.S. Department of Health and Human Services, Public

Health Service, National Institutes of Health, and National Institute on Alcohol Abuse and Alcoholism.

Allen, J. P., Maisto, S., & Connors, G. J. (1995). Self-report screening tests for alcohol problems in primary care. *Archives of Internal Medicine, 155,* 1726–1730.

Bachman, J., Wadsworth, K. N., O'Malley, P. M., Johnston, L. D., & Schulenberg, J. E. (1997). *Smoking, drinking and drug use in young adulthood.* Mahwah, NJ: Erlbaum.

Baer, J. S. (1994). Effects of college residence on perceived norms for alcohol consumption: An examination of the first year in college. *Psychology of Addictive Behaviors, 8,* 43–50.

———. (2002). Student factors: Understanding individual variation in college drinking. *Journal of Studies of Alcohol* (Suppl. 14), 40–53.

Baer, J. S., Kivlahan, D. R., & Marlatt, G. A. (1995). High-risk drinking across the transition from high school to college. *Alcoholism: Clinical and Experimental Research, 19*(1), 54–61.

Barnes, G. M., Welte, J. W., & Dintcheff, B. (1992). Alcohol misuse among college students and other young adults: Findings from a general population study in New York State. *International Journal of the Addictions, 27,* 917–934.

Benton, S. L., Schmidt, J. L., Newton, F. B., Shin, K., Benton, S. A., & Newton, D. W. (2004). College student protective strategies and drinking. *Journal of Studies on Alcohol, 65*(7), 11–21.

Billingham, R. E., Parrillo, A. V., & Gross, W. C. (1993). Reasons given by college students for drinking: A discriminant analysis investigation. *International Journal of the Addictions, 28,* 793–802.

Bisson, J., Nadeau, L., & Demers, A. (1999). The validity of the CAGE scale to screen for heavy drinking and drinking problems in a general population survey. *Addiction, 94*(5), 715–722.

Blane, H. T., & Hewitt, L. E. (1977). *Alcohol and youth: An analysis of the literature, 1960–1975.* Springfield, VA: National Technical Information Service.

Borsari, B., & Carey, K. (1999). Understanding fraternity drinking: Five recurring themes in the literature, 1980–1998. *Journal of American College Health, 48,* 30–37.

Boyd, C. J., McCabe, S. E., & d'Arcy, H. (2003). Ecstasy use among college undergraduates: Gender, race and sexual identity. *Journal of Substance Abuse Treatment, 24*(3), 209–215.

———. (2004). Collegiate living environments: A predictor of binge drinking, negative consequences and risk-reducing behaviors. *Journal of Addictions Nursing, 15*(3), 111–118.

Cantor, N., Norem, J. K., Niedenthal, P. M., Langston, C. A., & Brower, A. M. (1987). Life tasks, self-concept ideals, and cognitive strategies in a life transition. *Journal of Personality and Social Psychology, 53,* 1178–1191.

Carey, K. B., & Correia, C. J. (1997). Drinking motives predict alcohol-related problems in college students. *Journal of Studies on Alcohol, 58*(1), 100–105.

Cashin, J. R., Presley, C. A., & Meilman, P. W. (1998). Alcohol use in the Greek system: Follow the leader. *Journal of Studies on Alcohol, 59*(1), 63–70.

Chan, A. W., Pristach, E. A., Welte, J. W., & Russel, M. (1993). Use of the TWEAK test in screening for alcoholism/heavy drinking in three populations. *Alcoholism in Clinical and Experimental Research, 17*(6), 1188–1192.

Cherpitel, C. J. (1999). Screening for alcohol problems in the US general population: A comparison of the CAGE and TWEAK by gender, ethnicity and service utilization. *Journal of Studies on Alcohol, 60*(5), 705–711.

Davis, J. L., & Hunnicut, D. M. (1991). Community college alcohol abuse: An assessment. *Community College Review, 19,* 43–47.

DeBord, K. A., Wood, P. K., Sher, K. J., & Good, G. E. (1998). The relevance of sexual orientation to substance abuse and psychological distress among college students. *Journal of College Student Development, 39,* 157–168.

Delk, E. W., & Meilman, P. W. (1996). Alcohol use among college students in Scotland compared with norms from the United States. *Journal of American College Health, 44*(6), 274–281.

Dowdall, G., & Wechsler, H. (2002). Studying college alcohol use: Widening the lens, sharpening the focus. *Journal of Studies of Alcohol* (Suppl. 14), 14–22.

Eggleston, A. M., Woolaway-Bickel, K. W., & Schmidt, N. B. (2004). Social anxiety and alcohol use: Evaluation of the moderating and mediating effects of alcohol expectancies. *Anxiety Disorders, 18,* 33–49.

Eisenberg, M., & Wechsler, H. (2003). Substance use behaviors among college students with same-sex and opposite-sex experience: Results from a national study. *Addictive Behaviors, 28,* 899–913.

Engs, R. C. (1990). Family background of alcohol abuse and its relationship to alcohol consumption among college students: An unexpected finding. *Journal of Studies on Alcohol, 51,* 542–547.

Evans, D. M., & Dunn, N. J. (1995). Alcohol expectancies, coping responses and self-efficacy judgments: A replication and extension of Cooper et al.'s 1988 study in a college sample. *Journal of Studies on Alcohol, 56*(2), 186–193.

Fager, J. H., & Malnyk, B. M. (2004). The effectiveness of intervention studies to decrease alcohol use in college undergraduate students: An integrative analysis. *Worldviews on Evidence-based Nursing, 1*(2), 102–119.

Finn, P. (1996). *Preventing alcohol-related problems on campus: Substance-free residence halls.* Washington, DC: Abt Associates.

Gassman, R. A., Demone, H. W., & Wechsler, H. (2002). College students' drinking: Masters in social work compared with undergraduate students. *Health and Social Work, 27*(3), 184–192.

Gfroerer, J. C., Greenblatt, J. C., & Wright, D. A. (1997). Substance abuse in the college-age population: Differences according to educational status. *American Journal of Public Health, 87,* 62–65.

Glantz, M., & Pickens, R. (1992). *Vulnerability to drug abuse.* Washington, DC: American Psychological Association.

Goldstein, A. L., Wall, A., McKee, S. A., & Hinson, R. E. (2004). Accessibility of alcohol expectancies from memory: Impact of mood and motives in college drinkers. *Journal of Studies on Alcohol, 65*(10), 95–104.

Hanson, D. J., & Engs, R. C. (1992). College students' drinking problems: A national study, 1982–1991. *Psychological Reports, 71,* 39–42.

Harford, T. C., Wechsler, H., & Muthen, B. O. (2002). The impact of current residence and high school drinking on alcohol problems among college students. *Journal of Studies on Alcohol, 63*(3), 271–279.

Hastings, R. (1936). *The universities of Europe in the Middle Ages.* Oxford: Clarendon Press.

Heck, E. J., & Williams, M. D. (1995a). Using the CAGE to screen for drinking-related problems in college students. *Journal of Studies on Alcohol, 56,* 282–286.

————. (1995b). Criterion variability in problem-drinking research on college students. *Journal of Substance Abuse, 7*(4), 437–447.

Herman, A., I, Philbeck, J., Vasilopoulos, N. L., & Paolo, B. (2003). Serotonin transporter promoter polymorphism and differences in alcohol consumption behavior in a college student population. *Alcohol and Alcoholism, 38*(5), 446–449.

Hingson, R. W., Heeren, T., Zakocs, R. C., Kopstein, A., & Wechsler, H. (2002). Magnitude of alcohol-related mortality and morbidity among U.S. college students ages 18–24. *Journal of Studies of Alcohol, 63*(2), 136–144.

Hingson, R., Heeren, T., Zakocs, R., Winter, M., & Wechsler, H. (2003). Age of first intoxication, heavy drinking, driving after drinking and risk of unintentional injury among U.S. college students. *Journal of Studies on Alcohol, 64*, 23–31.

Jessor, R., & Jessor, S. (1977). *Problem behavior and psychosocial development.* New York: Academic Press.

Johnson, T. J. (2002). College students' self-reported reasons for why drinking games end. *Addictive Behaviors, 27*, 145–153.

Johnston, L. D., & O'Malley, P. M. (1986). Why do the nation's students use drugs and alcohol? Self-reported reasons from nine national surveys. *Journal of Drug Issues, 16*, 29–66.

Johnston, L. D, O'Malley, P. M., & Bachman, J. G. (1986–2002). *Drug use among American high school students, college students, and other young adults: National trends through 1985* (DHHS Pub. No. ADM 86–1450). Rockville, MD: National Institute on Drug Abuse.

————. (1999). *Drug use among American high school seniors, college students, and young adults, 1975–1998* (Vols. 1–2). Rockville, MD: National Institute on Drug Abuse.

————. (2003). *Monitoring the future national survey results on drug use, 1975–2002: Vol. 2. College students and adults ages 19–40* (NIH Pub. No. 3-5376). Bethesda, MD: National Institute on Drug Abuse.

Johnston, L. D., O'Malley, P. M., & Eveland, L. K. (1978). Drugs and delinquency: A search for causal connections. In D. G. Kandel (Ed.), *Longitudinal research on drug use: Empirical findings and methodological issues* (pp. 137–156). Washington, DC: Hemisphere Publishing.

Kandel, D. B. (1975). Reaching the hard-to-reach: Illicit drug use among high school absentees. *Addictive Diseases, 1*, 465–480.

Keefe, K., & Newcomb, M. D. (1996). Demographic and psychosocial risk for alcohol use: Ethnic differences. *Journal of Studies on Alcohol, 57*, 521–530.

Knight, J. R., Wechsler, H., Kuo, M., Seibring, M., Weitzman, E. R., & Schuckit, M. A. (2002). Alcohol abuse and dependence among U.S. college students. *Journal of Studies on Alcohol, 63*, 263–270.

Kokotailo, P. K., Egan, J., Gangnon, R., Brown, D., Mundt, M., & Fleming, M. (2004). Validity of the Alcohol Use Disorders Identification Test in college students. *Alcoholism: Clinical and Experimental Research, 28*(6), 914–920.

Kypri, K., Saunders, J. B., & Gallagher, S. J. (2003). Acceptability of various brief intervention approaches for hazardous drinking among university students. *Alcohol, 38*, 626–628.

Labouvie, E. (1996). Maturing out of substance use: Selection and self-correction. *Journal of Drug Issues, 26*, 457–476.

Labouvie, E., Bates, M. E., & Pandina, R. J. (1997). Age of first use: Its reliability and predictive utility. *Journal of Studies on Alcohol, 58*, 638–643.

Lawyer, S. R., Karg, R. S., Murphy, J. G., & McGlynn, F. D. (2002). Heavy drinking among college students is influenced by anxiety sensitivity, gender, and contexts for alcohol use. *Anxiety Disorders, 16*, 165–173.

Leichliter, J. S., Meilman, P. W., Presley, C. A., & Cashin, J. R. (1998). Alcohol use and related consequences among students with varying levels of involvement in college athletics. *Journal of American College Health, 46*(6), 257–262.

Lo, C. C., & Globetti, G. (1995). The facilitating and enhancing roles Greek associations play in college drinking. *International Journal of the Addictions, 30*(10), 1311–1322.

Luczak, S. E., Wall, T. L., Shea, S. H., Byun, S. M., & Carr, L. G. (2001). Binge drinking in Chinese, Korean, and White college students: Genetic and ethnic group differences. *Psychology of Addictive Behaviors, 15*(4), 306–309.

Lundahl, L. H., Davis, T. M., Adesso, V. J., & Lukas, S. E. (1997). Alcohol expectancies: Effects of gender, age and family history of alcoholism. *Addictive Behaviors, 22*(1), 115–125.

Maggs, J. L. (1997). Alcohol use and binge drinking as goal-directed action during the transition to postsecondary education. In J. Schulenberg, J. L. Maggs, & K. Hurrelmann (Eds.), *Health risks and developmental transitions during adolescence* (pp. 345–371). New York: Cambridge University Press.

Maisto, S., Connors, G., & Allen, J. (1995). Contrasting self-report screens for alcohol problems: A review. *Alcoholism: Clinical and Experimental Research, 19*(6), 1510–1516.

Maney, D. W. (1990). Predicting university students' use of alcoholic beverages. *Journal of College Student Development, 31*, 23–32.

Mayfield, D., McLeod, G., & Hall, P. (1974). The CAGE questionnaire: Validation of a new alcoholism screening instrument. *American Journal of Psychiatry, 131*, 1121–1123.

McCabe, S. E., Boyd, C. J., Couper, M. P., Crawford, S., & d'Arcy, H. (2002). Mode effects for collecting alcohol and other drug use data: Web and U.S. mail. *Journal of Studies on Alcohol, 63*(6), 755–761.

McCabe, S. E., Boyd, C., Hughes, T. L., & d'Arcy, H. (2003). Sexual identity and substance use among undergraduate students. *Substance Abuse, 24*(2), 77–91.

McCabe, S. E., Knight, J. R., Teter, C. J., & Wechsler, H. (2005). Nonmedical use of prescription stimulants among college students: Prevalence and correlates from a national survey. *Addiction, 100*(1), 96–106.

McCabe, S. E., Teter, C. J., & Boyd, C. J. (2005). Illicit use of prescription pain medication among college students. *Drug and Alcohol Dependence, 77*(1), 37–47.

Meilman, P. W. (1993). Alcohol-induced sexual behavior on campus. *Journal of American College Health, 42*(1), 27–31.

Meilman, P. W., Burwell, C., Smith, K. E., Canterbury, R. J., Gressard, C. G., Pryor, J. H., et al. (1993). Using survey data to capture students' attention: Three institutions look at alcohol-induced sexual behavior. *Journal of College Student Development, 34*, 72–73.

Meilman, P. W., Cashin, J. R., McKillip, J., & Presley, C. A. (1998). Understanding the three national databases on collegiate alcohol and drug use. *Journal of American College Health, 46*(6), 159–162.

Meilman, P. W., Leichliter, J. S., & Presley, C. A. (1998). Analysis of weapon carrying among college students, by region and institution type. *Journal of American College Health, 46*(6), 291–292.

————. (1999). Greeks and athletes: Who drinks more? *Journal of American College Health*, 47(4), 187–190.

Meilman, P. W., Presley, C. A., & Cashin, J. R. (1995). The sober social life at historically black colleges. *Journal of Blacks in Higher Education*, 9, 98–100.

Meilman, P. W., Presley, C. A., & Lyerla, R. (1994). Black college students and binge drinking. *Journal of Blacks in Higher Education*, 4, 70–71.

Mohler-Kuo, M., Dowdall, G. W., Koss, M. P., & Wechsler, H. (2004). Correlates of rape while intoxicated in a national sample of college women. *Journal of Studies on Alcohol*, 65, 37–45.

Mohler-Kuo, M., Lee, J. E., & Wechsler, H. (2003). Trends in marijuana and other illicit drug use among college students: Results from 4 Harvard School of Public Health College Alcohol Study Surveys: 1993–2001. *Journal of American College Health*, 52, 17–24.

Morison, S. E. (1936). *Harvard College in the seventeenth century*. Cambridge, MA: Harvard University Press.

Myerholtz, L., & Rosenberg H. (1998). Screening college students for alcohol problems: Psychometric assessment of the SASSI-2. *Journal of Studies on Alcohol*, 59(4), 439–446.

Naimi, T. S., Brewer, R. D., Mokdad, A., Denny, C., Sedula, M. K., & Marks, J. S. (2003). Binge drinking among US adults. *Journal of the American Medical Association*, 289(1), 70–75.

O'Hare, T., & Tran, T. (1997). Predicting problem drinking in college students: Gender differences and the CAGE questionnaire. *Addictive Behaviors*, 22(1), 13–21.

O'Malley, P., & Johnston, L. (2002). Epidemiology of alcohol and other drug use among American college students. *Journal of Studies on Alcohol* (Suppl. 14), 23–39.

Pascarella, E. T., & Terenzini, P. T. (1991). *How college affects students: Findings and insights from twenty years of research*. San Francisco: Jossey-Bass.

Perkins, H. W. (2002). Surveying the damage: A review of research on consequences of alcohol misuse in college populations. *Journal of Studies on Alcohol* (Suppl. 14), 91–100.

Perkins, H. W., & Berkowitz, A. D. (1991). Collegiate COAs and alcohol abuse: Problem drinking in relation to assessment of parent and grandparent alcoholism. *Journal of Counseling and Development*, 69(3), 237–240.

Perkins, H. W., Meilman, P. W., Leichliter, J. S., Cashin, J. S., & Presley, C. A. (1999). Misperceptions of the norms for the frequency of alcohol and other drug use on college campuses. *Journal of American College Health*, 47, 253–258.

Perry, B. L., Miles, D., & Svikis, D. S. (2004). *Risk factors for problem drinking in college women*. Poster presented at Research Society on Alcoholism, Vancouver, Canada.

Presley, C. A., Meilman, P. W., & Cashin, J. R. (1996). *Alcohol and drugs on American college campuses: Use, consequences, and perceptions of the campus environment, 1992–1994* (Vol. 4). Carbondale, IL: Core Institute.

————. (1997). Weapon carrying and substance abuse among college students. *Journal of American College Health*, 46(1), 3–8.

Presley, C. A., Meilman, P. W., & Lyerla, R. (1994). Development of the Core Alcohol and Drug Survey: Initial findings and future directions. *Journal of American College Health*, 42(6), 248–255.

Presley, C., Meilman, P. W., Lyerla, R., & Karmos, J. (1995). University policies and consequences of drinking. *College Student Journal*, 29, 304–307.

Saunders, J. B., Kypri, K., Scott, T. W., Laforge, R. G., & Larimer, M. (2004). Approaches to brief intervention for hazardous drinking in young people. *Alcoholism: Clinical and Experimental Research, 28*(2), 322–329.

Schulenberg, J., Bachman, J. G., O'Malley, P. M., & Johnston, L. D. (1994). High school educational success and subsequent substance use: A panel analysis following adolescents into young adulthood. *Journal of Health and Social Behavior, 35,* 45–62.

Schulenberg, J., & Maggs, J. (2002). Developmental perspective on alcohol use and heavy drinking during adolescence and the transition to young adulthood. *Journal of Studies on Alcohol* (Suppl. 14), 54–70.

Schulenberg, J. Maggs, J. L., Long, S. W., Gothman, H. J., Baer, J. S., Kivlahan, D. R., et al. (2001). Problem of college drinking: Insights from a developmental perspective. *Alcoholism: Clinical and Experimental Research, 25,* 473–477.

Schulenberg, J., O'Malley, P. M., Bachman, J. G., Wadsworth, K. N., & Johnston, L. D. (1996). Getting drunk and growing up: Trajectories of frequent binge drinking during the transition to young adulthood. *Journal of Studies on Alcohol, 57,* 289–304.

Schulenberg, J., Wadsworth, K. N., O'Malley, P. M., Bachman, J. G., & Johnston, L. D. (1996). Adolescent risk factors for binge drinking during the transition to young adulthood: Variable- and pattern-centered approaches to change. *Developmental Psychology, 32*(4), 659–674.

Straus, R., & Bacon, S. (1953). *Drinking in college.* New Haven, CT: Yale University Press.

Strote, J., Lee, J. E., & Wechsler, H. (2002). Increasing MDMA use among college students: Results from a national survey. *Journal of Adolescent Health, 30,* 64–71.

Teter, C. J., McCabe, S. E., Boyd, C. J., & Guthrie, S. K. (2003). Illicit methylphenidate use in an undergraduate student population. *Pharmacotherapy, 23*(5), 609–617.

Thombs, D. L. (1993). The differentially discriminating properties of alcohol expectancies for female and male drinkers. *Journal of Counseling and Development, 71,* 321–325.

U.S. Department of Education. (2002). American College Testing Program, unpublished tabulations, derived from statistics collected by the U.S. Bureau of the Census; and U.S. Department of Labor, College Enrollment of High School Graduates, various years. Retrieved July 30, 2004, from http://nces.ed.gov/pubs2002/digest2001/tables/dt185.asp

Wechsler, H., Davenport, A., Dowdall, G., Moeykens, B., & Castillo, S. (1994). Health and behavioral consequences of binge drinking in college: A national survey of students at 140 campuses. *Journal of the American Medical Association, 272,* 1672–1677.

Wechsler, H., Dowdall, G. W., Davenport, A., & Castillo, S. (1995). Correlates of college students binge drinking. American *Journal of Public Health, 85,* 921–926.

Weschsler, H., Dowdall, G. W., Maenner, G., Gledhill-Hoyt, J., & Lee, H. (1998). Changes in binge drinking and related problems among American college students between 1993 and 1997. *Journal of American College Health, 47,* 57–68.

Wechsler, H., & Isaac, N. (1992). "Binge" drinkers at Massachusetts colleges: Prevalence, drinking style, time trends, and associated problems. *Journal of the American Medical Association, 267,* 2929–2931.

Wechsler, H., Kuh, G., & Davenport, A. E. (1996). Fraternities, sororities and binge drinking: Results from a national study of American colleges. *NASPA Journal, 33,* 260–279.

Wechsler, H., Lee, J. E., Gledhill-Hoyt, H., & Nelson, T. F. (2000). Alcohol use and problems at colleges banning alcohol: Results of a national survey. *Journal of Studies on Alcohol, 62*(2), 13–141.

Wechsler, H., Lee, J. E., Hall, J., Wagenaar, A. C., & Lee, H. (2002). Secondhand effects of student alcohol use reported by neighbors of colleges: The role of alcohol outlets. *Social Science and Medicine, 55*(3), 425–435.

Wechsler, H., Lee, J. E., Kuo, M., & Lee, H. (2000). College binge drinking in the 1990's: A continuing problem. *Journal of American College Health, 48*(10), 199–210.

Wechsler, H., Lee, J. E., Kuo, M., Seibring, M., Nelson, T. F., & Lee, H. (2002). Trends in college binge drinking during a period of increased prevention efforts. Findings from 4 Harvard School of Public Health College Alcohol Study surveys: 1993–2001. *Journal of American College Health, 50,* 203–217.

Wechsler, H., Lee, J. E., Nelson, T. F., & Kuo, M. (2002). Underage college students' drinking behavior, access to alcohol, and the influence of deterrence policies: Findings from the Harvard School of Public Health College Alcohol Study. *Journal of American College Health, 50*(5), 223–236.

Wechsler, H., Lee, J. E., Nelson, T. F., & Lee, H. (2001). Drinking levels, alcohol problems, and secondhand effects substance-free college residences: Results of a national study. *Journal of Studies on Alcohol, 62,* 23–31.

Wechsler, H., & Nelson, T. F. (2001). Binge drinking and the American college student: What's five drinks? *Psychology of Addictive Behaviors, 15*(4), 287–291.

Wechsler, H., Nelson, T. F., Lee, J. E., Seibring, M., Lewis, C., & Keeling, R. P. (2003). Perception and reality: A national evaluation of social norms marketing interventions to reduce college students' heavy alcohol use. *Journal of Studies on Alcohol, 64,* 484–494.

Weitzman, E. R., Nelson, T. F., & Wechsler, H. (2003). Taking up binge drinking in college: The influences of person, social group and environment. *Journal of Adolescent Health, 32,* 26–35.

Williams, J., Chaloupka, F. J., & Wechsler, H. (2002). Are there differential effects of price and policy on college students' drinking intensity? *National Bureau of Economic Research, 1,* WP 8702.

Wood, P. K., Sher, K. J., Erickson, D. J., & DeBord, K. A. (1997). Predicting academic problems in college from freshman alcohol involvement. *Journal of Studies on Alcohol, 58*(2), 200–210.

Yu, J., & Shacket, R. W. (2001). Alcohol use in high school: Predicting students' alcohol use and alcohol problems in four-year colleges. *American Journal of Drug and Alcohol Abuse, 27,* 775–793.

Chapter 7

Alcohol Misuse, Abuse, and Addiction in Young and Middle Adulthood

Sandra M. Handley and Peggy Ward-Smith

ABSTRACT

This chapter reviews research on alcohol misuse, abuse, and addiction in young and middle adulthood. Young adulthood is defined as ages 21 to 35 and middle adulthood as ages 36 to 65.

The authors searched the Cumulative Index of Nursing and Allied Health Literature (CINAHL) and other databases for the years 1992 through 2004 using the terms alcohol abuse, alcoholism, and alcohol dependence, then hand-searched for the inclusion of age as a variable. The search was limited to research and English-language publications. Unpublished dissertation studies were excluded, as were topics that were reviewed in other chapters of this volume. When possible, articles for review were limited to alcohol only, as compared with other drugs of abuse. Research articles were selected for review if they contained the variables alcohol misuse, abuse, or alcohol addiction or dependence and age. The review included both nurse- and non-nurse-investigators and was comprised of 50 studies.

The results are in four content areas across the global area of alcohol misuse, abuse, and dependence in young and middle adulthood: incidence and prevalence, developmental changes, the work setting, and the family setting. Few articles used a developmental framework, although in some studies, the framework was implicit.

Nurse-investigators were more likely to produce qualitative studies, although the studies varied dramatically in size of sample, research design, and variables. Overall, there was greater breadth than depth.

The use of adult developmental theory was limited despite its potential explanatory potential in this field. There is a need for more nurse-researchers to explore adult developmental theory and pay increased attention to age and developmental stage as explanatory variables.

Keywords: alcohol misuse, alcohol abuse, alcohol addiction, alcohol dependence, young adulthood, middle adulthood, adult development, developmental stages

The purpose of this chapter is to review and critique the research on alcohol misuse, abuse, and addiction in young and middle adulthood. For the purposes of this review, young adulthood is defined as ages 21 to 35 and middle adulthood as ages 35 to 65. The age span covered in this review, 21 to 65, spans the bulk of adulthood.

Alcohol misuse, abuse, and addiction in young and middle adulthood are areas of interest for scientists and clinicians alike due to their widespread social, health, and economic consequences. According to the National Institute on Alcohol Abuse and Alcoholism (NIAAA), "as many as one-third of Americans may engage in drinking practices that place them at heightened risk for the medical disorders of alcohol dependence (alcoholism) and alcohol abuse" (NIAAA, 2003). More than half of American adults have a close family member who has or has had alcoholism (Dawson & Grant, 1998). Those who misuse alcohol suffer consequences that reflect negatively on their health, family, friends, work, and community. Given the extent of alcohol misuse, abuse, and addiction, it is an important topic for nurses in clinical practice and nurse-scientists alike, as many patients and colleagues in young and middle adulthood are likely to be affected by alcohol misuse, abuse, and addiction either personally or through relatives or friends.

THEORETICAL PERSPECTIVE

Dividing adulthood into two stages, young and middle adulthood, is logical from both a developmental and a health perspective. Although developmental theorists have differentiated distinct tasks for each stage of the life span, the tasks have been most fully developed in childhood as compared to adulthood. One of the early and influential developmental theorists to include adulthood was Erik Erickson (1963). The developmental tasks of Erikson focused on the development of an individual identity (adolescence), intimacy (young adult-hood), and generativity (middle adulthood and the remainder of the life span). Levinson (1978) updated and refined the tasks of young and middle adulthood, such as leaving the family (16 to 24 years old), forming and solidifying a life structure (24 to 35 years old), becoming one's own person (35 to 42 years old), midlife transition (the early 40s), and restabilization (45 years old and older). Although adult development theorists have been working toward increasing the understanding of the adult life span, the stage of middle adulthood has been extended far past 45 years and needs further refinement as people's life span increases well into their 80s and 90s.

Within the alcohol research field, there has been an interest in using a developmental framework to explain alcohol misuse over the life span. This framework is used to explicate three developmental themes that have emerged from research. Those themes are (1) the great variability in individual drinking patterns, (2) changes in drinking variability over the life span, and (3) variability of pressures to drink over the life span (NIAAA, 2000). Therefore, this chapter will focus on alcohol misuse, abuse, and addiction in young and middle adulthood, with a particular focus on developmental issues.

METHOD

The CINAHL and Medline databases were searched for articles from 1992 to 2004 about alcohol abuse and alcohol dependence (*alcohol misuse* was not a useful search term). The year 1992 was selected because a review of research by nurses on alcohol and other drugs of abuse from 1980 through 1991 appeared previously in the *Annual Review of Nursing Research* (Sullivan & Handley, 1993). Other terms such as *alcohol consumption, alcohol drinking, standard drink, problem drinking, heavy drinking, ethanol analysis, work and alcoholism,* and *work and alcohol abuse* were also searched for relevant articles. The parameters of this search were limited to research and English-language publications, but articles by both nursing and nonnursing investigators were included. Unpublished dissertation studies and topics that were reviewed in other chapters of this volume were excluded. The results were then hand-searched for studies with age as a variable because age-related search terms were not productive. When possible, articles for review were limited to alcohol only as opposed to other drugs of abuse. Fifty research articles were selected for review because they contained the variables of alcohol misuse, abuse, or addiction and were age defined so that young and middle adulthood could be distinguished.

For definitions of the terms *alcohol misuse, alcohol abuse,* and *alcohol depen-dence* see Table 2.1 in Chapter 2. In this chapter, the terms *alcohol addiction, alcoholism,* and *alcohol dependence* will be used interchangeably. Four content areas across the global area of alcohol misuse, abuse, and dependence in young and middle adulthood were identified: incidence and prevalence, developmental changes, the work setting, and the family setting.

INCIDENCE AND PREVALENCE OF ALCOHOL MISUSE, ABUSE, AND ADDICTION IN YOUNG AND MIDDLE ADULTHOOD

Six studies were identified that addressed the epidemiology of alcohol consumption using age as a variable of concern (see Table 7.1 for study details). Most of these studies included both young and middle adults in their samples.

Two teams of investigators studied levels of drinking and related them to alcohol-related problems (Clapp & Segars, 1993) and health problems (Perreira & Sloan, 2002). Both found an association with heavy drinking and alcohol-related adverse events. Clapp and Segars (1993) found that young males age 18 to 25 (young adulthood) had the highest percentage of heavier drinkers (14%; $p < .01$) as compared with other age groups and experienced more acute problems such as intoxication and fighting. Males over age 35 experienced more driving under the influence of alcohol (DUI) citations (35% of DUIs reported) and reported more family problems.

These age groupings closely represented the definitions of young and middle adulthood as laid out at the beginning of this chapter, and the results seem to indicate that young and older adults differ in the types of alcohol-related problems they experience. Because one cannot determine onset of drinking in many of these studies, it is difficult to determine whether the alcohol-related adverse events were related to the length of the problem's existence or the age of the subject. In addition, the sample was drawn randomly from one urban county in California, rendering the findings limited in generalizability.

Perreira and Sloan (2002) analyzed drinking data from the National Health and Retirement Survey. In men age 51 to 61 at baseline and 6 years later, the heaviest drinkers (five drinks or more daily) had an increased risk of functional impairment ([odds ratio] OR = 4.21, 95%; [confidence interval] CI = 1.67, 10.6), depression (OR = 1.45, 95%; CI = 0.46, 4.60), and mortality (OR = 1.71, 95%; CI = 1.14, 2.56). Problem drinkers (CAGE $\geq$ 2) were at increased risk for psychiatric problems (OR = 2.15, 95%; CI = 1.47, 3.13). Drinking status did not significantly increase the risk for cardiovascular problems. Heavier drinking subjects were more likely to be lost to follow-up than their lighter drinking counterparts.

Holdcraft and Iacono (2002) found that in subjects ages 40 to 59 (middle adulthood), alcohol dependence was greater in younger women and men with an early onset of drinking. Although the study had a limited age range and the

TABLE 7.1 Studies on Incidence and Prevalence of Alcohol Misuse, Abuse, and Dependence in Young and Middle Adulthood

Authors	Sample and design	Age (years)	Variables	Alcohol variable measurement	Results
Banks et al. (2000)	$N = 198,296$ ($n = 1,853$ treatment; $n = 196,443$ comparison) White; males discharged from treatment program. Compared mortality to statewide sample	18–29, 30–49, 50–79	Mortality	Alcohol-related diagnoses or problem assessment	• Treated subjects had higher mortality in all age groups 18–29 years $RR = 4.3$ (95%, $CI = 2.2$, 7.6) 30–49 years $RR = 2.5$ (95%, $CI = 1.1$, 4.8) 50–79 years $RR = 1.5$ (95%, $CI = 1.1$, 2.4)
Clapp & Segars (1993)	$N = 1,656$ Alcohol use in one county in adults over 18; random phone calls.	18–25, 26–35, 36+	4 categories of drinking: quantity/frequency, alcohol problems, acute, and chronic	Abstinence, light, moderate, and heavy drinking	• Heaviest drinkers were males 18–25 • Males 18–25 had more acute problems • Men over 35 had more driving under the influence citations and more family problems

(continued)

217

TABLE 7.1 *(continued)*

Authors	Sample and design	Age (years)	Variables	Alcohol variable measurement	Results
Hisnanick (1992)	Review of hospital discharge records of Native Americans	4–19, 20–34, 35–49	Period prevalence by gender and age	Alcohol-related discharge diagnosis	• Period prevalence (total) 20–34 = 32.91 35–49 = 49.87 50–64 = 25.16 • Ratio of men to women ranged from 2.14 to 2.50
Holdcraft & Iacono (2002)	$N = 600$ (468 men, 132 women) Parents in twin study who met interview criteria for lifetime alcohol dependence, sample compared by gender and median birth year (1952)	40–59	Cohort effects on alcohol use	*DSM-III-R* lifetime dependence based on diagnostic interview	• Gender effect ($Z = -11.21$, $p < .0001$) • Cohort effect ($Z = -2.91$, $p < 0.0004$) • Higher dependence rate in later born men ($X^2 = 5.35$, $p = .021$) and later born women ($X^2 = 23.7$, $p = .001$) • Prevalence in later born women 11.7% greater than earlier born women

TABLE 7.1 *(continued)*

Authors	Sample and design	Age (years)	Variables	Alcohol variable measurement	Results
Perreira & Sloan (2002)	$N = 4,545$ Health and retirement study with national representative sample of men	51–61 at baseline, 57–67 at outcome	Health variables	2+ on CAGE was equated to problem drinking; quantity of alcohol	• 5+ per day drinkers had higher risk of functional impairment ($OR = 4.21$, 95%; $CI = 1.67$, 10.6) and depression ($OR = 1.45$, 95%; $CI = 0.46$, 4.60) • Problem drinkers had increased risk of psychiatric disorder ($OR = 2.15$, 95%; $CI = 1.46$, 3.13)
Ross et al. (1998)	$N = 854$ Women veterans	< 30, 30–39, 40–49, 50–59, > 59	Treatment received	DSM-III-R diagnosis of alcohol dependence	49% between 30 and 39; 47% received treatment; age × treatment effect ($X^2 = 46.8$, $df = 12$, $p < .001$); 60+ less likely to receive treatment, < 30 more likely to complete treatment

CI = confidence interval, DSM-III-R = *Diagnostic and Statistical Manual of Mental Disorders* (3rd ed., rev.), OR = odds ratio, RR = relative risk age was divided according to median age of the group rather than using a developmentally based or more standardized age ranges, the findings suggested cohort differences in drinking patterns.

Three studies drew samples from health records. Banks, Pandiani, Schacht, and Gauvin (2000) found that male subjects discharged from a community treatment program had higher mortality than the general population in all age groups (18–29, 30–49, 50–79). The relative risk (RR) of mortality was 4 times greater in young adults (18–25) (RR = 4.3; CI = 2.2, 7.6). Hisnanick (1992) calculated period prevalence rates (the number of cases during a designated period) of alcohol-related discharge diagnoses in a Native American and Alaska Native population. He used a hospital discharge database that spanned a period of 8 years. The numerical incidence was highest in young adults (20–34), and prevalence per 1,000 was highest in middle adults (35–49, period prevalence = 49.87). The ratio of men to women was approximately 2 to 1 in all age groupings. Among males, the greatest prevalence was in the 35 to 49 age group (period prevalence = 70.64).

Ross, Fortney, Lancaster, and Booth (1998) studied women veterans and found that the highest incidence of alcohol-related diagnoses was in 30- to 39-year-olds (young to middle adulthood, 49%). Women younger than age 30 were more likely to receive and complete treatment for alcohol abuse/dependence, whereas women over age 60 were less likely to receive treatment ($p < .001$). Overall, 47% of the sample received and 34% completed treatment. Although the generalizability of this study is limited by its sample of women veterans, the study did provide interesting data about the treatment of alcohol dependence in women related to age.

Summary and Critique

This wide-ranging group of studies all included age as a study variable. Although the studies do not build on each other, they do contribute a list of characteristics of alcohol misuse, abuse, and dependence in young adulthood or middle adulthood.

Each study used slightly different age groupings, although the range of 20 to mid-30s (the period of young adulthood as designated by this review) is used in two of the six studies (Clapp & Segars, 1993; Hisnanick, 1992). Middle adulthood (defined as ages 35 to 65 in this review) is variously represented as age 36+ years (Clapp & Segars, 1993), age 35 to 49 (Hisnanick, 1992), and age 57 to 67 (Perreira & Sloan, 2002), and an even more narrow age breakdown by Ross et al. (1998). Several investigators measured alcohol variables using diagnostic criteria, and others used quantity/frequency data (Banks et al., 2000; Hisnanick, 1992; Holdcraft & Iacono, 2002; Ross et al., 1998), making the outcomes difficult to compare. All measures were supportable if not comparable, but it is important to note that subjects who met the criteria for an alcohol-related diagnosis were generally further along the alcohol abuse–alcohol dependence continuum than those who report heavy or problem drinking, hence making population comparisons problematic.

The interaction of age and gender was apparent from data in several studies. The incidence and prevalence of drinking and alcohol dependence were lower in women as compared with men (Hisnanick, 1992; Holdcraft & Iacono, 2002), which is a usual finding across multiple studies. Holdcraft and Iacono found that later born cohorts of women had higher incidence of alcohol dependence and earlier onset of drinking than earlier born cohorts; however, this finding is mitigated by the narrow age range of the sample population overall (age 40–59) and the arbitrary age by which the sample was divided.

The findings for young adulthood (age 21–35) suggested that (1) males between age 18 and 25 had the highest proportion of heavy drinkers and the most acute alcohol-related problems (Clapp & Segars, 1993), (2) women under age 30 were more likely to complete treatment (Ross et al., 1998), and (3) there was increased mortality compared to other ages for post-treatment subjects (Banks et al., 2000). In studies of middle adulthood (age 35 to 65), (1) men had a higher rate of driving under the influence and family problems (Clapp & Segars, 1993); (2) men had the highest period prevalence rate of alcohol-related problems in a Native American sample (Hisnanick, 1992); and (3) men had an increased risk of functional impairment, depression, and other psychiatric disorders (Perreira & Sloan, 2002).

There are a limited number of focused epidemiological studies using age or developmental stage as a primary variable, and none were conducted by nurse-investigators. A more complete understanding of alcohol misuse, abuse, and addiction by age and developmental stage would help target high-risk groups and focus a primary prevention message to appropriate groups.

RESEARCH ON DEVELOPMENTAL CHANGES IN ALCOHOL MISUSE, ABUSE, AND ADDICTION

Themes in this segment included changes in alcohol misuse, abuse, and dependence over the life span. Table 7.2 describes both qualitative (some conducted by nurse-researchers) and quantitative studies in the area of developmental change.

Qualitative Studies

Investigators using qualitative methods have studied the processes of becoming alcohol dependent, mechanism for resolving alcohol dependence, and the unique qualities of the lives of women and men with alcohol misuse, abuse, and depen-

TABLE 7.2 Developmental Changes in Alcohol Misuse, Abuse, and Dependence

Authors	Sample and design	Age (years)	Variables	Alcohol variable measurement	Results
Bishof et al. (2003)	$N = 178$ with natural recovery	35–63	Adverse consequences, social support, social pressure, age of drinking onset	Severity scale, alcohol dependence, quantity/frequency of drinking	• Cluster analysis revealed clusters: age of onset, consequences, alcohol dependence, social pressures, and social support
Boyd & Mackey (2000a)	$N = 14$ Grounded theory, purposive sampling in women	26–53	Process of alcohol dependence	In treatment	• Basic psychosocial problem is alienation from self and others
Boyd & Mackey (2000b)	$N = 14$ Grounded theory, purposive sampling in women	26–53	Strategies for addressing alienation	In treatment	• Isolation via drinking • Secrets • Early onset drinking • Lack of problem-solving skills
Chen & Kandel (1995)	$N = 1,160$ Longitudinal study begun during high school years, with 19-year follow-up	34–35	Alcohol and other drug use	Drug/alcohol history	• Little new use occurred after age 29 • Age 18 was peak year for onset of alcohol use • Lifetime use for men was 99.2% and for women was 98.8%

TABLE 7.2 (*continued*)

Authors	Sample and design	Age (years)	Variables	Alcohol variable measurement	Results
Chilcoat & Breslau (1996)	$N = 1{,}007$ Interview	21–30	Parenthood, marriage, alcohol use	*DSM-III-R* diagnosis	• At baseline 21% met diagnostic criteria • Parenthood and marriage decreased alcohol use • Divorce has RR of 3.76 (95%; CI = 0.73, 19.46) for *DSM* diagnosis • No children had RR of 3.13 (95%; CI = 0.91, 10.8) for *DSM* diagnosis
Crum et al. (1993)	$N = 11{,}871$ Epidemiologic	—	Education, alcohol abuse and dependence	*DSM-III-R*	RR for alcohol abuse or dependence in the following populations: • College, no degree: RR 3.01 (95%; CI = 1.22, 7.38) • High school dropout: RR 6.34 (95%; CI = 2.42, 16.61) • Age of intoxication before 18 years: RR 5.92 (95%; CI = 3.14. 11.11)

(*continued*)

TABLE 7.2 (*continued*)

Authors	Sample and design	Age (years)	Variables	Alcohol variable measurement	Results
Finfgeld (1999)	N = 26 (14 women, 12 men) Grounded theory	24–66	Self-resolution process	AUDIT score	• Intrapersonal vs. interpersonal processes, self-vision threatened
Finfgeld & Lewis (2002)	N = 12 (7 women, 5 men) Grounded theory	19–26	Self-resolution process	AUDIT score	• Precarious footings • Seeking solid grounds • Standing on solid ground
Gotham et al. (1997)	N = 288 College seniors	~24	Personality model, role transition variables, alcohol involvement	SMAST Frequency of intoxication	• Correlation of frequency of intoxication with full-time employment ($r = -0.14$), marriage ($r = -0.22$), and parenthood ($r = -0.06$)
Grant (1998)	N = 27,616 National survey	13–21 at first drink	Age at drinking onset, family history	Lifetime alcohol dependence, DSM-IV criteria	• Age at drinking onset (age 13–21) related to greater risk of lifetime dependence not related to family history

TABLE 7.2 *(continued)*

Authors	Sample and design	Age (years)	Variables	Alcohol variable measurement	Results
Greenfield et al. (2003)	N = 101 Prospective study 1 year after hospitalization	Mean age by education: high school 47.6 college 42.2	Education, drinking outcomes, time to relapse	DSM diagnosis	• Subjects with high school education or less had more relapse and more drinking days
Mosher-Ashley & Rabon (2001)	N = 160 (73 men, 87 women) Members of Alcoholics Anonymous	< 39, 40–59, 60+	Depression, emotional support, loneliness, life satisfaction	Self-reported recovery	• Subjects age 39 differed significantly from those over 60 in emotional support, loneliness, depression, and life satisfaction ($p < .05$)
Paris & Bradley (2001)	N = 3 Narrative case studies	27, 43, 52	Stage of adult development	History	• Turning points in events and developmental changes assisted in drinking cessation

(continued)

TABLE 7.2 (continued)

Authors	Sample and design	Age (years)	Variables	Alcohol variable measurement	Results
Tucker et al. (1994)	N = 39 (21 abstinent, 18 nonabstinent)	Abstinent mean age 49.3, nonabstinent 41.6	Life events	MAST	• Life events and changes motivate abstinence and maintain resolution • Primary reasons for resolution: health problems, family problems, work problems • Primary maintenance factors: self-control, health, role of spouse
Wiseman & Souder (1996)	N = 46 (male Veterans Administration patients in treatment)	Older group mean age 62, younger group mean age 45	Denial	Treatment setting DSM criteria	• No difference between deniers based on age (p = .49)
Zakrzewski & Hector (2004)	N = 7 (Alcoholics Anonymous men) Existential-phenomenological method	32–65	Experience of alcohol addiction	Self-report	• Four themes: emotions, control, awareness of others, the turning point

AUDIT = Alcohol Use Disorders Identification Test, CI = confidence interval, DSM = *Diagnostic and Statistical Manual of Mental Disorders*, MAST = Michigan Alcoholism Screening Test, OR = odds ratio, RR = relative risk, SMAST = Shortened Michigan Alcoholism Screening Test dence. Qualitative studies allow the researcher to look more closely at individual psychological and developmental processes that are specific to alcohol use, misuse, and dependence and are particularly appropriate to the study of developmental issues.

Nurse-researchers Boyd and Mackey (2000a) interviewed rural women about the process of becoming alcohol dependent and used grounded theory to describe the underlying psychological process of alienation. Drinking was one strategy the subjects used to respond to alienation from oneself and others, although drinking became increasingly out of control during the process of alienation. Other themes were the lack of emotional support in childhood and abuse during childhood; this neglect and abuse were hypothesized to lead to stunted development of adult-level problem-solving skills. Zakrzewski and Hector (2004) interviewed males participating in Alcoholics Anonymous (AA) and used phenomenological interviewing to elicit four themes: emotions, control, awareness of others, and the turning point. One researcher was in recovery from alcohol dependence, and although he took care to bracket his own experience and validate his findings with co-investigators, the impact of this personal experience on the study's credibility cannot be determined.

Paris and Bradley (2001) used a narrative case study approach to detail the alcohol-related processes of three college women over time. The women were interviewed at ages 27, 43, and 52 (young and middle adulthood), and the investigators used Erikson's (1963) developmental tasks to review their developmental progress. Although this study is primarily a case study, it is a good example of the use of developmental theory. The results of the study paralleled the findings of Boyd and Mackey (2000a) by describing lack of emotional support during childhood. Each subject had a turning point in adulthood that led to abstinence from drinking and renewed progress in meeting developmental tasks and stages, but the adolescent developmental stage of identity was a stage these women found particularly difficult due to their own drinking behaviors and family problems. Although identity development is considered an adolescent developmental task, subjects with alcohol misuse, abuse, or addiction may find themselves dealing with this task in young or middle adulthood. The findings from these studies suggested that one impact of alcohol misuse, abuse, and addiction is that development tasks may be delayed, especially if the alcohol misuse begins early in life. Elements of developmental theory are apparent in the reports of stunted development (Boyd & Mackey, 2000a) and unresolved adolescent identity (Paris & Bradley, 2001).

Nurse-researchers Finfgeld (1999) and Finfgeld and Lewis (2002) used grounded theory to elucidate the process of recovery from alcohol abuse or dependence without formal treatment. They interviewed both men and women in two studies about what they termed the "self-resolution process." In the earlier study, Finfgeld (1999) found that subjects started the process of self-resolution due to intrapersonal rather interpersonal processes. That is, the driving force was information that threatened the subject's self-vision or self-view rather than information that revealed difficulties with other people. In the later study, Finfgeld and Lewis (2002) interviewed subjects in their young adult years (ages 19–26) and distilled the data into stages they metaphorically labeled as precarious footing, loss of footing, seeking solid ground, and standing on solid ground. The phenomenon of recovery without treatment has also been addressed quantitatively (see Bischof et al., 2003).

Quantitative Studies of Young Adult Subjects

In the body of research described below, developmental processes were defined quantitatively using age, and the investigators studied the effect of increasing age on alcohol misuse, abuse, and addiction. One effect of age on alcohol misuse is often described as the "maturational hypothesis," which involves a rapid rise in alcohol misuse and abuse in early adulthood with later decrease in consumption (NIAAA, 2000).

Chilcoat and Breslau (1996) and Gotham, Sher, and Wood (1997) investigated the marker events of young adulthood (marriage, parenthood, and role transition) and related those events to alcohol misuse. Both studies involved young adults (ages 21–30, mean age = ~ 24) who were interviewed at baseline and 3 to 4 years later. Chilcoat and Breslau (1996) found that marriage resulted in decreased risk of alcohol misuse or abuse and a reduced number of alcohol-related problems. Among subjects who were divorced or childless, the risk of alcohol misuse and alcohol-related problems increased (RR for divorced = 5.98, 95%; CI = 2.02, 17.75; RR for childless = 2.50, 95%; CI = 0.92, 6.77). Gotham et al. (1997) found that subjects reported decreased frequency of intoxication three years after college graduation ($F(4,1,120) = 16.21, p < .001$). The investigators found a negative association between frequency of intoxication and fulltime employment ($r = -.14; p < .05$), marriage ($r = -.22; p < .05$), and parenthood ($r = -.06$; n.s.). In a regression analysis of single variables, only full-time work was significant ($B = -.13$).

Chen and Kandal (1995) analyzed data from the Monitoring the Future study, a 19-year longitudinal study that began when subjects were in high school. Investigating alcohol and other drug use over time, they noted that few subjects initiated the use of any new substance after age 29 and that the major risk period for initiation of alcohol peaked at age 18. The highest use peaked between ages 19 and 21, but by ages 34 and 35, 8.3% of men and 16.3% of women had stopped drinking. Lifetime prevalence of alcohol use was 99.2% for men and 98.8% for women.

Quantitative Studies of Middle Adult Subjects

Tucker, Vuchinich, and Gladsjo (1994) reviewed life events in adult subjects (ages 30–61) who were recovering from alcohol abuse or dependence ($n = 21$) or actively drinking ($n = 18$). They found that some events motivated individuals with alcohol abuse and dependence toward abstinence, and other events reinforced continued abstinence or maintenance. The presence of health problems was a primary motivator for abstinence, and improved health was a primary reenforcer of continued sobriety. Although the sample was small, the investigators used collateral sources to corroborate self-reported data. Bischof et al. (2003) used measures of age at onset, severity of dependence, consequences of use, social support, and social pressure to develop three clusters of natural remitters, one with early onset (mean age = 28.8), high dependency, and low support; the second cluster with early onset (mean age = 26.8), high dependency, and medium support; and the third cluster with late onset (mean age = 37), low consequences, and high support. The sample was small ($N = 178$), considering that cluster analysis was performed. Subjects were recruited through newspaper ads, but accessing subjects with natural recovery is problematic.

The studies reviewed above focused on the types and degrees of resources and stressors experienced by alcohol abusers and how the balance between resources and stressors can affect the course of alcohol abuse. The findings have important implications for treatment and other community alcohol programs, as resources and stressors are potentially modifiable elements.

Longitudinal Studies with Young and Middle Adulthood Subjects

Grant (1998), in a review and analysis of the National Longitudinal Alcohol Epidemiologic Survey, concluded age at onset of drinking was a primary risk factor for lifetime alcohol dependence. He found that subjects who began drinking between the ages of 13 and 21 had a prevalence of lifetime alcohol dependence that increased as age of first alcohol use decreased. A family history of alcohol disorders added to this risk. For subjects who first used alcohol at age 13 or younger, the prevalence of lifetime alcohol dependence was 57.3% for those with a family history and 26.4% with no family history. For subjects who first used alcohol at age 21, the prevalence of lifetime alcohol dependence was 15.6% for those with a family history and 6.5% with no family history. These data are relevant when exploring alcohol abuse in the youngest group of adults who are 21 years of age.

Crum, Helzer, and Anthony (1993) interviewed adult subjects at baseline and 1 year later to compare alcohol use over the year. Alcohol use was compared to educational achievement in a partial analysis of data from a large prospective study, the Epidemiologic Catchment Area Study. Risk for alcohol-related diagnoses was 6 times as high among high school dropouts (RR = 6.34, 95%; CI = 0.73, 19.46; p < .001) and 3 times as high among college dropouts (RR = 3.01, 95%; CI = 1.22, 7.38; p = .016) compared with college graduates. Other factors that contributed to alcohol diagnoses were male gender, single status, and alcohol intoxication before age 18. Greenfield et al. (2003) found that post-treatment relapse differed by educational attainment. In a sample of post-treatment subjects recovering from alcohol abuse and dependence (n = 101), the researcher found that subjects with a high school education or less education relapsed more often (p = 0.11) and sooner (p = .007) than subjects with some college or higher levels of education.

Mosher-Ashley and Rabon (2001) surveyed a convenience sample of AA members about subjective well-being variables, including depression, life satisfaction, emotional support, and feelings of loneliness. Overall, the youngest group (≤ age 39) differed significantly from the ≥ age 60 group by reporting less support ($F(2,152)$ = 2.0, p = .015), more loneliness ($F(2,152)$ = 4.128, p = .01), more mild depression ($F(2,147)$ = 8.237, p = .0001), and less life satisfaction ($F(2,148)$ = 5.155, p = .007). The investigators suggested that subjects in recovery became more satisfied over time. The differences across age groups could also be due to increased stability of recovery or maturity or both. Wiseman and Souder (1996), the latter a nurse-researcher, studied denial of alcohol-related problems in Veterans Administration patients and found no difference between older and younger patients in degree of denial, although denial was considered to interfere with recovery. This study had a small number of subjects (n = 46) and a convenience sample, which limited its generalizability.

Summary and Critique

Qualitative findings indicated decreased emotional support, and decreased problem-solving skills were associated with alienation and increased alcohol misuse. Across several studies using phenomenological methods, a process-oriented series of steps emerged that include predrinking behaviors, drinking behaviors, and resolution of drinking. Zakrzewski and Hector (2004) noted that, without prompting, subjects organized the information around their drinking in these steps.

In young adulthood, the failure to meet developmental marker events such as employment, marriage, and parenthood increased the risk of alcohol misuse and abuse. Young adults who waited longer to initiate alcohol use have fewer alcohol-related problems throughout adulthood. Peak alcohol use occurred from ages 19 to 21, which supported the hypothesis of the "maturing out" of alcohol use (NIAAA, 2000). It also suggests that meeting and mastering the developmental tasks of young adulthood may provide protection from alcohol abuse.

Study samples drawn from middle adulthood populations more often represent those who have been in alcohol treatment or have been diagnosed with alcohol abuse or dependence (Bischof et al., 2003; Mosher-Ashley & Rabon, 2001; Tucker et al., 1994). Subjects who have resolved their alcohol abuse or dependence without treatment identified stressors and supports that created a balance for individuals with alcohol abuse or dependence and that predict abstinence or alcohol use.

Investigators implementing longitudinal studies identified onset of first alcohol use as a predictor of lifetime dependence, and education provided protection from alcohol abuse and dependence. Higher educational status decreased the risk of alcohol abuse and dependence and increased the likelihood of sustained recovery after treatment. Older AA members were more satisfied and less lonely and depressed than younger members. The findings collectively suggest differences between the issues that face young adults and adults in middle adulthood.

RESEARCH ON ALCOHOL MISUSE, ABUSE, AND DEPENDENCE IN WORK SETTINGS

A major time investment of young and middle adulthood is associated with occupation. Alcohol misuse, abuse, and dependence are of concern in work settings, particularly from the standpoints of productivity and safety. Work stress and alcohol use have been comprehensively reviewed by Frone (1999) and will not be included in this review.

Six studies summarized in Table 7.3 addressed work-related concerns. Because the majority of subjects were presumed to be within young or middle adulthood, leeway was used in their inclusion for this review. For inclusion, the investigators had to provide a mean age with standard deviation that fell into young and middle adulthood.

Veazie and Smith (2000) studied young adults, ages 24 to 32, to investigate the relationship between occupational injury and drinking. They found the odds for injury were only slightly increased with both heavy drinking (OR = 1.2, 95%; CI = 0.7, 2.1) and with alcohol dependence (OR = 1.1, 95%; CI = 0.7, 1.8).

Conrad, Furner, and Qian (1999) studied the relationship between exposure to occupational hazards, binge drinking, and drinking and driving by using the National Health Interview Survey (a household interview). They found that subjects in middle adulthood who were exposed to environmental hazards had slightly increased odds for binge drinking (OR = 1.36, 95%; CI = 1.24, 1.5) and drinking and driving (OR = 1.36, 95%; CI = 1.21, 1.53). This study was among the few that included a nurse researcher.

Ettner (1997) used the same dataset and found that unemployment slightly decreased alcohol consumption and dependence symptoms in individuals age

TABLE 7.3 Studies on Alcohol Misuse, Abuse, and Dependence in Young and Middle Adulthood in Work Settings

Authors	Sample and design	Age (years)	Variables	Alcohol variable measurement	Results
Conrad et al. (1999)	N = 15,907 National Health Interview Survey	Mean age = 37.7; SD = 11.6	Exposure to occupational hazards, drinking and driving	Binge drinking, days in past year with 5+ drinking	• Exposure to hazards 60% • Binge drinking 31% • Binge drinking with hazard exposure, OR = 1.35 (95%; CI = 1.24, 1.5) • Drinking and driving with hazard exposure, OR = 1.36 (95%; CI = 1.21, 1.53)
Ettner (1997)	N = 32,012 National Health Interview Survey	18–64	Work, not work; voluntary, not voluntary	Average daily consumption, alcohol dependence	Regression coefficients: • Effect of not working on alcohol consumption: −0.01 • Effect of not working on dependence: 0.01 • Effect of involuntary unemployment on alcohol consumption: 0.04 • Effect of involuntary unemployment on dependence symptoms: 0.86

TABLE 7.3 *(continued)*

Authors	Sample and design	Age (years)	Variables	Alcohol variable measurement	Results
Fisher et al. (2000)	$N = 5,389$ (heavy drinkers, $n = 2,242$; light drinkers, $n = 3,147$) Military personnel, probability sampling	NA	Lateness, leaving early, low performance, injury, missed work due to illness	Quantity/frequency, heavy or light drinking	• Light drinkers: 19.4% • Heavy drinkers: 13.9% • Late for work and leaving early, higher rates for heavy drinkers
Guppy & Maarsden (1997)	$N = 104$ Employees referred to employee assistance program (EAP) for screening, longitudinal follow-up at 6 months	Mean age = 42.2; SD = 10.2	Job satisfaction, job commitment, self-rating of work performance, supervisor's rating of work performance, work problems, mental health, absenteeism	None	• After EAP referral increased client work rating, increased supervisor work rating, decreased absences, improved mental health

(continued)

TABLE 7.3 (*continued*)

Authors	Sample and design	Age (years)	Variables	Alcohol variable measurement	Results
Veazie & Smith (2000)	$N = 8,569$ National Longitudinal Survey of Youth, secondary analysis	24–32	Occupational injury	Frequent heavy drinking, alcohol dependence	• 191 injuries • Heavy drinking did not increase injury risk (OR = 1.2, 95%; CI = 0.7, 2.1) • Dependence did not increase injury risk (OR = 1.1, 95%; CI = 0.7, 1.8)
Westrup et al. (2003)	$N = 187$ Internet-based assessment and intervention at one company	22–77 Mean age = 40.9; SD = 11.5	Alcohol consumption, stress, social readjustment, coping	High, medium, or low risk for alcohol-related problems	• 23% high risk • 31% moderate risk • 61% low risk • High and moderate risk rated interest in topic higher • High risk spent more time on Web site

AUDIT = Alcohol Use Disorders Identification Test, CI = confidence interval, DSM = *Diagnostic and Statistical Manual of Mental Disorders*, MAST = Michigan Alcoholism Screening Test, OR = odds ratio; RR = relative risk, SMAST = Shortened Michigan Alcoholism Screening Test

18 to 64. Job loss, defined as involuntary unemployment, increased alcohol consumption and dependence symptoms in the sample. Fisher, Hoffman, Austin-Lane, and Kao (2000) examined work characteristics and drinking in a military sample. Both light and heavy drinkers were more likely to be late for work (light drinkers $RR = 1.41$, 95%; $CI = 1.21$, 1.63; $p = .05$; heavy drinkers $RR = 1.90$, 95%; $CI = 1.32$, 2.72; $p = .05$), and leave early (light drinkers $RR = 1.29$, 95%; $CI = 1.17$, 1.43; $p = .05$; heavy drinkers $RR = 1.67$, 95%; $CI = 1.35$, 2.07; $p = .05$). In a surprising finding, light drinkers were more likely than heavy drinkers to exhibit low performance (light drinkers $RR = 1.52$, 95%; $CI = 1.36–1.70$; $p = .05$). These studies were all derived from large datasets, including the National Health Interview Survey (Conrad et al., 1999; Ettner, 1997) and the National Longitudinal Survey of Youth (Veazie & Smith, 2000).

Two smaller studies focus on assessment and interventions in the workplace for alcohol abuse among workers in middle adulthood. Westrup et al. (2003) tested an Internet-based assessment and intervention program in which subjects were stratified as low (61% of sample), moderate (17% of sample), or high risk (23% of sample) for alcohol dependence. Low- and moderate-risk subjects received either a randomly assigned limited individualized feedback or full individualized feedback. High-risk subjects were assigned a full individualized feedback intervention. Overall, subjects responded well to the Web-based program, and 8% reported a change in drinking behavior. High-risk subjects spent a greater amount of time using the Internet program and reported greater interest. The greatest concern of the subjects was confidentiality.

Guppy and Maarsden (1997) measured work variables in subjects who were referred to an employee assistance program (EAP) and followed afterward for 6 months. The subjects significantly increased their personal work ratings (paired $t = -6.8$, $p < .001$) and those of their supervisors (paired $t = -7.26$, $p < .001$). They also decreased absence periods (paired $t = 6.57$, $p < .001$) and absence days (paired $t = 7.52$, $p < .001$), and also improved their mental health (paired $t = 7.07$, $p < .001$). Both of these studies (Guppy & Maarsden, 1997; Westrup et al., 2003) supported the use of work-based alcohol intervention programs. The latter study was conducted in the United Kingdom, and it is unclear whether a similar study could be easily conducted in the United States, given the subjects' concerns about confidentiality.

Summary and Critique

The first four studies investigated the occupational setting and drinking from the point of view of work productivity and injury (Conrad et al., 1999; Ettner, 1997; Fisher et al., 2000; Veazie & Smith, 2000). The sample sizes of the studies were relatively large, but the findings for the most part did not show significant differences in the outcome variables among light, moderate, and heavy drinkers.

The use of secondary data analyses also limited the research findings. Though smaller in size and scope, the intervention studies (Guppy & Maarsden, 1997; Westrup et al., 2003) made a significant contribution to responding to alcohol misuse, abuse, and dependence in work settings by testing interventions.

RESEARCH ON ALCOHOL MISUSE, ABUSE, AND DEPENDENCE AMONG WOMEN AND FAMILIES

Women recovering from alcohol dependence and who began drinking prior to becoming a young or middle adult reported high rates of childhood sexual abuse (Wiechelt & Sales, 2001). The incidence of childhood sexual abuse among women with alcohol dependence is 34% to 77% (Wilsnack et al., 1997). The association between alcohol and child sexual abuse would imply that this is a serious societal problem, but there is very little research that evaluates differences between sexually abused females who misuse alcohol and those who do not. The studies that were found (Goodale & Stoner, 1994; Hall, 1996) lacked comparison groups, enrolled a small number of participants, and included persons with other psychological disorders.

Three research studies evaluated alcohol misuse in women and included family as a study variable, although the phenomenon of concern for each study was quite different. Wiechelt and Sales (2001) compared the recovery experience of female members ($N = 53$) of AA who reported a history of childhood sexual abuse (68%) with those who did not. A significant relationship was found between shame and measures of difficulties in recovery problems, but experiences of child sexual abuse did not predict difficulty in recovery. Pastor and Evans (2003) administered the Alcohol Expectancy Questionnaire (AEQ) to 85 women between ages 19 and 35. The AEQ is an empirically derived self-report instrument used to assess anticipated experiences associated with alcohol use, such as sexual enhancement and social and physical pleasure. Women with a confirmed parental history of alcohol dependence ($n = 41$) had higher composite scores on the AEQ than the 44 women with a negative family history of alcohol dependence. Women with a family history of alcohol misuse not only had an increased risk for alcohol abuse but also had more negative drinking outcomes if they were heavy drinkers.

Rush (2002) used the Social Support Network Inventory (SSNI) to assess perceived group, personal, and overall social support among 125 female AA members. Results indicated that perceived reciprocal support, as assessed and defined by the SSNI, contributed 67% of the variance related to group participation and maintaining sobriety. The availability and sponsorship from other women were important components of maintaining a supportive environment for women.

Research focusing specifically on women, in particular that which considered the family impact of alcohol misuse, was limited. Pastor and Evans (2003) and Rush (2002) found that women from families of alcoholics have an increased risk for alcohol abuse. The results from these studies shed light on how one might develop interventions that would be successful. When working with women who misuse alcohol, nurses should understand that this group requires continuous social support to deal with the availability of alcohol.

Intimate Relationships

One developmental goal of young adulthood is the achievement of an intimate relationship. Individuals who abuse alcohol have difficulties with boundaries, which limits their success toward developing exclusive relationships (Sullivan, 1995). The precise role of alcohol's impact on intimate partner violence is under investigation. Leonard (1993) suggested that alcohol use often preceded or accompanied acts of marital aggression. Male partner drinking has been significantly associated with intimate partner violence, although this effect is reduced when adjusted for associated female partner drinking. Female partner drinking was not associated with intimate partner violence (Leonard & Quigley, 1999). Research by Cunradi, Caetano, and Schafer (2002) replicated these findings. The relationship between alcohol and the developmental task of intimacy warrants further exploration, but studies to date suggest that alcohol interferes with meeting the task of intimacy.

Family Impact

The idea that alcohol dependence runs in families has been documented since a 1944 study by Roe, with studies from the 1970s supporting this fact (Cotton, 1979). The question of whether this occurs because children learn to drink from alcoholic parents or because of inheriting a gene that predisposes them to alcohol dependence has not been answered. The Collaborative Study on the Genetics of Alcoholism (CSGA) is a federally funded effort that aims to identify and characterize genetic factors associated with alcohol dependence. Thus far, analyses from this effort have identified regions on several chromosomes that are associated with traits correlated to alcohol dependence (Bierut et al., 2002). With or without the availability of genetic testing, a family history of alcohol abuse is a well-established risk factor for alcohol dependence and the adverse consequences of drinking.

Investigators have found associations among poor parenting, poor family environment, and the development of alcohol misuse (Zucker et al., 1996). Blanton et al. (1997) concluded that families with parents who abused alcohol have poor parent–child relationships. This finding is supported by the work of Curran, Stice, and Chassin (1997). The results of these studies indicate that children of families who abuse alcohol do not develop adequate emotional and behavioral self-regulation skills. The lack of adequate emotional-behavioral skills, along with the lack of social skills, increases the risk of peer-group rejection during young adulthood for these individuals (Baer, Novick, & Hummel-Schluger, 1995). Thus, poor parenting, combined with poor social skills, seemed to create a high-risk situation that favored alcohol misuse and abuse.

Long and Mullen (1994) studied Irish women's perceptions of the major factors that contributed to their alcohol abuse. The findings indicated that each participant could identify specific life events and crises that contributed to increased alcohol intake. Replicating this study across a number of populations would provide data with greater generalizability among ethnic populations and demonstrate the contributions of life stressors to alcohol misuse.

Role of Genetics

Twin studies have consistently reported the role of genetic risk among men (Caldwell & Gottesman, 1991). Shared environmental factors appeared to play a role in the development of alcoholic difficulties among women (Heath, Slutske, & Madden, 1998). Current knowledge includes the fact that approximately 50% to 60% of the risk for developing alcoholism is genetic (NIAAA, 2000). Genetic epidemiological research breaks new ground each day, and the hope is that future molecular studies will assist in resolving the impact of genetic versus family factors in the development of alcoholic abuse. As the genetics of alcohol dependence unfolds, it will have clinical implications for genetic counseling, gene therapy, and pharmacological approaches toward treatment (Hesselbrock et al., 2004). In addition to analyzing the DNA sequence of those who misuse alcohol, evaluating their mRNA levels may provide information about the activity levels of the DNA among different environmental conditions (Ehringer & Sikela, 2002).

In evaluating the available research on the genetic role in the development of alcohol misuse, the data are irrefutable. A genetic component may explain why some persons have alcohol problems at an early age or with only a few years of alcohol use. Although these data may be useful to identify those at risk for alcohol problems, a greater value may be in developing interventions that incorporate the genetic factor into the interventions themselves.

Although studies on family issues are quite varied, they highlight common themes. One is the commonality of sexual abuse in women with alcohol abuse and dependence. Difficult parenting and environmental conditions also contribute to the risk of alcohol misuse and abuse. The genetic underpinnings of alcohol abuse are not yet clearly defined, but a family history of alcohol abuse or dependence is a major risk factor for alcohol abuse in the individual.

CONCLUSION

The research reviewed in this chapter is quite varied and reflects numerous areas affected by alcohol misuse, abuse, and addiction in young and middle adulthood. There is more breadth than depth in many areas, little cohesion, and a dearth of replication. Little research by nurse-investigators was found despite the fact that the developmental perspective is consistent with nursing theory. This problem is of great concern because individuals with alcohol misuse problems are found commonly in health care settings and are a population at risk for a myriad of health problems.

Subjects

Subjects tended to come from three major sources: national surveys, treatment settings, and AA. Investigators using national prospective surveys with representative samples were usually longitudinal in nature and well designed statistically. Studies drawn from the treatment population accessed them during treatment or upon discharge. Investigators using treatment samples had more difficulty getting a random selection, and the subjects were usually from the alcohol-dependence end of the spectrum. AA provides a ready source of subjects, but it is impossible to randomize due to the anonymous nature of the organization. Also, subjects from AA tend to share the theoretical perspective of the organization, thus providing a limited worldview of the phenomenon under consideration.

Research Design

Studies with large databases produce findings that may be generalizable, but secondary analyses do not allow the researchers to manipulate variables or follow up new findings that were not part of the original design. The findings from these studies, though statistically significant, may not be clinically significant. Smaller, more flexible studies are needed to address some of the more subtle research questions in young and middle adulthood. Little experimental or treatment research was found. Qualitative studies are important for their ability to create a new level of understanding and data that may triangulate or further explicate quantitative studies, but the movement to interventions was clearly absent.

Content

Longitudinal studies reveal changes in alcohol misuse, abuse, and addiction over the life span, with a particular ability to capture developmental changes. Studies on natural recovery, that is, recovery without treatment, are an important source of information about a phenomenon only recently uncovered. This research broadens the understanding of recovery beyond traditional treatment settings. Research distinguishing variables that contribute to sobriety and its maintenance is warranted so that practical implications for treatment may evolve. Data about the significance of family history of alcohol abuse as a risk factor need further exploration. The combination of family history data and genetic markers provides an opportunity in the future to predict and potentially change risk of negative outcomes from alcohol.

Age and Developmental Stage

Alcohol-related research has made little use of age and developmental status as explanatory variables. To consider age from a developmental framework, an agreement on standard age ranges is warranted to allow comparisons across studies and emergence of stages of adulthood to emerge. The idea of changes in alcohol misuse between generational cohorts is interesting and merits further investigation.

Implications for Further Research

Most research focuses on either end of the misuse–dependence continuum, with population samples on one end and treatment samples on the other. The same limited focus occurs on the ends of the age continuum, with a large body of research on adolescence and older adulthood, and little on how individuals move back and forth on the alcohol use continuum during middle adulthood. Further work is also required to determine the upper limits of middle adulthood, to explore the age that transition to older adulthood occurs, and the role of alcohol in both.

There is also little work on the effect of age and developmental stage. A rich potential exists to use adult developmental stages to determine how prevention, early intervention, and treatment may affect individuals differently. Nurses are uniquely placed to do this work because of their understanding of the developmental stages, as well as their expertise in behavioral interventions.

REFERENCES

Baer, J. S., Novick, N. J., & Hummel-Schluger, A. O. (1995). Task persistence after alcohol consumption among children of alcoholics. *Alcoholism: Clinical and Experimental Research, 19*, 955–960.

Banks, S. M., Pandiani, J. A., Schacht, L. M., & Gauvin, L. M. (2000). Age and mortality among white male problem drinkers. *Addiction, 95,* 1249–1254.

Bierut, L. J., Saccone, N. L., Rice, J. P., Goate, A., Foroud, T., Edenberg, H., et al. (2002). Defining alcohol-related phenotypes in humans: The Collaborative Study on the Genetics of Alcoholism. *Alcohol Health and Research World, 26,* 208–213.

Bischof, G., Rumpf, H. J., Hapke, U., Meyer, C., & John, U. (2003). Types of natural recovery from alcohol dependence: A cluster analytic approach. *Addiction, 98,* 1737–1746.

Blanton, H., Gibbons, E. X., Gerrard, M., Conger, K. J., & Smith, G. E. (1997). Role of family and peers in the development of prototypes associated with substance use. *Journal of Family Psychology, 11*(3), 271–288.

Boyd, M. R., & Mackey, M. C. (2000a). Alienation from self and others: The psychosocial problem of rural alcoholic women, part 1. *Archives of Psychiatric Nursing, 14,* 134–141.

Boyd, M. R., & Mackey, M. C. (2000b). Running away to nowhere: Rural women's experiences of becoming alcohol dependent, part 2. *Archives of Psychiatric Nursing, 14,* 142–149.

Caldwell, C. B., & Gottesman, I. I. (1991). Sex differences and the risk for alcoholism: A twin study. *Behavior Genetics, 21,* 563–572.

Chen, K., & Kandel, D. B. (1995). The natural history of drug use from adolescence to the mid-thirties in a general population sample. *American Journal of Public Health, 85,* 41–47.

Chilcoat, H. D., & Breslau, N. (1996). Alcohol disorders in young adulthood: Effects of transitions into adult roles. *Journal of Health and Social Behavior, 37,* 339–349.

Clapp, J. D., & Segars, L. B. (1993). Alcohol consumption patterns and related problems: Results of a county survey. *Journal of Community Health, 18,* 153–161.

Conrad, J. M., Furner, S. E., & Qian, Y. (1999). Occupational hazard exposure and at risk drinking. *AAOHN Journal, 47,* 9–16.

Cotton, N. S. (1979). The familiar incidence of alcoholism: A review. *Journal of Advanced Studies on Alcohol, 40,* 89–116.

Crum, R. M., Helzer, J. E., & Anthony, J. C. (1993). Level of education and alcohol abuse and dependence in adulthood: A further inquiry. *American Journal of Public Health, 83,* 830–837.

Cunradi, C. B., Caetano, R., & Schafer, J. (2002). Alcohol-related problems, drug use and male intimate partner violence severity among U.S. couples. *Alcoholism: Clinical and Experimental Research, 26,* 493–500.

Curran, P. J., Stice, E., & Chassin, L. (1997). The relationship between adolescent alcohol use and peer alcohol use: A longitudinal random coefficients model. *Journal of Consulting and Clinical Psychology, 65,* 130–140.

Dawson, D. A., & Grant, B. F. (1998). Family history of alcoholism and gender: Their combined efforts on DSM-IV alcohol dependence and major depression. *Journal of Studies on Alcohol, 59,* 97–106.

Ehringer, M. A., & Sikela, J. M. (2002). Genomic approaches to the genetics of alcoholism. *Alcohol Research and Health, 26,* 181–192.

Erikson, E. (1963). *Childhood and society.* New York: Norton.

Ettner, S. L. (1997). Measuring the human cost of a weak economy: Does unemployment lead to alcohol abuse? *Social Science and Medicine, 44,* 251–260.

Finfgeld, D. L. (1999). Self-resolution of alcohol problems as a process of investing and re-investing in self. *Archives of Psychiatric Nursing, 13,* 212–220.

Finfgeld, D. L., & Lewis, L. M. (2002). Self-resolution of alcohol problems in young adulthood: A process of securing solid ground. *Qualitative Health Research, 12,* 581–592.

Fisher, C. A., Hoffman, K. J., Austin-Lane, J., & Kao, T. (2000). The relationship between heavy alcohol use and work productivity loss in active duty military personnel: A secondary analysis of the 1995 Department of Defense Worldwide Survey. *Military Medicine, 165,* 355–361.

Frone, M. R. (1999). Work stress and alcohol use. *Alcohol Research and Health, 23,* 284–292.

Goodale, T. S., & Stoner, S. B. (1994). Sexual abuse as a correlate of women's alcohol abuse. *Psychological Reports, 75*(3, part 2), 1596–1498.

Gotham, H. J., Sher, K. J., & Wood, P. K. (1997). Predicting stability and change in frequency of intoxication from the collge years to beyond: Individual-difference and role transition variables. *Journal of Abnormal Psychology, 106,* 619–629.

Grant, B. F. (1998). The impact of a family history of alcoholism on the relationship between age of onset of alcohol use and DSM-IV alcohol dependence. *Alcohol Health and Research World, 22,* 144–147.

———. (2000). Estimates of US children exposed to alcohol abuse and dependence in the family. *American Journal of Public Health, 90,* 112–115.

Greenfield, S. F., Sugarman, D. E., Muenz, L. R., Patterson, M. D., He, D. Y., & Weiss, R. D. (2003). The relationship between educational attainment and relapse among alcohol-dependent men and women: A prospective study. *Alcoholism: Clinical and Experimental Research, 27,* 1278–1285.

Guppy, A., & Maarsden, J. (1997). Assisting employees with drinking problems changes in mental health, job perceptions and work performance. *Work and Stress, 11,* 341–350.

Hall, J. M. (1996). Pervasive effects of childhood sexual abuse in lesbians' recovery from alcohol problems. *Substance Use and Misuse, 31,* 225–239.

Heath, A. C., Slutske, W., & Madden P. A. F. (1998). Gender differences in the genetic contribution to alcoholism risk and alcohol consumption patterns. In R. W. Wilsnack & S. C. Wilsnak (Eds.), *Gender and alcohol: Individual and social perspectives* (pp. 114–149). New Brunswick, NJ: Rutgers University Press.

Hesselbrock, V., Dick, D., Hesselbrock, M., Foroud, T., Schuckit, M., Edenberg, H., et al. (2004). The search for genetic risk factors associated with suicidal behavior. *Alcoholism: Clinical and Experimental Research, 28*(Supp. 5), 70S–76S.

Hisnanick, J. J. (1992). The prevalence of alcohol abuse among American Indians and Alaska natives. *Health Values, 16,* 32–37.

Holdcraft, L. C., & Iacono, W. G. (2002). Cohort effects on gender differences in alcohol dependence. *Addiction, 97,* 1025–1036.

Jackson, K. M., Sher, K. J., & Wood, P. K. (2000). Trajectories of current substance use disorders: A developmental, typological approach to comorbidity. *Alcoholism: Clinical and Experimental Research, 24,* 902–913.

Leonard, K. (1993). Drinking patterns and intoxication in martial violence: Review, critique and future directions for research. In S. Martin (Ed.), *Alcohol and interpersonal violence: Fostering interdisciplinary research* (NIAAA Research Monograph No. 24, NIH Pub. No. 93-3496). Rockville, MD: National Institutes of Health.

Leonard, K., & Quigley, B. M. (1999). Drinking and marital aggression in newlyweds: An event-based analysis of drinking and the occurrence of husband marital aggression. *Journal of Studies on Alcohol, 60,* 537–545.

Levinson, D. J. (1978). *The seasons of a man's life*. New York: Ballantine.

Long, A., & Mullen, B. (1994). An exploration of women's perceptions of the major factors that contributed to their alcohol abuse. *Journal of Advanced Nursing, 19*, 623–639.

Mosher-Ashley, P. M., & Rabon, C. E. (2001). A comparison of older and younger adults attending alcoholics anonymous. *Clinical Gerontologist, 24*, 27–37.

National Institute on Alcohol Abuse and Alcoholism (NIAAA). (2000). *10th special report to the U.S. Congress on alcohol and health* (NIH Pub. No. 00-1583). Rockville, MD: National Institutes of Health.

————. (2003, April 2). 5th National Screening Day to focus Americans on alcohol and health—NIAAA analysis suggests one-third of adults are "risky" drinkers. News release retrieved from www.niaaa.gov/press/2003/Screeningday03.htm

Paris, R., & Bradley, C. L. (2001). The challenge of adversity: Three narratives of alcohol dependence, recovery, and adult development. *Qualitative Health Research, 11*, 647–667.

Pastor, A. D., & Evans, S. M. (2003). Alcohol outcomes expectancies and risk for alcohol use problems in women with and without a family history of alcoholism. *Drug and Alcohol Dependence, 70*, 201–214.

Perreira, K. M., & Sloan, F. A. (2002). Excess alcohol consumption and health outcomes: A 6-year follow-up of men over age 50 from the health and retirement study. *Addiction, 97*, 301–310.

Prescott, C. A. (2002). Sex differences in the genetic risk for alcoholism. *Alcohol Research and Health, 26*, 264–273.

Roe, A. (1944). The adult adjustment of children of alcoholic parents raised in foster homes. *Quarterly Journal of Studies on Alcohol, 5*, 378–393.

Ross, R., Fortney, J., Lancaster, B., & Booth, B. M. (1998). Age, ethnicity, and comorbidity in a national sample of hospitalized alcohol-dependent women veterans. *Psychiatric Services, 49*, 663–668.

Rush, M. M. (2002). Perceived social support: Dimensions of social interaction among sober female participants in Alcoholics Anonymous. *Journal of the American Psychiatric Nurses Association, 8*, 114–119.

Sullivan, E. J. (1995). *Nursing care of clients with substance abuse*. St. Louis: Mosby.

Sullivan, E. J., & Handley, S. M. (1993). *Annual Review of Nursing Research* (Vol. 11). New York: Springer.

Tucker, J. A., Vuchinich, R. E., & Gladsjo, J. A. (1994). Environmental events surrounding natural recovery from alcohol-related problems. *Journal of Studies on Alcohol, 55*, 401–411.

Veazie, M. A., & Smith, G. S. (2000). Heavy drinking, alcohol dependence, and injuries at work among young workers in the US labor force. *Alcoholism: Clinical and Experimental Research, 24*, 1811–1819.

Westrup, D., Futa, K. T., Whitsell, S. D., Mussman, L., Wanat, S. F., Koopman, C., et al. (2003). Employees' reactions to an interactive website assessing alcohol use and risk for alcohol dependence, stress level and coping. *Journal of Substance Use, 8*, 104–111.

Wiechelt, S. A., & Sales, E. (2001). The role of shame in women's recovery from alcoholism: The impact of childhood sexual abuse. *Journal of Social Work Practice in the Addictions, 1*, 101–116.

Wilsnack, S. A., Vogeltanz, N. D., Klassen, A., & Harris, T. R. (1997). Childhood sexual abuse and women's substance abuse: National survey findings. *Journal of Studies on Alcohol, 58*, 264–271.

Wiseman, E. J., & Souder, E. (1996). Age and denial of alcoholism severity. *Clinical Gerontologist, 17,* 55–57.

Zakrzewski, R. F., & Hector, M. A. (2004). The lived experiences of alcohol addiction: Men of alcoholics anonymous. *Issues in Mental Health Nursing, 25,* 61–77.

Zucker, R. A., Kincaid, S. B., Fitzgerald, H. E., & Bingham, C. R. (1996). The development of alcoholic subtypes: Risk variation among alcoholic families during the childhood years. *Alcohol Health and Research World, 20,* 46–54.

Chapter 8

Alcohol Use, Misuse, Abuse, and Dependence in Later Adulthood

Joanne Sabol Stevenson

ABSTRACT

Considerable research has focused on alcohol problems in older adults, but the clinical utilization of this knowledge has lagged at least 3 decades behind the scientific developments. This unfortunate situation takes on added significance as the "baby boomer" generation ages because more of them drink more often in larger quantities than previous generations. This chapter focuses more on the ramifications of use, misuse, and abuse than on chronic dependence because the prevalence in the former categories far outweighs the latter.

Older alcohol misusers and abusers are at excess risk for myriad physical problems and premature death because alcohol interacts with the natural aging process in negative ways to increase risks for injuries, hypertension, cardiac dysrhythmic events, cancers, gastrointestinal problems, neurocognitive deficits, bone loss, and emotional challenges, most notably depression. Low volume and less than daily alcohol consumption appear to be protective against blood clots in the coronary and brain vessels, bone loss and falls, and cognitive decline compared with current abstainers. At higher levels, alcohol has the opposite effect.

Research findings strongly support positive outcomes of case finding, referral, and treatment of older adults who are misusing or abusing alcohol. However, there

245

is ample evidence that health care providers across the spectrum of primary, acute, and long-term care ignore the signs and symptoms of alcohol misuse and abuse in their older patients and treat symptoms and sequelae of the abuse rather than confronting the abuse itself. Recommendations for changes in practice are made together with ideas for additional research in several areas where the current state of knowledge is inadequate, conflicting, or based on narrowly homogeneous samples.

Keywords: alcohol misuse, alcohol abuse, alcoholism, older adult, elderly drinkers, late onset alcoholism

In the foreword to the National Institute on Alcohol and Alcoholism (NIAAA) 1998 monograph *Alcohol Problems and Aging*, then director Enoch Gordis acknowledged a growing public health concern about alcohol-related problems among older adults (defined as persons over age 65). The "baby boomer" population drinks more than previous generations and is expected to continue drinking during later adulthood. Indeed, North Americans born after World War II reportedly drink more than persons born during the 1920s or 1930s, reflecting a cohort effect influenced by the prevailing societal attitudes toward alcohol during their respective childhoods (Beresford, 1995). National data collected between 1997 and 2001 from respondents ages 60 to 85+ showed that 52.8% of men and 37.2% of women were current drinkers (Breslow, Faden, & Smothers, 2003). Older drinkers are more vulnerable than younger ones to a wide variety of negative alcohol sequelae, including deleterious effects of decades of alcohol use or abuse on organ systems; mixing alcohol with prescription drugs, or over-the-counter (OTC) drugs, which can prolong or inhibit their effects; decreased body water to muscle and fat ratio and reduced physiological tolerance for alcohol, with resulting risks for accidents, falls, and other harm to self or others; and psychological problems such as depression or suicide (Fink, Hays, Moore, & Beck, 1996; Waern, Spak, & Sundh, 2002).

Screening, one-on-one assessment, case finding, intervention, and referral for treatment are exceptionally challenging issues for those who care for and about elders. There are two dominant prevailing myths that stymie family members and care providers alike: One is the myth that alcohol use is a fitting reward for a lifetime of hard work and should not be curtailed in later adulthood; the second is the erroneous belief that older abusers or dependents cannot or will not change, and therefore attempts at intervention and treatment will be fruitless (McInnes & Powell, 1994).

This review attempts to clarify the state of the science about alcohol use, misuse, abuse, and dependence among older adults of both sexes. Excluded from the review were topics such as advanced alcoholic dementia, cirrhosis and other diseases of chronic alcoholism, and care during terminal stages of lifelong alcohol addiction. Rather, the review focuses on alcohol use, misuse, abuse, and dependence that are amenable to change at the individual, family, health care system (particularly primary care and acute care), and larger community levels. Health care providers have been documented over at least the last 20 years as being sublimely negligent about assessing older primary care (Arndt, Schultz, Turvey, & Petersen, 2002) and acute care patients (Schneekloth et al., 2001) for alcohol misuse and abuse. This negligence must be reversed.

METHOD

The literature search was set up to collect peer-reviewed reports of studies in these categories: epidemiologic surveys on prevalence of alcohol use in those over age 65 in the community, primary care, and acute care (long-term care was excluded from this review), including differences between men and women. Also reviewed were studies of the differences in alcohol tolerance and physiological and psychological effects among older adults, including gender differences. The sources that were systematically searched included the Cumulative Index of Nursing and Allied Health Literature (CINAHL), Medline, PsychINFO, EM-BASE, and the NIAAA and Substance Abuse and Mental Health Services Administration (SAMHSA) Web sites. In most instances, the literature from 1990 through July 2004 is reported, but in some instances older sources provided the only known work on a particular topic. Relevant reviews and meta-analyses from the general literature and the Cochrane Collaboration database also were used to increase understanding. Keywords used were *alcoholism, alcohol abuse, alcohol consumption, aging, older adult, elderly, late life,* and *treatment.*

PREVALENCE OF ALCOHOL USE AMONG THE OLDER ADULT POPULATION

In general, older adults report less alcohol intake compared with younger age groups. Other investigators reported conflicting data about whether or not heavy drinkers significantly decrease their alcohol use as they age. Because cross-sectional surveys do not follow the same people over time, these data do not capture the long-term behavioral integrity of drinkers. Longitudinal panel studies have shown considerable consistency in drinking over the life course (Kerr, Fillmore, & Bostrom 2002; Welte & Mirand, 1994), especially among heavy drinkers (Walton, Mudd, Blow, Chermack, & Gomberg, 2000). Longitudinal data from the Australian Twin Study (initiated in 1979) support the case for consistent drinking over adulthood until at least the mid-70s (Bucholz et al., 1998).

National surveys in the United States, including the N. Hanes Survey (Moore, Hays, Greendale, Damesyn, & Reuben, 1999), have consistently documented that between 40% and 62% of the older population drink alcohol, with older men consuming about twice as much as older women (Adams, Barry, & Fleming, 1996; Mirand & Welte, 1996). Heavy drinking (multiple definitions) ranged from 13% to 17% among older men and between 2% and 9% among older women (Graham, Carver, & Brett, 1996; Moore et al.; National Center on Addiction and Substance Abuse [NCASA], 1998; Sangwan, Damesyn, Reuben, Greendale, & Moore, 1997). Breslow and colleagues (2003) found lower and tighter figures in three national surveys. Heavy drinking among elderly men was 9.2% to 10.1% (CI [confidence interval] = 7.2–11.5), and among women it was 2.2% to 2.4% (CI = 1.4–3.3). Importantly, this study combined those from age 65 and older, including fairly large numbers of respondents who were age 85 and older, whereas earlier investigators made clear that their findings of steady intake persisted to age 70, but they could not discern intake beyond that. So the change in incidence may be due to the inclusion of many who were 80+ years old.

A problem with large survey studies that include elders is measurement error from quantity and frequency questions that may be answered in different ways by elders compared with younger persons; measurement error may occur if survey instruments used to determine problem drinking consist of items that focus on situations that are much more relevant to young and middle-age adults rather than older adults. Examples of young and middle-age adult foci include marital discord, coworker conflicts, drunk driving, employment difficulties, and financial problems (Fillmore et al., 1998; Temple et al., 1991). Hence, the surveys probably underestimate alcohol-related problems in elders who live alone or with spouses who are resigned to the drinking habits, only drive during earlier/ nonrush hours of the day or within the local community, and are retired and living on automatic monthly income checks. Furthermore, older adulthood covers almost 4 decades; within this population there are several cohorts with different alcohol expectancies and experiences. Gero-sensitive instruments are needed that include questions to differentiate among the young-old, middle-old, and old-old; between men and women; between Whites and several ethnic minorities; and between lifelong abstainers, "sick quitters," and treated dependents in remission in order to garner more valid data about incidence and prevalence of alcohol use and drinking problems among older adults. Screening items relevant to elder alcohol abuse or dependence include years of alcohol use, past and current quantity/frequency, mixing alcohol with medications, sleep quantity and quality, gastrointestinal symptoms, fine motor movement, problem-solving ability, and short-term memory testing.

THE PHENOMENON OF EARLY- AND LATE-ONSET ALCOHOL ABUSE

The concept of early- versus late-onset alcohol abuse and dependence emerged in the 1960s (Droller, 1964) and was firmly placed into the vernacular by Schuckit in 1977. Early onset generally refers to consistent alcohol abuse or dependence that manifested before age 36, and late onset is arbitrarily defined as alcohol abuse or dependence that began sometime after that (Schuckit, 1977). However, in more recent studies, late onset has been designated as occurring after retirement or at least after age 50 or 55 (Gomberg, Hegedus, & Zucker, 1998).

According to the American Medical Association (1996), about two thirds of elderly alcohol abusers and dependents are early onset, and the other one third are late onset. Older women are more often late-onset alcohol abusers/dependents than are men. In a study from the 1980s, Hurt, Finlayson, Morse, and Davis (1988) found the late onsets to be 46% of women compared to 39% of men, while later figures (Barrick & Connors, 2002; Brennan & Moos, 1991) showed analogous but smaller proportions of 33% women and 25% men.

Prospective and longitudinal studies of older adults who are multidecade alcohol abusers (early onset) indicate that compared to nonabusers, they come from lower socioeconomic backgrounds, have less education, are long-term smokers, were heavier drinkers in early adulthood or adolescence, experienced drinking in their families or socialized with drinkers, are more often single or divorced and estranged from family, use avoidance coping strategies for stress and problems, have histories of interpersonal or legal problems, but, paradoxically, have fewer comorbid (physical) medical conditions (Dawson, 2000b; Schonfeld & Dupree, 1991; Schutte, Brennan, & Moos, 1998). In fact, Nakamura et al. (1990) found that older drinkers, who retain their physical capabilities over the long term, are more likely to drink heavily. The Chou and Pickering (1992) data showed that 42.2% of early onset drinkers (mainly men) experienced alcohol-related lifestyle problems. Grant (1998) found a strong association between early-onset smoking and lifetime alcohol abuse or dependence. Stevenson and Masters (in review) found that lifetime smoking behavior and coffee drinking were strong predictors of heavier and longer-term alcohol use among older women.

In contrast, late-onset alcohol abusers have higher education and income levels and more family and social support systems in place. Investigators have attributed late-onset alcohol abuse to negative life events, including retirement, illness or death of a spouse, relocation, loss of lifelong friends, increasing social isolation, financial worries, degenerating health and functional ability, and depression (Brennan, Schutte, & Moos, 1999; Schutte et al., 1998; Wetterling, Veltrup, John, & Driessen, 2003). In one prospective 7-year study, risk factors for late-onset alcohol abuse included heavier lifelong drinking quantities, presence of chronic stressors, more social isolation or losses, and an avoidance coping style compared with abstainers and lifelong moderate drinkers (Brennan & Moos, 1996). Recently, these findings were corroborated by a 10-year prospective cohort study (Moos, Schutte, Brennan, & Moos, 2004; Schutte, Nichols, Brennan, & Moos, 2003). Perhaps late-onset drinkers always had the potential to use alcohol as a negative coping strategy, but they did not succumb to abuse or dependence until they crossed over some invisible line when their work schedule, family and social supports, or physical or mental health no longer helped keep their drinking behavior under control. It may also be that late-onset dependents have weaker genetic predispositions for the disease (Dawson, 2000b; Whitfield, Madden, Neale, Health, & Martin, 2004) than early onsets.

Late-onset male problem drinkers were found to have better overall health; better psychological functioning; more positive family, occupational, and social relationships; and were less likely to have been in alcohol treatment compared with early-onset male drinkers (Atkinson, 1994; Liberto & Oslin, 1995). In one of the few studies of late-onset older women, they were found to consume much less alcohol than men, but they were more depressed and used more psychoactive medications along with the alcohol (Brennan, Moos, & Kim, 1993) than late-onset men.

The late-onset group is more likely to complete treatment and have better long-term outcomes than their early-onset counterparts (Brennan et al., 1996a; Liberto & Oslin, 1995). Schutte, Brennan, and Moos (1994) found an overall 21% stable remission rate (abstinence) among treated late-onset alcohol abusers 4 years after treatment; this was double the 4-year remission rate for the treated early-onset group. Once older adults are engaged in treatment, it may appeal to them because it solves two problems: The alcohol problem is being solved, but, in addition, the prevalent inpatient and outpatient treatment models are social network enhancers. The programs introduce a new social world that includes a sponsor, attendance at meetings comprised of sincere and friendly people, helpful phone calls between meetings, transportation to meetings, and pre- and postmeeting social interactions. These activities can help fill the needs of older adults—especially late-onset isolated drinkers, widows/widowers, and the old-old—for repeopling their lives and gaining a new network of social support. In this process, they can find positive alternatives to the loneliness and isolation that some investigators posit as having led them to cross the line from moderate drinking to alcohol abuse or dependence.

Early-onset abusers, on the other hand, often find that remaining abstinent after treatment requires that they reject old drinking partners and places. Their job and/or place of residence may be in an area surrounded by temptation. They are often heavy smokers, and this may pose additional temptations to keep a drink in the opposite hand. They may feel ill at ease with the new social milieu of aftercare or Alcoholics Anonymous (AA) meetings. In addition, their biological addiction may be more advanced because it has been in process longer, or their genetic predisposition may be stronger. There are many reasons, both physiologic and psychosocial, why early onset problem drinkers would have more difficulty with post-treatment life compared to late-onset problem drinkers.

Interesting research lines of inquiry about early-onset alcohol dependents merit attention: first is uncovering genetic predispositions to alcohol dependence and using these finding to prevent early onset (and also late or delayed onset) addiction; second is developing and testing treatments for early-onset dependents that make use of genetic discoveries to ameliorate the brain chemical imbalances and simultaneously deal with the personal, social, cognitive, emotional, and physical problems resulting from decades of alcohol abuse.

ALCOHOL ABUSE OR DEPENDENCE, EXCESS MORTALITY, AND GENETICS

Early-onset alcohol abusers and dependents die about 10 years earlier than age-comparable abstainers and low-volume drinkers (Fried et al., 1998; Thun et al., 1997). The causes of death include heart and vessel diseases and stroke, several cancers, liver cirrhosis, pancreatitis, diabetes, kidney disease, pneumonia, car crashes or other trauma, victims or perpetrators of violence, suicide, and dementias (Corrao, Bagnardi, Zambon, & Arico, 1999; Corrao, Bagnardi, Zambon, & LaVecchia, 2004; Hanna, Chou, & Grant, 1997). Although both genders are equally prone to some of these diseases as sequelae of alcohol abuse (i.e., cancers of the mouth, pharynx, and esophagus, and liver cancer and cirrhosis), women have significantly more relative risk (RR) for hemorrhagic stroke compared with men ($RR = 7.98$ vs. 2.38), and slightly more for coronary heart disease ($RR = 1.12$ vs. 1.00) and diabetes ($RR = 1.13$ vs. 0.73). On the other hand, men are more prone to hypertension ($RR = 4.10$ vs. 2.00) and to ischemic stroke ($RR = 1.65$ vs. 1.06) (Bagnardi, Blangiardo, La Vecchia, & Corrao, 2001; Corrao et al., 1999; Corrao, Rubbiati, Bagnardi, Zambon, & Poikolainen, 2000). The risk of breast cancer for women drinkers over age 45 is between 1.14 and 1.62, depending on quantity/frequency, compared with abstainers (Smith-Warner et al., 1998).

Throughout adulthood, men are significantly more likely than women to comprise definite and likely categories of early-onset alcohol abuse/dependence, and thus men die prematurely in much larger numbers. Data on the ultimate effects of alcohol abuse from 10,268 persons (> age 65) in the longitudinal Canadian Study of Health and Aging showed an odds ratio (OR) of 1.56 (95%, CI 13.5–16.1) for early death after adjusting for age, sex, and dementia. This represented a 56% additional risk of death for the definite and probable alcohol abuser groups combined (Thomas & Rockwood, 2001).

Reportedly, alcohol abuse, even in late-onset drinkers, is associated with excess mortality (Li, Smith, & Baker, 1994). Dawson (2000a, 2001) matched the 1988 National Health Interview Survey—Alcohol Supplement dataset to the National Death Index for 1988–1995 and adjusted for several relevant demographic and other variables. Light and moderate drinkers did exhibit a slightly reduced risk of death ($OR = 0.68$ and 0.96, respectively). In contrast, heavy drinkers and dependent drinkers had significantly increased risk of excess mortality ($OR = 1.56$ and 1.65, respectively). Both groups were compared to abstainers and low-volume infrequent drinkers.

According to several twin studies, alcohol heritability accounts for 50% to 60% of the variance in development of alcohol dependence (Prescott, Aggen, & Kendler, 1999; Reich et al., 1998), although the results are much more consistent in early-onset males and in identical twins of both sexes. Genetics seems to play a role in early- versus late-onset alcohol dependence (Dawson, 2000b), perhaps explaining why female twin studies are less definitive than male twin studies about the heritability factor. Studies of male late-onset alcohol dependents also failed to show the strong heritability factor compared with early-onset males; the investigators surmised that late-onset men were genetically more like women dependents.

One hypothesis is that women need to have a higher level of inherited risk compared with men (perhaps an evolutionary protection for child bearing) before the disease becomes manifest. Conversely, data have shown that relatives of female dependents are at higher risk than are relatives of male dependents. Prescott (1999) conducted a meta-analysis on all types of pairs; data came from four twin studies, two adoption studies, and seven family studies. Across all samples there was a 40% greater risk for relatives of female alcohol dependents compared with male dependents. Studies of the genetics of alcohol dependence are at an early stage, but currently evidence favors a preeminent role for genetics in the development of alcohol dependence.

Gender Differences and the Special Case of Older Women

Alcohol abuse and dependence in older women take on added importance in older adulthood. One reason is the larger proportion of women in the older cohort; they outnumber men in all the decades after age 60, and this gender disproportion accelerates each decade thereafter (U.S. Bureau of the Census, 2000). Second, women are more often late-onset alcohol abusers or dependents (Hurt et al., 1988), and they may continue to drink more than one standard drink per day into late adulthood (Breslow et al., 2003). Third, women are more often widowed, and they experience loneliness, isolation, and depressive symptoms (Blow & Barry, 2002). Fourth, women are more vulnerable to the deleterious effects of alcohol in fewer drinking years and with less alcohol intake per episode compared with men (Chou & Dawson, 1994; Gomberg, 1995). Fifth, older women are unlikely to seek or be referred for treatment without external pressure or referral (Dawson, 1996). However, older women have shown long-term positive outcomes from treatment (Schutte, Byrne, Brennan, & Moos, 2001), so early case finding and treatment are worthwhile. Sixth, older women present to health care providers more frequently and in larger numbers than older men; hence, informed health care providers have more opportunities to detect alcohol problems before damage is irreversible.

Women drink only about 50% to 60% as much as men in most national surveys, but they become intoxicated at a lower dose (Eckardt et al., 1998; Taylor, Dolhert, Friedman, Mumenthaler, & Yesavage, 1996) and appear to experience physiological damage earlier in their drinking history and with more severe short- and long-term effects (Gambert & Katsoyannis, 1995; Li, Beard, Orr, Kwo, & Ramchandani, 1998). Women who abuse alcohol experience more overall physical harm in fewer years of harmful drinking and have death rates 50% to 100% higher than their male counterparts; they die earlier from cardiac and circulatory disorders, liver disease, and suicides (Fried et al., 1998; Thun et al., 1997). Women have less overall weight and less lean (muscle) weight in proportion to fat weight than men. Thus, women have a smaller volume of body water in which to distribute the alcohol compared with men (Thomasson, 1995). Dawson and Archer (1992) showed that, whereas men drank about twice as much as women, after accounting for differences in total body water, weight, body composition, and alcohol dehydrogenase (ADH) differences, the blood alcohol level was essentially the same. This conclusion seems to have formed the basis for the accepted formula that 1.0 standard drink for a man equals 0.5 standard drink for a woman (U.S. Department of Agriculture & Department of Health and Human Services, 2000; NIAAA, 2004).

Because women do experience more biological damage from fewer drinks per drinking episode and a shorter drinking history, recommendations for safe consumption levels are half those for men during young and middle adulthood (Anderson, Cremana, Paton, Turner, & Wallace, 1993). Interestingly, the NIAAA guideline of one drink per day (2004) is the same for older men and women. This seems at odds with the data about alcohol effects on women of all ages, but for the rationale we turn to information about the effects of aging on men. As men age, they lose lean muscle mass and body water; hence, they increase their body fat to lean mass and water ratio. Moreover, they produce less ADH and consequently experience decreased first-pass alcohol metabolism. The outcome is increased sensitivity to alcohol, and eventually older men appear to become essentially as sensitive as age-matched women (Pozzato et al., 1995).

PHYSIOLOGIC AND PSYCHOLOGIC EFFECTS OF ALCOHOL IN OLDER MEN AND WOMEN

Elders of both sexes experience important physiologic and psychological effects from consuming alcohol. The general finding is that low-volume consumption may have positive effects, but positive and deleterious effects may occur simultaneously in different body systems even with moderate intake.

Physiologic Effects

Cardiovascular Effects

Low-volume alcohol intake is associated with positive health outcomes and increased longevity (Camargo, Stampfer, Glynn, Grodstein, & Graziano, 1997; Dawson, 2000a; Fuchs et al., 1995; Thun et al., 1997). Reasons include slower blood clotting and less plaque formation, thus decreasing the risk of myocardial infarction (MI) and (ischemic) stroke (Wannamathee & Shaper, 1996; White, 1999).

Unfortunately, the definition and criteria of what constitutes low-volume drinking are anything but consensual. Some investigators used the NIAAA definition of moderate drinking for young and middle adults (two for men, one for women per day), and others (see chapter 2, Table 2.1) set it at a maximum of four or three (four for men, three for women) drinks per week. The NIAAA guideline of one standard drink per day for men and women over 65 was not mentioned as the criterion in the studies. Besides defining the maximum amount of alcohol intake, there must be a minimum because one drink per month was shown to have the same cardiovascular risk as total abstinence (Klatsky, 1999). Dufour (1999) offered one of the few definitions in the literature but called it light drinking: 0.01 to 0.21 fl oz of pure alcohol per day or 1 to 13 standard drinks per week. White (1999) concluded from a meta-analysis that all-cause mortality was lowest at 69.3 g (5.0 standard drinks) per week for U.S. men and 22.33 g (1.5 standard drinks) per week for U.S. women.

In the previously cited study by Stevenson et al. (in review), older women drinkers had higher levels of regular exercise, lower levels of low-density lipoprotein (LDL) cholesterol, and higher levels of high-density lipoprotein (HDL) cholesterol than abstainers, but they also had increased mean corpuscular volume (MCV) and serum glutamyltransferase. Bittner and colleagues (2000) found that, among women, older age, alcohol consumption, and prior estrogen use were each independently associated with higher HDL cholesterol levels. Mukamal and Rimm (2001) and Mukamal et al. (2003) found decreased coronary heart disease (CHD) among male moderate drinkers. Rimm and colleagues' (Rimm, Williams, Fosher, Criqui, & Stumplar, 1999) meta-analysis of 42 studies showed that two drinks per day raised triglyceride levels by 5.7%, which translates to a 4.6% increase in CHD risk. They also found a 7.5 mg/dl decrease in fibrinogen; this equates to a 12.5% decreased risk of MI, plus alcohol appeared to inhibit platelet aggregation. Thus, they concluded that when looked at in total, the differences in HDL cholesterol, triglycerides, and fibrinogen from low-volume alcohol intake appeared to result in a 24.7% reduction in risk of CHD for older women and men.

Other investigators have shown that low-volume drinkers differ from abstainers in other important health-related behaviors. Dufour's (1994) analysis of national survey data revealed that low-volume drinkers more often slept 7 to 8 hours per night, maintained ideal weight, and exercised regularly; Wannamethee and Shaper (1999) and Smothers and Bertolucci (2001) also uncovered healthy lifestyle behaviors as confounders of low-volume benefits. Hence, there may be interaction effects of these healthy behaviors that impact clotting and other protective factors and thus confound the moderate alcohol effect. Also, ingestion or noningestion of daily low-dose aspirin (81 mg) or alternative remedies and herbals that affect clotting were not addressed in any of these surveys. The Fillmore et al. (1998) meta-analysis showed that once "sick quitters" were removed from the abstainer groups, no difference remained between long-term abstainers and low-volume drinkers.

Some data suggest that even light and moderate drinking over many years is associated with increases in injuries (e.g., car crashes and falls) (Higgins, Wright, & Wrenn, 1996; Mukamal, Mittleman, et al., 2004; O'Loughlin, Robitaille, Boivin, & Suissa, 1993), hemorrhagic stroke, cirrhosis, breast cancer, and bowel cancer (Bagnardi et al., 2001; Corrao et al., 1999; Palomaki & Kaste, 1993). There also are data that implicate even low-volume alcohol with perturbations in heart rate variability, cardiac arrhythmias, and potential risk of sudden cardiac death (Masters & Stevenson, 2003; Masters, Stevenson, & Schaal, 2004). More research is needed to clarify the role of low-volume alcohol use in health protection and risk and to more precisely specify the quantity, frequency, and length of drinking history that distinguishes protection from harm for older adults. The concept of "net outcome" was proposed by Dufour (1996) to shed light on this question, but she admits the awesome difficulty posed by trying to partition out positive from negative alcohol effects, given the multiple confounding variables, including genetics, gender, quantity/frequency, length of drinking history, nutritional status, normal aging, coexisting chronic conditions, and health behaviors.

Inflammatory process is important in myocardial infarction. Some investigators have observed that moderate drinkers have lower levels of inflammation biomarkers, such as C-reactive protein (Imhof et al., 2001; Mukamal, Cushman, et al., 2004; Ridker, Buring, Shih, Matias, & Hennekens, 1998), thus implying possible protection from MI. Others have found higher levels of other markers, such as homocysteine, that would indicate increased risk of blood clots in the vessels (Jacques et al., 2001). These findings conflict, and so nothing can be concluded at this time. This area of research is at an immature stage, and much more work is required before definitive evidence can be reported.

The influence of low volume and frequency of alcohol intake on blood pressure is not clear, even though many studies have addressed the issue (Camargo & Rimm, 1996). Initially, alcohol dilates blood vessels and lowers blood pressure. On the other hand, longer-term consumption of two or more drinks per day in women and three or more drinks per day in men was associated with increases in blood pressure (Keil, Liese, Filipiak, Swales, & Grobbee, 1998). Alcohol abuse and dependence are generally related to hypertension in both men and women (Beilin, 1995; Seppa, Laippala, & Sillanaukee, 1994; Wanna-methee & Shaper, 1996). This finding seems to be contrary to the knowledge that alcohol relaxes smooth muscle and thus dilates blood vessels and lowers internal pressures. Some investigators have shown that blood pressure actually rises between drinking episodes rather than during the time that alcohol is in the bloodstream, so the implication is that alcohol withdrawal rather than alcohol in the bloodstream is to blame. Blood pressure seesawed in these experiments; it decreased in the evening shortly after a drinking episode but had risen by morning after a night of abstinence (Kawano et al., 1996). The role of circadian rhythm in these studies was not adequately explained; however, the findings are consistent with the observation that sympathetic nerve activity increases in the presence of acute alcohol withdrawal (Denison, Jern, Jagenburg, Wendestam, & Walllerstedt, 1997).

It is well accepted that alcohol has a deleterious effect on heart muscle and increases risk of cardiomyopathy (Shanmugan & Regan, 1996); indeed, this condition is more common in women. For unknown reasons, older women drinkers are more susceptible to cardiomyopathy than older men, and it occurs with shorter alcohol histories, lower lifetime consumption, and lower daily doses compared with men (Fernandez-Sola et al., 1997; Urbano-Marquez et al., 1995). Women alcohol abusers often present with rhythm disturbances, and this may be the first sign of alcohol abuse available to the health care provider. Indeed, it has been suggested that alcohol ingestion may account for one third of all new cases of atrial fibrillation (Lip, Beevers, Singh, & Watson, 1995) and should be a red flag for health care providers—especially when assessing older women patients.

Data from autopsies showed that sudden death due to ventricular arrhythmias occurred more often in alcohol abusers between drinking episodes rather than while alcohol was in the bloodstream (Clark, 1988; Wannamethee & Shaper, 1992, 1999). Investigators found that among 62 alcohol dependents undergoing inpatient alcohol withdrawal, nearly 50% had prolonged QT intervals that returned to normal after successful detoxification (Otero-Anton, Gonzalez-Quintela, Saborido, Torre, & Virgos, 1997). Abnormally high adrenaline and noradrenaline levels also have been found during detoxification, as have depleted stores of magnesium and potassium (Denison et al., 1997); all of these changes increase the chances for arrhythmias. Even after inpatient medical detoxification, some patients die (Hurt et al., 1996). These findings suggest that older people who try to stop drinking on their own may be at risk for arrhythmias and even sudden cardiac death. This finding also has implications for outpatient and inpatient detoxification, and also surgeries if medical detoxification is not done first. Considerably more research is needed in this area not only on larger samples of men and women but in animal models to determine the fundamental mechanisms that are involved. In addition, more attention needs to be paid to development and testing of safe and effective detoxification protocols for older adults with comorbid chronic conditions.

The data about cardiovascular effects of alcohol use and abuse are complex and often contradictory. Knowledge development should go forward to sort out more clearly (1) the true role of low-volume intake on prevention of MI and ischemic stroke and how alcohol interfaces with inflammation in blood vessels; (2) the precise effects of acute alcohol intake on blood pressure and arrhythmias versus the effects of acute (unmedicated) withdrawal; and (3) how and why older women develop arrhythmias and cardiomyopathies much more often than age-matched men, even though they drink about half as much as men and are more often late-onset alcohol abusers.

Gastrointestinal Effects

Alcohol's passage from the mouth through the gastrointestinal (GI) tract affects every tissue along the way. It can impair the muscles that separate the esophagus from the stomach (gastric reflux results in heartburn) (Bode & Bode, 1997, 2003). In the stomach, alcohol interferes with gastric acid secretion and weakens the muscles surrounding the stomach; this effect can lead to marked mucosal damage and inflammation (gastritis, gastric ulcers, and GI bleeding) (Bienia, Sodolski, & Luchowska, 2002; Chari, Teysson, & Singer, 1993). Alcohol can impair the muscles of the small and large intestine (sets up conditions for diarrhea); it also induces mucosal injuries in the duodenum and jejunum. These injured areas result in significantly increased permeability, allowing large molecules (endotoxins and bacterial toxins) to pass into the blood and lymph (Maier, Bode, Fritz, & Bode, 1999), resulting in bacterial overgrowth with liver damage, weight loss, and malnutrition (Adachi, Moore, Bradford, Gao, & Thurman, 1995; Schafer, Schips, Landig, Bode, & Bode, 1995).

Alcohol inhibits absorption of many nutrients (certain amino acids, fatty acids, carbohydrates, thiamine, folic acid, sodium, and water) (Pfeiffer, Schmidt, Vidon, Pehl, & Kaess, 1992). Bergheim and colleagues (2003) compared 76 alcohol abusers at various stages of alcoholic liver disease and 22 nondrinkers on nutrient intake and absorption. There were no differences in intake, but the alcohol consumers had significantly lower blood levels ($p < .05$) of several micronutrients (vitamin C, retinal, lycopene, alpha- and gamma-carotene, selenium, and zinc).

Neurocognitive Effects

Some investigators have found that low-volume alcohol consumption by older women resulted in fewer falls, better mobility, and improved physical functioning compared with abstainers (Mukamal, Mittleman, et al., 2004). In the same vein, Pfefferbaum, Rosenbloom, Servanti, and Sullivan (2002) and Mukamal (2004) found that older female drinkers were more resistant to some brain structure changes compared with older male drinkers. However, higher amounts and longer drinking histories showed opposite outcomes. Older alcohol-dependent women had more abnormal brain morphology than either age-matched female abstainers or male dependents (Hommer et al., 1996; Hommer, Momenan, Kaiser, & Rawlings, 2001; Pfefferbaum, Rosenbloom, Deshmukh, & Sullivan, 2001). Additionally, female alcohol dependents perform more poorly on recall and psychomotor tests compared with male dependents (although the men consumed 2 times more alcohol), and women drinkers (at levels of intake from moderate through heavy) are at higher risk for Alzheimer's disease and other dementias (Cupples et al., 2000; Orgogozo et al., 1997; Ruitenberg et al., 2002).

A nonlinear relationship between alcohol intake and neurocognitive deficits has been found in retrospective studies of older women drinkers. Intake of less than three standard drinks per day was correlated with improved cognitive ability, whereas three or more drinks per day showed the opposite effect (Zuccala et al., 2001). A prevailing hypothesis regarding the switchover from protective to detrimental effects of alcohol for women pinpoints the protective action of estrogen. A J-shaped curve is posited wherein up to three drinks per day seems to be covered by natural estrogen in younger women and by estrogen replacement therapy (ERT) in older women subjects. Beyond three drinks per day, estrogen effects are overpowered, and women experience increased risk for neurological damage (Cupples et al., 2000; Orgogozo et al., 1997; Pfefferbaum et al., 2002; Ruitenberg et al., 2002). Although the above data all came from retrospective descriptive human studies, some prospective animal studies also have shown the neuroprotective action of estrogen. One prospective human study showed that ERT starting before menopause decreased the risk of Alzheimer's disease (Tang et al., 1996). Apparently estrogen therapy works prophylactically (but not therapeutically once damage has occurred) by protecting blood supply to the brain during assaults from noxious substances such as alcohol (Dubal et al., 1998; Simpkins et al., 1997). Assuming this hypothesis holds up in future studies, the current movement of many postmenopausal women away from ERT would appear to have ramifications for more neurocognitive deficits among older women drinkers in the future.

Effects on Bone Density

Some epidemiological data showed that low-volume alcohol intake appeared to have a positive effect on bone density in postmenopausal women (Felson, Zhang, Hannan, Kannel, & Kiel, 1995; Naves-Diaz, O'Neill, & Silman, 1997), but chronic alcohol abuse is associated with substantially decreased bone density

(Hannan et al., 2000) and high risk for fractures (Feskanich, Korrick, Greenspan, Rosen, & Colditz, 1999). It has been suggested that low-volume alcohol produces either an increased estradiol release or a slowing of its degradation. Furthermore, alcohol may increase blood estradiol levels in ERT. The Hannan group (2000) (Framingham Osteoporosis Study (FOS)) found that ERT protected against loss of bone density and fractures. Once the quantity of alcohol moved above the protective threshold level, however, the bone density protective effects of estrogen were apparently overwhelmed. Data from the FOS showed that older women who drank three or more drinks per day (age range 67–90) had significantly more bone loss than age-matched women with minimal alcohol intake. For clarification of the fundamental mechanism, adult female rat studies showed that bone formation suffers more than resorption of old bone in the presence of alcohol (Hogan, Argueta, Moe, Nguyen, & Sampson, 2001).

Drinkers smoke more often than nondrinkers (75% more likely), and smokers are more likely to drink (86% more likely); the combination of smoking and drinking greatly increases the risk of bone loss and subsequent osteoporosis, especially among women (Shiffman & Balabanis, 1995). Kiel, Baron, Anderson, Hannan, and Felson (1992) suggested that smoking speeds the breakdown of estrogen and hence leads to more bone loss. Certainly more research is needed in this area to disentangle the separate contributions to bone sparing or loss of estrogen, smoking, and alcohol intake. However, it seems clear that older women smokers who present with significant bone loss should routinely be queried about the quantity and frequency of their alcohol intake. Positive findings about alcohol misuse or abuse should be addressed with an alcohol intervention, because in this situation, even moderate drinking is problem drinking.

Psychologic Effects

In a large home-based interview study of 826 older adults (Graham & Schmidt, 1998), nurse-interviewers found that poorer interpersonal relationships, decreased physical functioning, depression, and poorer psychological well-being correlated with heavier drinking per episode, but not with frequency of drinking episodes. There were no gender differences in the effects, although alcohol use was higher among cohorts of males, especially the younger-old group (age 65–74).

The relationship between depression and drinking behavior appears stronger for women than men. Schutte, Hearst, and Moos (1997) discovered that less depression at treatment intake predicted continued remission at 1 year equally for men and women, but higher levels of depression at intake among women predicted relapse before 1 year. Also, Skaff, Finney, and Moos (1999) showed that alcohol-abusing women not only had a higher incidence of depression than a comparison group of men, but also depended much more on friendships and social support. Findings across these and other studies are fairly consistent that women problem drinkers have more short- and long-term depressive symptoms than men (Krause, 1995; Schutte, Brennan, & Moos, 1995). Mining longitudinal data from a national representative sample of women, Graham and Wilsnack (2000) found a strong relationship between current use of tranquilizer drugs and alcohol problems in the past. Women appear to be more prone to negative emotional sequelae in general, and women alcohol abusers and dependents seem at risk during the active drinking period, during the treatment and early recovery period, and even years after continuous abstinence (Grant & Harford, 1995; Waern et al., 2002).

In contrast, Hasin and Grant (2002) analyzed data from the National Longitudinal Alcohol Epidemiologic Survey. Their sample consisted of 6,050 men and women former drinkers who had not smoked or used alcohol in the previous 12 months. The group was divided into those who had been moderate drinkers and those who had been alcohol dependent according to *Diagnostic and Statistical Manual of Mental Disorders* (4th ed.) criteria (*DSM-IV* American Psychiatric Association, 1994). The two groups were compared for current major depression using *DSM-IV* criteria. Linear logistic regression showed that the abstinent alcohol-dependent group had a fourfold risk of major depression when controlling for several intervening variables. Men and women had equally high associations between prior alcohol dependence and current depression.

The collective findings from this corpus of studies suggest that recovering alcohol abusers and dependents of both sexes are at excess risk of major depression long after they become abstinent. Unfortunately, the investigators did not collect information on possible intervening variables: degree of participation in AA; marital status, family relationships, friendships, and social support; exercise and nutritional status, perceived health status, and religiosity/spirituality; and use of psychoactive drugs. Research needed in the future includes genetic studies and brain metabolic studies to clarify whether alcohol abuse causes depression or whether genetics explains both conditions.

MIXING ALCOHOL WITH OVER-THE-COUNTER AND PRESCRIPTION DRUGS

There are two types of interactions between alcohol and medications, whether prescription, over-the-counter (OTC) drugs, herbal remedies, or illegal drugs: pharmacokinetic—alcohol interferes with the metabolism of the other drug—or pharmacodynamic—alcohol enhances the effects, usually central nervous system (CNS), of the other drug (Weathermon & Crabb, 1999). Pharmacokinetic interactions usually occur in the liver or stomach, where alcohol and other drugs vie for the same metabolic enzymes, prolonging the half-life of both substances; examples include drugs for stomach ulcers and heartburn. Pharmacodynamic interactions typically prolong the action of the drug, enhance its CNS depressant effects, and prolong the decrement in motor skills. The most common types of the latter are sedating antihistamines, barbiturates, nonnarcotic pain relievers, antidepressants, benzodiazepines, and herbal sleep aids (chamomile, valerian, and echinacea) (Adams, 1995; Forster, Pollow, & Stoller, 1993; Miller, 1998). Aspirin has the unique effect of increasing gastric emptying and thus increasing the blood alcohol level (BAL) from rapid alcohol absorption (Roine, Gentry, Hernandez-Munoz, Baraona, & Lieber, 1990). Older adults have exaggerated interaction effects due to less body water to dilute the substances and less liver and stomach ADH to metabolize the substances compared with younger persons.

Use of OTC drugs mixed with prescription drugs and alcohol is a common risk behavior among older adults (Fink et al., 2002; Solomon, Manepalli, Ireland, & Mahon, 1993). Among the 826 older adults in the Graham and Schmidt (1998) community study of alcohol effects in old age, antidepressant medication use was higher among all of the female age cohorts and one male cohort—the old-old males (75+)—compared with men under age 75. The 2-year National Center on Addiction and Substance Abuse (NCASA, 1998) national survey of older women found that 11% abused psychoactive drugs (7% abused alcohol). OTC drug use increases with age, especially among females, and two thirds of all elders take at least one OTC drug each day (Chrischilles et al., 1992; Forster et al., 1993). The most commonly used OTC drugs are analgesics, antacids/ digestive aids, laxatives, antihistamines, anticholinergics, and sleeping aids. The most commonly prescribed drugs for elders are cardiovascular medicines (22% of prescriptions), analgesics (20%), sedatives (10%), hypnotics (9%), tranquilizers (10%), and diuretics (9%) (Weathermon & Crabb, 1999). Combining prescription drugs with OTC drugs and alcohol is frequent, complex, and dangerous for older adults (Fink et al., 2002; Roeloffs, Fink, Unutzer, Tang, & Wells, 2001). According to the NCASA findings, older women are more likely than older men to mix alcohol with prescription psychoactive drugs.

Mixing alcohol and drugs during old age is exceptionally dangerous because aging results in decreases in lean body mass and body water, with resultant increases in body fat. Lipid-soluble drugs (e.g., psychotropics such as benzodiazepines) become stored in fat, resulting in prolonged half-lives. Toxic levels of drugs also can accumulate in the blood because serum albumin levels are reduced 10% to 20% in older adults, making it less available to bind with the drugs and thus leading to slower metabolic and excretion rates of the drugs (Bressler & Katz, 1993). Alcohol enhances or retards the metabolism of many drugs. Several vie with alcohol for dehydrogenase, so the half-lives of both substances are prolonged and the next dosage is taken while the previous dosage is still active (Thomas & Regan, 1990). This problem compounds itself with subsequent dosages of the drug and more alcohol consumption.

Numerous studies documenting that elders mixed alcohol with OTC and prescription drugs were published throughout the 1970s, 1980s, and 1990s

(Chrischilles et al., 1992; Finlayson, 1994; Forster et al., 1993). Early 21st-century research shows similar behaviors (Fink et al., 2002; Roeloffs et al., 2001). This continuance of risky drug–drug mixing and drug–alcohol mixing over at least 30 years indicates a failure among health care providers and public health officials to educate and warn older adults about the dangers of these practices. In fact, the problem today is no doubt much worse than the studies indicate because the studies did not incorporate herbal and folk remedies into the mix of drugs. Sales of herbal and other natural remedies have been escalating exponentially over the past decade. Future studies must address this deficit in the survey instruments and develop valid measures of the prevalence of mixing all three types of drugs with each other and with alcohol.

In addition, the health care community must find a way to intervene at the national, local, and individual level to educate the public about this preventable cause of excess morbidity. One hopeful sign is the partnership effort between the American Association of Retired Persons (AARP) and the Hazelden Foundation, a not-for-profit alcohol treatment facility in Minnesota. In 1995 they collaborated on publication and distribution of a pamphlet entitled *Alcohol, Medications, and Older Adults*. Because simply telling people not to perform a risky action is rarely successful in changing habituated behaviors, more research is needed to find successful approaches to decrease and eliminate mixing of OTCs, prescription drugs, and other substances with alcohol among the older adult population.

Challenges of Case Finding, Treatment, and Outcomes

One of the most persistent and troubling challenges surrounding alcohol abuse and dependence among older adults is the continued apathy about it among health care professionals. They overlook it, ignore the symptoms, and avoid diagnosing it.

Screening in Primary Care

The American Medical Association (1996), the American Nurses Association (1984), and the U.S. Preventive Services Task Force (2004) have all strongly recommended that patients be screened for both alcohol and drug abuse. Nevertheless, a long list of studies conducted over the past 20 years consistently has shown that adult problem drinkers of all ages, and older adults in particular, have very little chance of being assessed for alcohol problems or of being referred for alcohol treatment by their health care providers (Schneekloth et al., 2001). An analysis of 23,349 adults in the Centers for Disease Control and Prevention Behavioral Risk Factor Surveillance System—1997 showed that primary care practitioners rarely queried patients about their alcohol intake. White males, middle-adult women, older women, and widows were least likely to have alcohol usage mentioned during primary care visits (Arndt et al., 2002). Given the high risk for physical problems among older drinkers, it is unfortunate that they have little chance of being screened for harmful alcohol intake (Lichtenberg, Gibbons, Nanna, & Blumenthal, 1993; Moore, Beck, Babor, Hays, & Reuben, 2002).

Case Finding and Referral to Treatment

Elders do not self-present for alcohol treatment. Furthermore, in light of their age and work status, they are not coerced into treatment by employers, judges, school authorities, or family members. Although behavioral clues are evident—self-neglect, weight loss, sleeplessness and sleep deprivation, falls, depression, and confusion—the family and health care providers too often relegate these behaviors to normal changes of old age (Bercsi, Brickner, & Saha, 1993).

Instead of being pressed to seek treatment, these older problem drinkers continue to consume alcohol until some attention-getting or life-threatening crisis occurs, such as an acute medical condition, an accident, a fall, a bout of major depression, or a suicide attempt (Bercsi et al., 1993). Older persons who have alcohol treatment needs often demonstrate prodromal symptoms before the definitive crisis that include tangential vague symptoms, complaints of pain or sleep problems, and minor injuries. These complaints are presented to primary care providers, emergency department personnel, mental health professionals, or religious advisers, who, unfortunately, fail to recognize the underlying alcohol problem (Khan, Davis, Wilkinson, Sellman, & Graham, 2002).

McInnes and Powell (1994) found that only one third of inpatient alcohol abusers were accurately assessed in their intake history and physical. Although the community prevalence of alcohol abuse among elders is somewhere between 3% and 15%, the prevalence in acute care hospitals is much higher (Adams, Yuan, Barboriak, & Rimm, 1993; Beckett, Kouimtsidis, Reynolds, & Ghodse, 2002; Kouimtsidis et al., 2003) because alcohol abuse is a risk factor for so many medical conditions and emergency events that lead to hospitalization. Myriad studies of the incidence of alcohol abuse and dependence among hospitalized medical and surgical patients have shown the incidence of alcohol abuse or dependence ranges from 25% to 30% of men and 5% to 12% of women (Adams & Cox, 1995), but less than 4% of men and only about 2% of women have relevant notations in their charts, and referrals/consults for alcohol treatment are even more rare; findings in the latter category generally are less than 1% (Hearne, Connally, & Sheehan, 2002; Schneekloth et al., 2001).

Admitting elderly inpatients without gathering information about their alcohol history is exceptionally dangerous. As one example, surgical teams need to be alert to the high risks associated with operative patients who are withdrawing (unmedicated) from alcohol. A study of 42 surgical patients who were detoxified of alcohol for 1 month prior to surgery showed significantly different operative and postoperative experiences compared with a comparable group of patients who drank continuously up to hospital admission and were not detoxified before surgery (Tonnesen et al., 1999). The intervention group had fewer episodes of myocardial ischemia (23% vs. 85%), arrhythmias (33% vs. 86%), nighttime hypoxemia (4 vs. 18 episodes on postop day 2), and fewer postoperative complications (31% vs. 74%, $p = .02$). Considerably more research in this vein is needed, as is training of health care providers to routinely obtain a precise alcohol history when interviewing older adult preoperative patients.

Challenges of Treatment for Older Adults

Brief Interventions

For older adults, harmful drinking can mean drinking within the one drink per day limits set by the NIAAA. Harm at this low level can occur when alcohol is taken together with prescription, OTC, or herbal drugs that interact with alcohol. Additionally, harmful drinking can mean moderate alcohol intake in the presence of chronic conditions, such as hypertension, heart disease, and diabetes. Elders appear to be amenable to brief interventions when delivered by an authority figure, such as a health care provider. The primary care setting is an ideal location for these interventions. Fleming and colleagues (Fleming, Manwell, Barry, Adams, & Stauffacher, 1999) conducted a study of brief interventions (Project GOAL) delivered by 43 primary care physicians to 158 older problem drinkers (screened from 6,073 records). Interveners used a scripted workbook during two 10- to 15-minute sessions. After 12 months, 146 subjects remained, with 93 men and 53 women. The experimental group reduced 7-day alcohol use ($t = 3.77$, $p < .001$), episodes of binge drinking ($t = 2.68$, $p < .005$), and bouts of excessive drinking ($t = 2.65$, $p < .005$) compared with the control group. Similar positive results were obtained in other intervention studies and meta-analyses (Blow & Barry, 2000; Poikolainen, 1999; Wilk, Jensen, & Havighurst, 1997). Studies of brief interventions with larger and more diverse samples of older adults should be conducted. It is a cost-effective intervention that could be used with that subset of older adults who do not require acute inpatient detoxification and treatment.

Inpatient and Outpatient Treatment

In general, older adults should be detoxified as inpatients because of their vulnerable physiological state and the risk of multitoxicity from medications and alcohol. Beyond detoxification, a major question is whether older adults benefit from alcohol treatment and aftercare.

The proportion of older male alcohol abusers and dependents that completed inpatient and aftercare treatment was twice that of younger males (Atkinson, 1995). Treatment studies of older women alcohol abusers are few, but they too appear to respond well once all the hurdles of getting them diagnosed and into treatment are traversed (Rice, Longabaugh, Beattie, & Noel, 1993).

Some investigators found that both older men and older women respond better to senior-tailored regimens, including individual one-on-one counseling rather than group sessions; nonconfrontational approaches; slower-paced informational sessions; medical and nursing attention to their comorbid conditions and any physical disabilities or frailties; higher levels of structure and less ambiguity about post-treatment behavior changes; and comprehensive 12-month aftercare (Atkinson, 1995; Blow, 2000; Rice et al., 1993). Blow and colleagues (Blow, Walton, Chermack, Mudd, & Brower, 2000) found that at 6-month follow-up, patients who were treated in elder-specific inpatient alcohol units had positive outcomes across a range of measures, including general health and well-being. Data are sparse on the long-term outcomes of elders in specialized treatment compared with younger persons, but some investigators found 50% abstinence in elders compared with only 25% in younger groups 6 months after completion of treatment (Fitzgerald & Mulford, 1992; Oslin, Pettinati, & Volpicelli, 2002).

Currently, few special programs for older adults exist (Schultz, Arndt, & Liesveld, 2003), and many people speak against segregated treatment programs for older adults. Atkinson's (1995) meta-analysis of 11 of the better studies of mixed-age treatment outcomes found that older adults do well in mixed-age programs, but some studies included persons aged 45 and up, outcome measures were weak, there were few people over age 65 in the samples, and follow-up periods were too short. Newer data, however, also showed positive outcomes (Barrick & Connors, 2002; Lemke & Moos, 2002, 2003a,b). Perhaps the most salient arguments against separate programs are: high cost and inadequate numbers of staff trained to administer specialized care to elders.

Outcomes of Treatment

Intervening variables play a role in better treatment outcomes among late-onset compared with early-onset abusers and dependents (Kashner, Rodell, Ogden, Guggenheim, & Karson, 1992; Moos, Brennan, & Mertens, 1994; Rice et al., 1993). Treatment compliance is better among late-onset drinkers who more often finish the regimen and do not leave against medical advice, as early-onset drinkers tend to do. Late-onset drinkers usually have a family support system, a home, transportation to aftercare, and previous adult life experiences without alcohol upon which to draw. In one study, 56% of elders who completed inpatient treatment and outpatient aftercare remained abstinent after 6 months and were healthier (Blow et al., 2000).

Schutte and colleagues (2003) followed 3 groups of treated elder drinkers for 10 years and found long-term remission was predicted by being female, and long-term abstinence resulted in levels of overall functioning akin to nonproblem drinkers. An 8-year follow-up study of four groups of treated elderly problem drinkers (Timko, Moos, Finney, Moos, & Kaplowitz, 1999) showed that those who went into formal treatment immediately after diagnosis/confrontation about the problem drinking participated in more outpatient treatment, had more consistent participation in AA, and had the best long-term outcomes. The conclusion was that allowing time to pass after the interventions permits the patient's denial system to kick in and weakens the resolve of the family members, so that the window of opportunity for treatment is lost.

CRITIQUE OF THE RESEARCH

Demographic Issues

Definitions of terms and concepts are always a challenge. What is an older adult? When does this phase of life begin? Many studies with the term *aging* or *older adult* or *elderly* in the title actually included persons who were 50 or even 45 years old, with no way to separate out younger subjects. At the very least, 65 or 60 should be the beginning age for this population, and whatever age is chosen, consistency among investigators would be very helpful in interpreting results across studies.

Gender is a high-priority issue. Although research on older women increased in recent years, more questions were raised than answered. Moreover, studies of older men continue to concentrate largely on early-onset chronic dependents. It would be useful for some of the focus to shift to late-onset heavy drinking and abuse so that we can learn more about this phenomenon and how to prevent it or intervene in the negative trajectory.

Few minorities were included in the studies, although some investigators oversampled to ensure inclusion of minorities. Simply including some percentage of people from one or more minority groups in the sample does little to advance the knowledge base about alcohol use and abuse in these subpopulations during later life. Future studies should include comparison groups of minorities so that particular issues about their drinking problems and treatment issues can become clearer. Also, studies that focus on one minority group at a time would most certainly be informative. It is not possible to uncover the interactions of cultural differences in drinking expectancies and behaviors or to find fundamental differences in biologic reactions to alcohol unless the minority group forms an entire sample or an entire comparison group.

Drinking Patterns

Early versus late onset made sense when it was introduced in 1964. But with the ever-elongating life span, the late-onset portion of the term is fast losing its usefulness. By using age 36 as the start of late-onset alcohol abuse or dependence, at age 70 a person could have been drinking in a problematic manner for 35 years; thus, the original intent of the concept is lost. Increasing the number of groupings wherein early onset would remain as defined originally (through age 35), middle adult onset would include the period between ages 36 and 65 (retirement), and older adult onset/late onset would mean onset around age 65 (Gomberg et al., 1998). The better question is whether the designations are useful at all. Though it seems logical that they are useful to make and test projections of organ damage and disability, they have not been used that way to date. A clearer definitional system and longitudinal studies could be enlightening.

The relatively consistent demographic differences between the current two categories of early- and late-onset problem drinking would be useful for planning treatment program options. The long-term utility of forming research comparison groups comprised of early- and late-onset adults might be useful for genetic research; there may be inborn differences between these groups. Certainly, this would add a new dimension to the extant alcohol research that seems tightly tied to the study of demographics and coping styles as the rationale for early- versus late-onset problematic drinking patterns.

Operationalization of Variables

There were considerable differences in the meaning of concepts and variables in the studies. For example, abstainers were sometimes lifelong nonusers, sometimes consistently very low volume users who drank no more than 11 standard drinks in the past 12 months, and sometimes persons who had not used in the past 12 months but were higher-level drinkers in previous years. The latter group could have included "sick quitters" and recovering abusers or dependents. Such mixing of abstainer groups makes them a poor comparison for current drinker groups and renders the findings of the studies suspect.

Heavy drinking and *binge drinking* were two other terms that often were treated in a cavalier manner and often not defined at all. Even in the more rigorous studies, the cut point for women versus men often was not differentiated. Terminology needs to be precise, used within the study, and defined in the report. Whenever possible, nationally (NIAAA) or internationally (World Health Organization) approved consensus terms and definitions should be used. In this way, data from multiple studies can be compared, the science can move forward, and evidence-based practice will become more viable.

Measurement Issues

Instrument sensitivity and specificity are major concerns in studies of older adults. Essentially all of the alcohol-screening instruments and most other categories of instruments and criteria were designed for young and middle adults. Items do not match the current life experiences of older adults. Given that the drinking behavior of older men and older women is quite different (i.e., more social for older men and more isolated/hidden for older women), it may be appropriate to create different screening instruments for each gender. There is a temptation to suggest it would be best to simply collect quantity and frequency over a designated time frame. Then a drinking pattern of more than one standard drink per day, seven or more standard drinks per week, would be considered abuse. In a research project, that subject goes into the abuser group, and in a clinical context that person merits attention from a health care provider.

This approach, however, overlooks the interactions of genetic, gender, biological age, the overlay of chronic medical conditions, length of years that persons have been abusing alcohol, and mixing alcohol with prescription drugs, OTCs, or herbal remedies. Much more research is needed on the actual impact of these powerful intervening variables in older adults. Only then will it be possible to create evidence-based guidelines about safe moderate alcohol use in older adult women and men.

Target Populations

Many of the samples or parts of the samples were drawn from Veterans Administration (VA) patient populations, and this could have had profound influences on the findings, not only because they were generally more than 90% men but also because this is a special population and may not generalize well to older adult men in the community as a whole. In the future, more of the intervention studies should be done in Medicare and fee-for-service populations. Also, minorities should be a focus of study.

CONCLUSION AND RECOMMENDATIONS

Studies conducted after 1995 show alcohol use findings slightly higher than studies conducted during the 1970s, 1980s, and early 1990s, so the older cohort of the early 21st century seems more comfortable with alcohol than previous cohorts. Unfortunately, findings from earlier and newer studies show no improvement over a span of 30 years in screening, case finding, intervention, or referrals to treatment of older alcohol abusers or dependents. The few experiments in which physicians and nurses were trained to assess older patients and use brief interventions showed promise both in the responses of the elders and in the 6- and 12-month persistence of the trained providers. This aspect of research should be substantially expanded with more RCTs.

On the matter of gender, women drink far less than men and are more likely to be late-onset abusers. Yet women have higher risk for untoward outcomes, both physical and mental. Until recently the overwhelming majority of alcohol research focused on men; hence, most of what we accept as the basic principles about alcohol effects and the major treatment models emanated from research on men. Alcohol and depression needs its own "women's health initiative" to parallel the emerging findings about women and disease from work sponsored by the National Institutes of Health on cardiovascular conditions, cancers, and other conditions.

Alcohol scientists ought to decide what alcohol research will be when it grows up. The research still suffers from too much focus on VA patients, chronic psychiatric patients, and other captive audiences. The majority of older adult drinkers live in the general community, where they continue to work or are retired. Many of them are women who are hiding in plain view and need to be discovered by those who see them but do not look at them in a discerning way. Ordinary people should be inducted into research studies on alcohol use, misuse, abuse, and dependence to move the science forward.

Psychosocial theories about the cause of alcohol abuse and dependence still dominate the literature. Scientists continues to ruminate about demographic variables, personality characteristics, coping styles, and the triad of loneliness, anxiety, and depression. Findings from the human genome project and recent brain-related biochemical research need to be used to shine a bright light into the dusty corners of alcohol theory and research. We need to find out why women tolerate alcohol less well, why some people have a high tolerance for alcohol, why aging produces the changes in alcohol tolerance that it does, and why some people turn to alcohol abuse in early life, whereas others either never do so or do so late in life.

Importantly, we must find solutions to the question of why health care providers are so extremely reluctant to view alcohol abuse as a medical problem. This may be a health care services research question rather than a clinical research question. The problem is systemic rather than individual, and health services researchers should be commissioned to address the puzzle. Their mission would be to determine what changes are needed in medical and nursing schools, primary care environments, and acute hospital environments to increase screening, diagnosis, and treatment of alcohol abuse in all patients during all phases of life, from early adolescence through young, middle, and older adulthood, and with equal attention to women and men.

REFERENCES

Adachi, Y., Moore, L. E., Bradford, B. U., Gao, W., & Thurman, R. G. (1995). Antibiotics prevent liver injury in rats following long-term exposure to ethanol. *Gastroenterology, 108*, 218–224.

Adams, W. L. (1995). Interactions between alcohol and other drugs. *International Journal of Addiction, 30*, 1903–1923.

Adams, W. L., Barry, K. L., & Fleming, M. F. (1996). Screening for problem drinking in older primary care patients. *Journal of the American Medical Association, 276*, 1964–1967.

Adams, W. L., & Cox, N. S. (1995). Epidemiology of problem drinking among elderly people. *International Journal of Addiction, 30*, 1693–1716.

Adams, W. L., Yuan, Z., Barboriak, J. J., & Rimm, A. A. (1993). Alcohol-related hospitalizations of elderly people: Prevalence and geographic variation in the United States. *Journal of the American Medical Association, 270*, 1222–1225.

American Medical Association. (1996). Alcoholism in the elderly. *Journal of the American Medical Association, 275*, 797–801.

American Nurses Association. (1984). *Addictions and psychological dysfunctions: The profession's response to the problem.* Washington, DC: Author.

American Psychiatric Association. (1994). *Diagnostic and Statistical Manual of Mental Disorders* (4th ed.). Washington, DC: Author.

Anderson, P., Cremana, A., Paton, A., Turner, C., & Wallace, P. (1993). The risk of alcohol. *Addiction, 88*, 1493–1508.

Arndt, S., Schultz, S. K., Turvey, C., & Petersen, A. (2002). Screening for alcoholism in the primary care setting: Are we talking to the right people? *Journal of Family Practice, 51*, 41–46.

Atkinson, R. M. (1994). Late onset problem drinking in older adults. *International Journal of Geriatric Psychiatry, 9*, 321–326.

———. (1995). Treatment programs for aging alcoholics. In T. P. Beresford & E. S. L. Gomberg (Eds.), *Alcohol and aging* (pp. 3–18). New York: Oxford University Press.

Atkinson, R. M., Tolson, R. L., & Turner, J. A. (1993). Factors affecting outpatient treatment compliance of older male problem drinkers. *Journal of Studies in Alcohol, 54*, 102–106.

Bagnardi, V., Blangiardo, M., La Vecchia, C., & Corrao, G. (2001). Alcohol consumption and the risk of cancer: A meta-analysis. *Alcohol Research and Health, 25*, 263–270.

Barrick, C., & Connors, G. J. (2002). Relapse prevention and maintaining abstinence in older adults with alcohol-use disorders. *Drugs and Aging, 19*, 583–594.

Beckett, J., Kouimtsidis, C., Reynolds, M., & Ghodse, H. (2002). Substance misuse in elderly general hospital in-patients. *International Journal of Geriatric Psychiatry, 17*(2), 193–194.

Beilin, L. J. (1995). Alcohol and hypertension. *Clinical and Experimental Pharmacology and Physiology, 22*, 185–188.

Bercsi, S. J., Brickner, P. W., & Saha, D. C. (1993). Alcohol use and abuse in the frail, homebound elderly: A clinical analysis of 103 persons. *Drug and Alcohol Dependence, 33*, 139–149.

Beresford, T. P. (1995). Alcoholic elderly: Prevalence, screening, diagnosis, and prognosis. In T. P. Beresford & E. S. L. Gomberg (Eds.), *Alcohol and aging* (pp. 3–18). New York: Oxford University Press.

Bergheim, I., Parlesak, A., Dierks, C., Bode, J. C., & Bode, C. (2003). Nutritional deficiencies in German middle-class male alcohol consumers: Relation to dietary intake and severity of liver disease. *European Journal of Clinical Nutrition, 57,* 431–438.

Bienia, A., Sodolski, W., & Luchowska, E. (2002). The effect of chronic alcohol abuse on gastric and duodenal mucosa. *Annales Universitatis Mariae-Curie Sklodowska [Med.], 57,* 570–582.

Bittner, V., Simon, J. A., Fong, J., Blumenthal, R. S., Newby, K., & Stefanick, M. L. (2000). Correlates of high HDL cholesterol among women with coronary heart disease. *American Heart Journal, 139,* 288–296.

Blow, F. (2000). Treatment of older women with alcohol problems: Meeting the challenge for a special population. *Alcoholism: Clinical and Experimental Research, 24*(8), 1257–1266.

Blow, F. C., & Barry, K. L. (2000). Older patients with at-risk and problem drinking patterns: New developments in brief interventions. *Journal of Geriatric Psychiatry and Neurology, 13*(3), 115–123.

———. (2002). Use and misuse of alcohol among older women. *Alcohol Research and Health, 26,* 308–315.

Blow, F. C., Walton, M. A., Chermack, S. T., Mudd, S. A., & Brower, K. L. (2000). Older adult treatment outcome following elder-specific inpatient alcoholism treatment. *Journal of Substance Abuse Treatment, 19*(1), 67–75.

Bode, C., & Bode, J. C. (1997). Alcohol's role in gastrointestinal tract disorders. *Alcohol Health and Research World, 21,* 76–83.

———. (2003). Effect of alcohol consumption on the gut. *Best Practice and Research Clinical Gastroenterology, 17,* 572–592.

Brennan, P. L., & Moos, R. H. (1991). Functioning, life context, and help-seeking among late-onset problem drinkers: Comparison with nonproblem and early-onset problem drinkers. *British Journal of Addiction, 86,* 1139–1150.

———. (1996a). Late-life drinking behavior: The influence of personal characteristics, life context, and treatment. *Alcohol Health Research World, 20,* 197–204.

———. (1996b). Late-life problem drinking: Personal and environmental risk factors for 4-year functioning outcomes and treatment seeking. *Journal of Substance Abuse, 8*(2), 167–180.

Brennan, P. L., Moos, R. H., & Kim, J. Y. (1993). Gender differences in the individual characteristics and life contexts of late-middle-aged and older problem drinkers. *Addiction, 88,* 781–790.

Brennan, P. L., Schutte, K. K., & Moos, R. H. (1999). Reciprocal relations between stressors and drinking behavior: A three-wave panel study of late middle-aged and older women and men. *Addiction, 94*(5), 737–749.

Breslow, R. A., Faden, V. B., & Smothers, B. (2003). Alcohol consumption by elderly Americans. *Journal of Studies in Alcohol, 64,* 884–892.

Bressler, R., & Katz, M. D. (1993). Drug therapy for geriatric depression. *Drugs and Aging, 3,* 195–219.

Bucholz, K. K., Heath, A. D., Madden, P. A., Slutske, W. S., Statham, M. A., Dunne, M. P., et al. (1998). Drinking in an older population: Cross-sectional and longitudinal data from the Australian Twin Registry. In E. S. L. Gomberg, A. M. Hegedus, & R. A. Zucker (Eds.), *Alcohol problems and aging* (Vol. 33, pp. 41–62). Bethesda, MD: NIAAA.

Camargo, C. A., & Rimm, E. B. (1996). Epidemiological research on moderate alcohol consumption and blood pressure. In S. Zakhari & M. Wassef (Eds.), *Alcohol and the cardiovascular system* (Vol. 31, pp. 25–62). Washington, DC: NIAAA.

Camargo, C. A., Stampfer, M. J., Glynn, R. J., Grodstein, F., & Graziano, J. M. (1997). Moderate alcohol consumption and risk for angina pectoris or myocardial infarction in U.S. male physicians. *Annals of Internal Medicine, 126,* 364–371.

Chari, S., Teyssen, S., & Singer, M. V. (1993). Alcohol and gastric acid secretion in humans. *Gut, 34,* 843–837.

Chou, S. P., & Dawson, D. A. (1994). A study of the gender differences in morbidity among individual diagnoses with alcohol abuse and/or dependence. *Journal of Substance Abuse, 6,* 381–392.

Chou, S. P., & Pickering, R. P. (1992). Early onset of drinking as a risk factor for lifetime alcohol-related problems. *British Journal of Addiction, 87,* 1199–1204.

Chrischilles, E. A., Foley, D. J., Wallace, R. B., Lemke, J. H., Semla, T. P., Hanlon, J. T., et al. (1992). Use of medications by persons 65 and over: Data from the established populations for epidemiologic studies of the elderly. *Journal of Gerontology, 47,* M137–M144.

Clark, J. C. (1988). Sudden death in the chronic alcoholic. *Forensic Science International, 36*(1–2), 105–111.

Corrao, G., Bagnardi, V., Zambon, A., & Arico, S. (1999). Exploring the dose-response relationship between alcohol consumption and the risk of several alcohol-related conditions: A meta-analysis. *Addiction, 95,* 1551–1573.

Corrao, G., Bagnardi, V., Zambon, A., & La Vecchia, C. (2004). A meta-analysis of alcohol consumption and the risk of 15 diseases. *Preventive Medicine, 38,* 613–619.

Corrao, G., Rubbiati, L., Bagnardi, V., Zambon, A., & Poikolainen, K. (2000). Alcohol and coronary heart disease: A meta-analysis. *Addiction, 95,* 1505–1523.

Cupples, L. A., Weinberg, J., Beiser, A., Auerbach, S. H., Wells, J., Growdon, J. H., et al. (2000). Effects of smoking, alcohol and ApoE genotype on Alzheimer's disease. *Alzheimer's Reports, 3*(2), 105–114.

Dawson, D. A. (1996). Gender differences in the probability of alcohol treatment. *Journal of Substance Abuse, 8,* 211–225.

———. (2000a). Alcohol consumption, alcohol dependence, and all-cause mortality. *Alcohol Clinical and Experimental Research, 24*(1), 72–81.

———. (2000b). The link between family history and early onset alcoholism: Earlier initiation of drinking or more rapid development of dependence? *Journal of Studies on Alcohol, 61,* 637–646.

———. (2001). Alcohol and mortality from external causes. *Journal of Studies on Alcohol, 62,* 790–797.

Dawson, D. A., & Archer, L. (1992). Gender differences in alcohol consumption: Effects of measurement. *British Journal of Addiction, 87*(1), 119–123.

Denison, H., Jern, S., Jagenburg, R., Wendestam, C., & Wallerstedt, S. (1997). ST-segment changes and catecholamine-related myocardial enzyme release during alcohol withdrawal. *Alcohol and Alcoholism, 32*(2), 185–194.

Droller, H. (1964). Some aspects of alcoholism in the elderly. *Lancet, 13,* 137–139.

Dubal, D. B., Kashon, M. L., Pettigrew, L. C., Ren, J. M., Finklestein, S. P., Rau, S. W., et al. (1998). Estradiol protects against ischemic injury. *Journal of Cerebral Blood Flow and Metabolism, 18,* 1253–1258.

Dufour, M. C. (1994). Are there net health benefits from moderate alcohol consumption? Morbidity and other parameters of health. *Contemporary Drug Problems*, 21(1), 163–183.

———. (1996). Risks and benefits of alcohol use over the life span. *Alcohol Health and Research World*, 20(3), 145–152.

———. (1999). What is moderate drinking? *Alcohol Research and Health*, 23(1), 5–14.

Eckardt, M. J., File, S. E., Gesse, G. L., Hoffman, P. L., Grant, K. A., Guerri, C., et al. (1998). Effects of moderate alcohol consumption on the central nervous system. *Alcoholism*, 22, 998–1040.

Felson, D. T., Zhang, Y., Hannan, M. T., Kannel, W. B., & Kiel, D. P. (1995). Alcohol intake and bone mineral density in elderly men and women: The Framingham Study. *American Journal of Epidemiology*, 142, 485–492.

Fernandez-Sola, J., Estruch, R., Nicolas, J. M., Pare, J. C., Scanella, E., Antunez, E., & Urbano-Marquez, A. (1997). Comparison of alcoholic cardio-myopathy in women versus men. *American Journal of Cardiology*, 80, 481–485.

Feskanich, D., Korrick, S. A., Greenspan, S. L., Rosen, H. N., & Colditz, G. A. (1999). Moderate alcohol consumption and bone density among postmenopausal women. *Journal of Women's Health*, 8(1), 65–73.

Fillmore, K. M., Golding, J. M., Graves, K. L., Kniep, S., Leino, E. V., Romelsjo, A., et al. (1998). Alcohol consumption and mortality: Characteristics of drinking groups. *Addiction*, 93, 183–203.

Fink, A., Hays, R. D., Moore, A. A., & Beck, J. C. (1996). Alcohol-related problems in older persons: Determinants, consequences, and screening. *Archives of Internal Medicine*, 156, 1150–1156.

Fink, A., Morton, S. C., Beck, J. C., Hays, R. D., Spritzer, K., Oishi, S., et al. (2002). The alcohol-related problems survey: Identifying hazardous and harmful drinking in older primary care patients. *Journal of the American Geriatric Society*, 50, 1717–1722.

Finlayson, R. F. (1994). Prescription drug dependence in the elderly population: Demographic and clinical features of 100 inpatients. *Mayo Clinic Proceedings*, 69, 1137–1145.

Fitzgerald, J. L., & Mulford, H. A. (1992). Elderly vs younger problem drinker treatment and recovery experiences. *British Journal of Addiction*, 87, 1281–1291.

Fleming, M. F., Manwell, L. B., Barry, K. L., Adams, W., & Stauffacher, E. A. (1999). Brief physician advice for alcohol problems in older adults: A randomized community-based trial. *Journal of Family Practice*, 48, 378–384.

Forster, L. E., Pollow, R., & Stoller, E. P. (1993). Alcohol use and potential risk for alcohol-related adverse drug reaction among community-based elderly. *Journal of Community Health*, 18, 225–239.

Fried, L. P., Kronmal, R. A., Newman, A. B., Bild, D. E., Mittelmark, M. B., Polak, J., et al. (1998). Risk factors for 5-year mortality in older adults: The Cardiovascular Health Study. *Journal of the American Medical Association*, 278, 585–592.

Fuchs, C. S., Stampfer, M. J., Colditz, G. A., Giovannucci, E. L., Manson, J. E., Kawachi, I., et al. (1995). Alcohol consumption and mortality among women. *New England Journal of Medicine*, 332, 1245–1250.

Gambert, S. R., & Katsoyannis, K. K. (1995). Alcohol-related medical disorders of older heavy drinkers. In T. P. Beresford & E. S. L. Gomberg (Ed.), *Alcohol and aging* (pp. 70–81). New York: Oxford University Press.

Gomberg, E. S. L. (1995). Older women and alcohol use and abuse. In M. Galanter (Ed.), *Recent developments in alcoholism* (Vol. 12, pp. 61–79). New York: Plenum Press.

Gomberg, E. S. L., Hegedus, A. M., & Zucker, R. A. (1998). Research issues and priorities. In E. S. L. Gomberg, A. M. Hegedus, & R. A. Zucker (Eds.), *Alcohol problems and aging* (Vol. 33, pp. 451–475). Bethesda, MD: National Institutes of Health.

Graham, K., & Schmidt, G. (1998). The effects of drinking on health of older adults. *American Journal of Drug and Alcohol Abuse, 24*(3), 465–481.

———. (1999). Alcohol use and psychological well-being among older adults. *Journal of Studies on Alcohol, 60,* 345–351.

Graham, K., Carver, V., & Brett, P. J. (1996). Alcohol and drug use by older women: Results of a national survey. *Canadian Journal of Aging, 14*(4), 769–791.

Graham, K., & Wilsnack, S. C. (2000). The relationship between alcohol problems and use of tranquilizing drugs: Longitudinal patterns among American women. *Addictive Behaviors, 25*(1), 13–28.

Grant, B. F. (1998). The impact of a family history of alcoholism on the relationship between age of onset of alcohol use and DSM-IV alcohol dependence: Results of the National Longitudinal Alcohol Epidemiologic Survey. *Alcohol Health and Research World, 22,* 144–147.

Grant, B. F., & Harford, T. C. (1995). Comorbidity between DSM-IV alcohol use disorders and major depression: Results of a national survey. *Drug and Alcohol Dependence, 39,* 197–206.

Hanna, E. Z., Chou, S. P., & Grant, B. F. (1997). The relationship between drinking and heart disease morbidity in the United States: Results from the National Health Interview Survey. *Alcoholism: Clinical and Experimental Research, 21,* 111–118.

Hannan, M. T., Felson, D. T., Dawson-Hughes, B., Tucker, K. L., Cupples, L. A., Kiel, D. P., et al. (2000). Risk factors for longitudinal bone loss in elderly men and women: The Framingham Osteoporosis Study. *Journal of Bone and Mineral Research, 15,* 710–720.

Hasin, D. S., & Grant, B. F. (2002). Major depression in 6050 former drinkers: Association with past alcohol dependence. *Archives of General Psychiatry, 59*(9), 794–800.

Hearne, R., Connolly, A., & Sheehan, J. (2002). Alcohol abuse: Prevalence and detection in a general hospital. *Journal of the Royal Society of Medicine, 95*(2), 84–87.

Higgins, J. P., Wright, S. W., & Wrenn, K. D. (1996). Alcohol, the elderly, and motor vehicle crashes. *American Journal of Emergency Medicine, 14,* 265–267.

Hogan, H. A., Argueta, F., Moe, L., Nguyen, L. P., & Sampson, H. W. (2001). Adult-onset alcohol consumption induces osteopenia in female rats. *Alcoholism: Clinical and Experimental Research, 254,* 746–754.

Hommer, D., Momenan, R., Kaiser, E., & Rawlings, R. (2001). Evidence for a gender-related effect of alcoholism on brain volumes. *American Journal of Psychiatry, 158,* 198–204.

Hommer, D., Momenan, R., Rawlings, R., Ragan, P., Williams, W., Rio, D., et al. (1996). Decreased corpus collosum size among alcoholic women. *Archives of Neurology, 53,* 359–363.

Hurt, R. D., Finlayson, R. E., Morse, R. M., & Davis, L. J., Jr. (1988). Alcoholism in elderly persons: Medical aspects and prognosis for 216 inpatients. *Mayo Clinic Proceedings, 63,* 753–760.

Hurt, R. D., Offord, K. P., Croghan, I. T., Gomez-Dahl, L., Kottke, T. E., Morse, R. M., et al. (1996). Mortality following inpatient addictions treatment. *Journal of the American Medical Association, 275,* 1097–1103.

Imhof, A., Froehlich, M., Brenner, H., Boeing, H., Pepys, M. B., & Koenig, W. (2001). Effect of alcohol consumption on systemic markers of inflammation. *Lancet, 357,* 763–767.

Jacques, P. F., Bostom, A. G., Selhub, J., Rich, S., Ellison, R. C., Eckfeldt, J. H., et al. (2001). Effects of polymorphisms of methionine synthase and methionine synthase reductase on total plasma homocysteine in the NHLBI Family Heart Study. *Atherosclerosis, 166,* 49–55.

Kashner, T. M., Rodell, D. E., Ogden, S. R., Guggenheim, F. G., & Karson, C. N. (1992). Outcomes and costs of two V. A. inpatient treatment programs for older alcoholic patients. *Hospital and Community Psychiatry, 43,* 985–999.

Kawano, Y., Abe, H., Imanishi, M., Kojima, S., Yoshimi, H., Takishita, S., et al. (1996). Pressor and depressor hormones during alcohol-induced blood pressure reduction in hypertensive patients. *Journal of Human Hypertension, 10,* 595–599.

Keil, U., Liese, A., Filipak, P., Swales, J. D., & Grobbee, D. E. (1998). Alcohol, blood pressure, and hypertension. *Novartis Foundation Symposium, 216,* 125–144.

Kerr, W. C., Fillmore, K. M., & Bostrom, A. (2002). Stability of alcohol consumption over time: Evidence from three longitudinal surveys from the United States. *Journal of Studies on Alcohol, 63,* 325–333.

Khan, N., Davis, P., Wilkinson, T. J., Sellman, J. D., & Graham, P. (2002). Drinking patterns among older people in the community: Hidden from medical attention? *New Zealand Medical Journal, 115*(1148), 72–75.

Kiel, D. P., Baron, J. A., Anderson, J. J., Hannan, M. T., & Felson, D. T. (1992). Smoking eliminates the protective effect of oral estrogens on the prevention of hip fractures among women. *Annals of Internal Medicine, 116,* 716–721.

Klatsky, A. L. (1999). Moderate drinking and reduced risk of heart disease. *Alcohol Research and Health, 23,* 15–23.

Kouimtsidis, C., Reynolds, M., Hunt, M., Lind, J., Beckett, J., Drummond, C., et al. (2003). Substance use in the general hospital. *Addictive Behavior, 28,* 483–499.

Krause, N. (1995). Stress, alcohol use, and depressive symptoms in late life. *Gerontologist, 35,* 296–307.

Lemke, S., & Moos, R. H. (2002). Prognosis of older patients in mixed-age alcoholism treatment programs. *Journal of Substance Abuse Treatment, 22,* 33–43.

———. (2003a). Outcomes of 1 and 5 years for older patients with alcohol use disorders. *Journal of Substance Abuse Treatment, 24*(1), 43–50.

———. (2003b). Treatment and outcomes of older patients with alcohol use disorders in community residential programs. *Journal of Studies on Alcohol, 64,* 219–226.

Li, G., Smith, G. S., & Baker, S. P. (1994). Drinking behavior in relation to cause of death among U.S. adults. *American Journal of Public Health, 84,* 1402–1406.

Li, T. K., Beard, J. D., Orr, W. E., Kwo, P. Y., & Ramchandani, V. A. (1998). Gender and ethnic differences in alcohol metabolism. *Alcoholism: Clinical and Experimental Research, 22,* 771–772.

Liberto, J. G., & Oslin, D. W. (1995). Early versus late onset of alcoholism in the elderly. *International Journal of the Addictions, 30,* 1799–1818.

Lichtenberg, P. A., Gibbons, T. A., Nanna, M., & Blumenthal, F. (1993). The effects of age and gender on the prevalence and detection of alcohol abuse in elderly medical inpatients. *Clinical Gerontologist, 13*(3), 17–27.

Lip, G. Y., Beevers, D. G., Singh, S. P., & Watson, R. D. (1995). ABC of atrial fibrillation: Aetiology, pathology, and clinical features. *British Medical Journal, 311*, 1245–1328.

Maier, A., Bode, C., Fritz, P., & Bode, J. C. (1999). Effects of chronic alcohol abuse on duodenal monomuclear cells in man. *Digestive Diseases and Sciences, 44*, 691–696.

Masters, J. A., & Stevenson, J. S. (2003). A theoretical model of the role of brain stem nuclei in alcohol-mediated arrhythmogenesis in older adults. *Biological Research for Nursing, 4*, 218–231.

Masters, J. A., Stevenson, J. S., & Schaal, S. F. (2004). The association between moderate drinking and heart rate variability in healthy community-dwelling older women. *Biological Research for Nursing, 5*, 222–233.

McInnes, E., & Powell, J. (1994). Drug and alcohol referrals: Are elderly substance abuse diagnoses and referrals being missed? *British Medical Journal, 308*, 444–446.

Miller, L. G. (1998). Herbal medicinals. *Archives of Internal Medicine, 158*, 2200–2211.

Mirand, A. L., & Welte, J. W. (1996). Alcohol consumption among the elderly in a general population, Erie County, New York. *American Journal of Public Health, 86*, 978–984.

Moore, A. A., Beck, J. C., Babor, T. F., Hays, R. D., & Reuben, D. B. (2002). Beyond alcoholism: Identifying older, at-risk drinkers in primary care. *Journal of Studies on Alcohol, 63*, 316–324.

Moore, A. A., Hays, R. D., Greendale, G. A., Damesyn, M., & Reuben, D. B. (1999). Drinking habits among older persons: Findings from the NHANES 1 Epidemiologic Follow-up Study (1982–84). *Journal of the American Geriatrics Society, 47*, 412–416.

Moos, R., Brennan, P. L., & Mertens, J. R. (1994). Diagnostic sub-groups and predictors of one-year re-admission among late-middle-aged and older substance abuse patients. *Journal of Studies on Alcohol, 55*, 173–183.

Moos, R. H., Schutte, K., Brennan, P. L., & Moos, B. S. (2004). Ten-year patterns of alcohol consumption and drinking problems among older women and men. *Addiction, 99*, 829–838.

Mukamal, K. J. (2004). Alcohol consumption and abnormalities of brain structure and vasculature. *American Journal of Geriatric Cardiology, 13*(1), 22–28.

Mukamal, K. J., Conigrave, K. M., Mittleman, M. A., Camargo, C. A., Jr., Stampfer, M. J., Willett, W. C., et al. (2003). Roles of drinking pattern and type of alcohol consumed in coronary heart disease in men. *New England Journal of Medicine, 348*, 109–118.

Mukamal, K. J., Cushman, M., Mittleman, M. A., Tracy, R. P., & Siscovick, D. S. (2004). Alcohol consumption and inflammatory markers in older adults in the Cardiovascular Health Study. *Atherosclerosis, 173*, 79–87.

Mukamal, K. J., Mittleman, M. A., Longstreth, W. T., Jr, Newman, A. B., Fried, L., & Siscovick, D. S. (2004). Self-reported alcohol consumption and falls in older adults: Cross-sectional and longitudinal analyses of the Cardiovascular Health Study. *Journal of the American Geriatric Society, 52*, 1174–1179.

Mukamal, K. J., & Rimm, E. B. (2001). Alcohol's effects on the risk for coronary heart disease. *Alcohol Research and Health, 25*, 255–261.

Nakamura, C., Molgaard, C. A., Stanfords, E., Peddecord, K. M., Morton, D. J., Lockery, S. A., et al. (1990). A discriminant analysis of severe alcohol consumption among older persons. *Alcohol and Alcoholism, 25*(1), 75–80.

National Center on Addiction and Substance Abuse (NCASA). (1998). *Under the rug: Substance abuse and the mature woman.* New York: Columbia University. Retrieved on September 15, 2004, from http://www.casa.columbia.org

National Institute on Alcohol Abuse and Alcoholism (NIAAA). (2004). Definition of a standard drink. Retrieved June 15, 2004, from http://www.niaaa.nih.gov/publications/niaaa-guide/standardDrinksChart.htm

Naves-Diaz, M., O'Neill, T. W., & Silman, A. J. (1997). The influence of alcohol consumption on the risk of vertebral deformity: European Vertebral Osteoporosis Study Group. *Osteoporosis International, 7*(1), 65–71.

O'Loughlin, J. L., Robitaille, Y., Boivin, J. F., & Suissa, S. (1993). Incidence and risk factors for falls and injurious falls among the community dwelling elderly. *American Journal of Epidemiology, 137,* 342–354.

Orgogozo, J. M., Dartigues, J. F., Lafont, S., Letenneur, L., Commenges, D., Salamon, R., et al. (1997). Wine consumption and dementia in the elderly: A prospective community study in the Bordeaux area. *Revue Neurologique (Paris), 153,* 185–192.

Oslin, D. W., Pettinati, H., & Volpicelli, J. R. (2002). Alcoholism treatment adherence: Older age predicts better adherence and drinking outcomes. *American Journal of Geriatric Psychiatry, 10,* 740–747.

Otero-Anton, E., Gonzalez-Quintela, A., Saborido, J., Torre, J. A., & Virgos, A. E. (1997). Prolongation of the QTc interval during alcohol withdrawal syndrome. *Acta Cardiologica, 52,* 285–294.

Palomaki, H., & Kaste, M. (1993). Regular light-to-moderate intake of alcohol and the risk of ischemic stroke: Is there a beneficial effect? *Stroke, 24,* 1828–1832.

Patterson, T. L., & Jeste, D. V. (1999). The potential impact of the baby-boom generation on substance abuse among elderly persons. *Psychiatric Services, 50,* 1184–1188.

Pfeiffer, A., Schmidt, T., Vidon, N., Pehl, C., & Kaess, H. (1992). Absorption of a nutrient solution in chronic alcoholics without nutrient deficiencies and liver cirrhosis. *Scandinavian Journal of Gastroenterology, 27,* 1023–1030.

Pfefferbaum, A., Rosenbloom, M., Deshmukh, A., & Sullivan, E. (2001). Sex differences in the effects of alcohol on brain structure. *American Journal of Psychiatry, 158*(2), 188–197.

Pfefferbaum, A., Rosenbloom, M., Servanti, K. L., & Sullivan, E. (2002). Corpus callosum, pons, and cortical white matter in alcoholic women. *Alcoholism: Clinical and Experimental Research, 26,* 400–406.

Poikolainen, K. (1999). Effectiveness of brief interventions to reduce alcohol intake in primary health care populations: A meta-analysis. *Preventive Medicine, 28*(5), 503–509.

Pozzato, G., Moretti, M., Franzin, F., Croce, L. S., Lacchin, T., Benedetti, G., et al. (1995). Ethanol metabolism and aging: The role of "first pass metabolism" and gastric alcohol dehydrogenase activity. *Journal of Gerontology, 50A,* B135–141.

Prescott, C. A., Aggen, S. H., & Kendler, K. S. (1999). Sex differences in the sources of genenic liability to alcohol abuse and dependence in a population-based sample of U.S. twins. *Alcoholism: Clinical and Experimental Research, 23,* 1136–1144.

Prescott, C. A. (1999). The genetic epidemiology of alcoholism: Sex differences and future directions. In D. P. Agarwal & H. K. Seitz (Eds.), *Alcohol in health and disease* (pp. 125–149). New York: Marcel Dekker.

Reich, T., Edenberg, H. J., Goate, A., Williams, J. T., Rice, K. P., Van Eerdewegh, P., et al. (1998). Genome-wide search for genes affecting the risk for alcohol dependence. *American Journal of Medical Genetics, 81,* 207–215.

Rice, C., Longabaugh, R., Beattie, M., & Noel, N. (1993). Age group differences in response to treatment for problematic alcohol use. *Addiction, 88,* 1369–1375.

Ridker, P. M., Buring, J. E., Shih, J., Matias, M., & Hennekens, C. H. (1998). Prospective study of C-reative protein and the risk of future cardiovascular events among apparently healthy women. *Circulation, 98,* 731–733.

Rimm, E. B., Williams, P., Fosher, K., Criqui, M. H., & Stampler, M. J. (1999). Moderate alcohol intake and lower risk of coronary heart disease: A meta-analysis of effects of lipids and haemostatic factors. *British Medical Journal, 319,* 1523–1528.

Roeloffs, C. A., Fink, A., Unutzer, J., Tang, L., & Wells, K. B. (2001). Problematic substance usc, depressive symptoms, and gender in primary care. *Psychiatric Services, 52,* 1251–1253.

Roine, R., Gentry, R. T., Hernandez-Munoz, R., Baraona, E., & Lieber, C. S. (1990). Aspirin increases blood alcohol concentration in humans after ingestion of ethanol. *Journal of the American Medical Association, 264,* 2406–2408.

Ruitenberg, A., van Sweiten, J. C., Witteman, J. C., Mehta, K. M., van Duijn, C. V., Hofman, A., et al. (2002). Alcohol consumption and risk of dementia: The Rotterdam Study. *Lancet, 359,* 281–286.

Sangwan, N., Damesyn, M., Reuben, D., Greendale, G., & Moore, A. (1997). Lifetime alcohol use and alcohol-related conditions in older persons. *Journal of the American Geriatrics Society, 45*(9), S5.

Schafer, C., Schips, I. Landig, J., Bode, J. C., & Bode, C. (1995). Tumor-necrosis-factor and interelukin-6 response of peripheral blood monocytes to low concentrations of lipopolysaccharide in patients with alcoholic liver disease. *Zut Gastroenterolgy, 33,* 503–508.

Schneekloth, T. D., Morse, R. M., Herrick, L. M., Suman, V. J., Offord, K. P., & Davis, L. J. (2001). Point prevalence of alcoholism in hospitalized patients: Continuing challenges of detection, assessment, and diagnosis. *Mayo Clinic Proceedings, 76,* 457–458.

Schonfeld, L., & Dupree, L. W. (1991). Antecedents of drinking for early-and late-onset alcohol abusers. *Journal of Studies on Alcohol, 52,* 587–592.

Schuckit, M. A. (1977). Geriatric alcoholism and drug abuse. *Gerontologist, 17,* 168–174.

Schultz, S. K., Arndt, S., & Liesveld, J. (2003). Locations of facilities with special programs for older substance abuse clients in the U.S. *International Journal of Geriatric Psychiatry, 18,* 839–843.

Schutte, K. K., Brennan, P. L., & Moos, R. H. (1994). Remission of late-life drinking problems: A 4-year follow-up. *Alcoholism: Clinical and Experimental Research, 18,* 835–844.

———. (1995). Depression and drinking behavior among women and men: A three-wave longitudinal study of older adults. *Journal of Consulting Clinical Psychology, 63,* 810–822.

———. (1998). Predicting the development of late-life-onset drinking problems: A 7-year prospective study. *Alcoholism: Clinical and Experimental Research, 22*(6), 1349–1358.

Schutte, K. K., Byrne, F. E., Brennan, P. L., & Moos, R. H. (2001). Successful remission of late-life drinking problems: A 10-year follow-up. *Journal of Studies on Alcohol, 62*(3), 322–334.

Schutte, K. K., Hearst, J., & Moos, R. H. (1997). Gender differences in the relations between depressive symptoms and drinking behavior among problem drinkers: A three-wave study. *Journal of Consulting Psychology, 65,* 392–404.

Schutte, K. K., Nichols, K. A., Brennan, P. L., & Moos, R. H. (2003). A ten-year follow-up of older former problem drinkers: Risk of relapse and implications of successfully sustained remission. *Journal of Studies on Alcohol, 64,* 367–274.

Seppa, K., Laippala, P., & Sillanaukee, P. (1994). Drinking pattern and blood pressure. *American Journal of Hypertension, 7,* 249–254.

Shanmugan, M., & Regan, T. J. (1996). Alcohol and cardiac arrhythmias. In S. Zakhari & M. Wassef (Eds.), *Alcohol and the cardiovascular system* (Vol. 31, pp. 159–172). Washington, DC: NIAAA.

Shiffman, S., & Balabanis, M. (1995). Associations between alcohol and tobacco. In J. B. Fertig & J. P. Allen (Eds.), *Alcohol and tobacco: From basic science to clinical practice* (pp. 17–36). Bethesda, MD: National Institutes of Health.

Simpkins, J. W., Rajakumar, G., Zhang, Y. Q., Simpkins, C. E., Greenwald, D., Bodor, N., et al. (1997). Estrogens may reduce mortality and ischemic damage caused by middle cerebral artery occlusion in the female rat. *Journal of Neurosurgery, 87,* 724–730.

Skaff, M. M., Finney, J. W., & Moos, R. H. (1999). Gender differences in problem drinking and depression: Different "vulnerabilities"? *American Journal of Community Psychology, 27*(1), 25–54.

Smith-Warner, S. A., Spiegelman, D., Yaun, S. S., van den Brandt, P. S., Folsom, A. R., Goldbohm, R. A., et al. (1998). Alcohol and breast cancer in women: A pooled analysis of cohort studies. *Journal of the American Medical Association, 279,* 535–540.

Smothers, B., & Bertolucci, D. (2001). Alcohol consumption and health-promoting behavior in a U.S. household sample: Leisure-time physical activity. *Journal of Studies on Alcohol, 62,* 467–476.

Solomon, K., Manepalli, J., Ireland, G. A., & Mahon, G. M. (1993). Alcoholism and prescription drug abuse in the elderly: St. Louis University grand rounds. *Journal of the American Geriatrics Society, 41,* 57–69.

Stevenson, J. S., & Masters, J. A. (in review). Indicators of alcohol misuse in community-dwelling older women.

Tang, M. X., Jacobs, D., Stern, Y., Marder, K., Schofield, P., Gurland, B., et al. (1996). Effect of oestrogen during menopause on risk and age at onset of Alzheimer's Disease. *Lancet, 348,* 429–432.

Taylor, J. L., Dolhert, N., Friedman, L., Mumenthaler, M. S., & Yesavage, J. A. (1996). Alcohol elimination and simulator performance of male and female aviators: A preliminary report. *Aviation Space and Environmental Medicine, 67,* 407–413.

Temple, M. T., Fillmore, K. M., Hartka, E., Johnstone, B., Leino, E. V., & Motoyoshi, M. (1991). A meta-analysis of change in marital and employment status as predictors of alcohol consumption on a typical occasion. *British Journal of Addiction, 86,* 1269–1281.

Thomas, B. A., & Regan, T. J. (1990). Interactions between alcohol and cardiovascular medications. *Alcohol Health and Research World, 14,* 333–339.

Thomas, V. S., & Rockwood, K. J. (2001). Alcohol abuse, cognitive impairment, and mortality among older people. *Journal of the American Geriatric Society, 49,* 415–420.

Thomasson, H. R. (1995). Gender differences in alcohol metabolism: Physiological responses to ethanol. In M. Galanter (Ed.), *Recent developments in alcoholism* (Vol. 12, pp. 163–179). New York: Plenum Press.

Thun, M. J., Peto, R., Lopez, A. D., Monaco, J. H., Henley, S. J., Heath, C. W., et al. (1997). Alcohol consumption and mortality among middle-aged and elderly US adults. *New England Journal of Medicine, 337,* 1705–1714.

Timko, C., Moos, R. H., Finney, J. W., Moos, B. S., & Kaplowitz, M. S. (1999). Long-term treatment careers and outcomes of previously untreated alcoholics. *Journal of Studies on Alcohol, 60*(4), 437–447.

Tonnesen, H., Rosenberg, J., Nielsen, H. J., Rasmussen, V., Hauge, C., Pederser, I. K., et al. (1999). Effect of preoperative abstinence on poor postoperative outcomes in alcohol misusers: Randomized controlled trial. *British Medical Journal, 318,* 1311–1316.

Urbano-Marquez, A., Estruch, R., Fernandez-Sola, J., Nicolas, J. M., Pare, J. C., & Rubin, E. (1995). The greater risk of alcoholic cardiomyopathy and myopathy in women compared with men. *Journal of the American Medical Association, 274,* 149–154.

U.S. Bureau of the Census. (2000). Population projections of the United States by age, sex, race, Hispanic origin, and nativity. Washington, DC: Author.

U.S. Department of Agriculture (USDA) & Department of Health and Human Services (HHS). (2000). *Nutrition and your health: Dietary guidelines for Americans* (5th ed.). Washington, DC: Author.

U.S. Preventive Services Task Force. (2004). Recommendations on alcohol misuse. Retrieved October 25, 2004, from http://www.ahrq.gov/clinic/uspsdrin.htm

Waern, M., Spak, F., & Sundh, V. (2002). Suicidal ideation in a female population sample: Relationship with depression, anxiety disorder, and alcohol dependence/abuse. *European Archives of Psychiatry and Clinical Neuroscience, 252*(2), 81–85.

Walton, M. A., Mudd, S. A., Blow, F. C., Chermack, S. T., & Gomberg, E. S. L. (2000). Stability in the drinking habits of older problem drinkers recruited from the community. *Journal of Substance Abuse Treatment, 18,* 169–177.

Wannamethee, S. G., & Shaper, A. G. (1992). Alcohol and sudden cardiac death. *British Heart Journal, 68,* 443–448.

———. (1996). Patterns of alcohol intake and risk of stroke in middle-aged British men. *Stroke, 27,* 1033–1039.

———. (1999). Type of alcoholic drink and risk of major coronary heart disease events and all-cause mortality. *American Journal of Public Health, 89,* 685–690.

Weathermon, R., & Crabb, D. W. (1999). Alcohol and medication interactions. *Alcohol Health and Research, 23*(1), 40–54.

Welte, J. W., & Mirand, A. L. (1994). Lifetime drinking patterns of elders from a general population survey. *Drug and Alcohol Dependence, 35,* 133–140.

Wetterling, T., Veltrup, C., John, U., & Driessen, M. (2003). Late onset alcoholism. *European Psychiatry, 18*(3), 112–118.

White, I. R. (1999). The level of alcohol consumption at which all-cause mortality is least. *Journal of Clinical Epidemiology, 54,* 537–540.

Whitfield, J. B. Z., Madden, P. A., Neale, M. C., Heath, A. C., & Martin, N. G. (2004). The genetics of alcohol intake and of alcohol dependence. *Alcohol: Clinical and Experimental Research, 28,* 1153–1160.

Wilk, A., Jensen, N. M., & Havighurst, T. C. (1997). Meta-analysis of randomized controlled trials addressing brief interventions in heavy alcohol drinkers. *Journal of General Internal Medicine, 12,* 274–283.

Zuccala, G., Onder, G., Pedone, C., Cesari, M., Landi, F., Bernabei, R., et al. (2001). Dose-related impact of alcohol consumption on cognitive function in advanced age: Results of a multicenter survey. *Alcoholism: Clinical and Experimental Research, 25,* 1743–1748.

PART III

Alcohol Challenges in
Selected Populations
and Situations

Chapter 9

Alcohol Use and Alcohol-related Problems Among Lesbians and Gay Men

Tonda L. Hughes

ABSTRACT

While a substantial amount is known about some of the risk factors for alcohol-related problems among lesbians and gay men, major gaps in knowledge exist. Epidemiological studies focusing on alcohol use rarely ask about sexual orientation, and broad-based studies of sexual minority population groups have only occasionally assessed alcohol use. Although the AIDS crisis has stimulated substantial research on alcohol and other substance use among gay men, only a handful of studies have systematically explored lesbians' use of alcohol. Further, existing research on sexual orientation and alcohol use is characterized by a plethora of methodological problems. Nevertheless, when viewed as a whole, this research suggests that lesbians and gay men are more likely than their heterosexual counterparts to drink alcohol and to report alcohol-related problems; differences based on sexual orientation are more pronounced for women than for men. Risks related to alcohol use do not stem from sexual orientation per se, but are more likely a consequence of cultural and environmental factors associated with being part of a stigmatized and marginalized population. Much of the research on alcohol use among sexual minorities has focused on White, middle-class, and well-educated lesbians and gay men. There is a clear need for more research with bisexual women and men and with sexual minority members of color. Longitudinal studies, including those that focus on treatment effectiveness, are particularly lacking.

Keywords: lesbian, gay, sexual orientation, sexual identity, sexual minority, alcohol use, substance use

The purported relationship between homosexuality and alcohol abuse has a long history. During much of the past century, adherents of Freudian theories attempted to explain alcohol abuse in terms of latent homosexuality—connecting alcoholism and homosexuality using psychoanalytic theories of oral fixation, oedipal conflicts, and incestuous drives (Israelstam & Lambert, 1983). Further, because many early studies used clinical samples from psychiatric settings, research findings tended to support the prevailing view of homosexuality as a form of mental illness. One notable exception was a study conducted in the 1950s by Evelyn Hooker (1957). Hooker's work challenged the pathology model and stimulated a paradigm shift that resulted in the removal of homosexuality from the *Diagnostic and Statistical Manual of Mental Disorders (DSM)* in 1973. Following the removal of homosexuality from the *DSM*, studies were increasingly conducted with nonclinical samples. However, because recruitment strategies relied heavily on mailing lists of organizations or on social settings where lesbians and gay men could be found in large numbers, research findings continued to reflect the characteristics of the populations from which the samples were drawn. Most research on lesbians' and gay men's alcohol use in the 1970s and early 1980s recruited some or all of the samples in gay bars (Fifield, Latham, & Phillips, 1977; Lohrenz, Connely, Coyne, & Spare, 1978; Saghir & Robins, 1973). Not surprisingly, these studies found high rates of alcohol use/abuse and related problems.

Research conducted since the mid-1980s—though also limited by methodological problems—suggests that rates of alcohol use and abuse among lesbians and gay men are substantially lower than in earlier studies but still higher than those of women and men in the general population.

METHODS OF RETRIEVAL

To prepare this integrated literature review, computer-assisted searches were conducted using the Medline, CINAHL, and PsychINFO databases. The keywords alcohol use/abuse, substance use/abuse, addiction/chemical dependency, homosexuality/homosexual, sexual orientation, sexual identity, sexual minority, lesbian, bisexual, and gay located studies published since 1985. The author also hand searched reference lists of new journal articles and publications related to sexual orientation and health (e.g., AJPH, 2001; GLMA & LGBT Experts, 2001; SAMHSA, 2001).

Articles reviewed were primarily databased reports of original research focusing on alcohol use or alcohol-related problems among adult lesbians, gay men, and bisexual women and men. Studies focusing on transgender women and men and adolescents[1] were excluded, as were studies that have human immunodeficiency virus/acquired immunodeficiency syndrome (HIV/AIDS) as a major focus. Studies from all disciplines published in the English language were reviewed.

This review (1) summarizes existing research on the prevalence and patterns of alcohol use and alcohol-related problems in lesbians and gay men (and, to a lesser extent, bisexual women and men),[2] (2) examines potential risk and protective factors associated with alcohol use/abuse in these population groups, (3) describes issues related to assessment and treatment, (4) summarizes methodological issues pertinent to research conducted with sexual minority groups, and (5) discusses future directions for research focusing on sexual minorities.

DEFINITION OF SEXUAL ORIENTATION

Researchers are only beginning to consider sexual orientation an important focus of health research and an important demographic variable for inclusion in studies of health (Sell & Becker, 2001). Like race/ethnicity and socioeconomic status, sexual orientation is a complex construct that is difficult to measure. Sexual orientation is most commonly described as including behavioral, affective (attraction or desire), and cognitive (identity) dimensions (Laumann, Gagnon, Michael, & Michaels, 1994). Although these dimensions are generally strongly correlated, they are not perfectly congruent. For example, women whose sex partners are primarily, or only, women may not identify as lesbian or bisexual. Similarly, women who identify as lesbian may have both female and male sexual partners or not be sexually active. Others define sexual orientation as a person's predisposition to experience sexual attraction or desire for persons of the same gender, the other gender, or both genders (Diamond, 2000; Jorm, Dear, Rodgers, & Christensen, 2003) and view sexual identity as the self-concept that an individual forms around this predisposition (Cass, 1984). Whereas sexual orientation is presumed to develop early and remain stable (Bell, Weinberg, & Hammersmith, 1981; Diamond, 2000; Money, 1988), sexual identity is thought to evolve in adolescence or adulthood and to vary as a result of social, historical, and cultural factors (Kitzinger & Wilkinson, 1995; Rust, 1993; Weinberg, Williams, & Pyror, 1994). The definition of sexual orientation used in this chapter is most consistent with the tridimensional conceptualization of Laumann et al. (1994). The terms *lesbian* and *gay* are used to refer to women and men, respectively, whose primary sexual and emotional attachments are to persons of the same gender. *Bisexual* refers to women or men who are sexually attracted or have emotional attachments to both genders. *Lesbian, gay,* and *bisexual* are also used to refer to self-identity. The term *sexual minority* includes lesbians, gay men, and bisexual women and men. It is important to distinguish sexual orientation (heterosexual, homosexual, and bisexual) from gender identity (masculine, feminine, androgynous, and transgender), and to recognize that transgender women and men may identify as heterosexual, lesbian, gay, or bisexual (American Public Health Association, 1999).

PREVALENCE OF LESBIANS, GAYS, AND BISEXUALS IN THE UNITED STATES

Most attempts to estimate prevalence are based on the assumption that homosexuality is a static and uniform attribute across individuals. Researchers and others routinely blur the distinction between sexual behavior and sexual identity, a factor that complicates efforts to understand the health of sexual minority groups. Published reports about the prevalence of sexual minorities commonly cite two major U.S. studies of sexuality and sexual behavior conducted nearly a half century apart: Kinsey's pioneering research in the mid-1900s (Kinsey, Pomeroy, & Martin, 1948; Kinsey, Pomeroy, Martin, & Gebhard, 1953) and the relatively recent National Health and Social Life Survey (NHSLS) (Laumann et al., 1994). Findings from these studies demonstrate that prevalence varies greatly depending on the sample, the definition of sexual orientation used, and the time frame assessed by individual questions. For example, using a large convenience sample of women and men from various parts of the United States, Kinsey and his colleagues found that 13% of women and 37% of men reported having at least one sexual experience since puberty with a same-gender partner that led to orgasm. A smaller percentage of respondents reported having only same-gender sex partners since puberty (1%–3% of women and 4% of men).

In comparison, same-gender sexual behavior was substantially lower in the NHSLS. In this national probability sample, approximately 4% of women and 9% of men reported having sex with a same-gender partner since puberty. Just over 2% of women and 4% of men reported same-gender sex partners in the past 5 years. Only 1.4% of women and 2.8% of men reported homosexual or bisexual identity. Nine percent of women and 10% of men reported at least one of the three dimensions of sexual orientation (behavior, attraction, or identity) since age 18. Responses to questions regarding the different dimensions of homosexuality varied based on respondents' age at the time of interview, birth cohort, race/ethnicity, educational level, religious affiliation, and geographic residence (Laumann et al., 1994).

Thus, variations in sampling, participation bias (e.g., reluctance to disclose same-gender behavior or nonheterosexual identity), demographic characteristics, historical and other factors that influence both identity development and willingness to disclose a minority sexual orientation, and measurement error (e.g., imprecise and inconsistent measures of sexual orientation) make it difficult to estimate the prevalence of sexual minorities.

ALCOHOL USE AND SEXUAL ORIENTATION

In the general population, rates and patterns of alcohol use vary according to a number of characteristics such as age, gender, race/ethnicity, education and employment, and other social roles. Although much less is known about these variations within sexual minorities, this section will summarize existing literature related to prevalence and patterns of alcohol use and alcohol-related problems in these groups.

Inclusion of Bisexual Women and Men

Much alcohol research conducted with sexual minority females has focused on lesbians. However, because of unclear study inclusion criteria and incomplete measurement of sexual orientation, it is likely that data from women who identify as bisexual and those who have sex with women (WSW) but do not identify as lesbian are often included in samples presumed to be lesbian. Even when bisexual women and WSW are explicitly included in studies of sexual minority women, their numbers are often too small to permit between-group comparisons.

Like bisexual women, bisexual men have not been a primary focus in alcohol research. However, bisexual men and men who have sex with men (MSM) are more often explicitly included as part of the sample in studies of gay men. One reason for this is the fact that many studies of sexual minority men have as a major aim greater understanding of risk factors associated with sexually transmitted diseases, including HIV, among MSM. Thus, it is sexual behavior rather than sexual identity that is of primary concern in most existing research on alcohol use among sexual minority men.

Alcohol Use and Alcohol-Related Problems

Studies done in the 1970s and early 1980s found high rates of alcohol use and abuse among lesbians and gay men (Fifield et al., 1977; Morales & Graves, 1983; Saghir & Robins, 1973). However, methodological limitations, such as small, homogeneous samples (which often overrepresented bar patrons) and lack of heterosexual comparison groups, raise questions about the validity of these findings. Later research suggests overall lower rates of heavy drinking (Bergmark,

1999; Bloomfield, 1993; Gruskin, Hart, Gordon, & Ackerson, 2001; Hughes, 2003; Hughes, Haas, Razzano, Cassidy, & Matthews, 2000; McKirnan & Peterson, 1989a; Skinner, 1994). Nonetheless, findings from these and several other studies (Cochran, Keenan, Schober, & Mays, 2000; Gilman et al., 2001; Stall & Wiley, 1988; Valanis, Bowen, Bassford, Whitlock, Charney, & Carter, 2000), suggest that, compared with heterosexuals, lesbians and gay men are more likely to drink and to report alcohol-related problems. In addition, differences between lesbians and heterosexual women are substantially larger than differences between gay and heterosexual men (Bergmark, 1999; Cochran et al., 2000; Cochran & Mays, 2000; Gilman et al., 2001; McKirnan & Peterson, 1989a; Meyer, 2003; Sandfort, Graaf, Bijl, & Schnabel, 2001). In contrast, a few studies have found either no difference between lesbians' and gay men's drinking when compared with demographically similar samples of heterosexual women and men (Jorm, Korten, Rodgers, Jacomb, & Christensen, 2002; Welch, Howden-Chapman, & Collings, 1998) or, modest, if any, differences between gay and heterosexual men.

As noted in the earlier discussion about prevalence estimates of sexual minorities, inconsistent findings related to alcohol use in the above studies can be partially explained by differences in study designs, samples, and definitions of sexual orientation. For example, only about one third of the studies cited above used probability sampling methods. In addition, the definition of sexual orientation varied substantially. A little more than half used sexual identity as a criterion for inclusion in the study or as the basis of group comparisons with heterosexuals; the remainder used sexual behavior. Recent findings suggest that health risks, including substance abuse, are higher in studies that use same-gender sexual behavior than in those that use gay or lesbian self-identity as a criterion for sample selection or analysis (Chng & Geliga-Vargas, 2000; Gomez, Garcia, Kegebein, Shade, & Hernandez, 1996; Markovic, Aaron, & Danielson, 2001; Scheer et al., 2003). Finally, because most studies include samples of lesbians and gay men that are predominantly White, younger (25–40 years old), well educated, and who live in or near larger cities, comparisons with national probability samples can lead to inconsistent or biased results and conclusions (Hughes, Wilsnack, & Johnson, in press).

In light of these limitations, it is somewhat surprising that several consistent patterns are apparent when findings across studies are considered as a whole. First, the relationship between some demographic characteristics and drinking behaviors differs by sexual orientation. For example, gender differences in drinking patterns and related problems are smaller between lesbians and gay men than between heterosexual women and men. Further, there appear to be fewer and smaller differences between gay and heterosexual men's drinking than between lesbians' and heterosexual women's drinking. Second, compared with heterosexual women and men, rates of drinking, heavy drinking, and problem drinking among lesbians and gay men seem to decline less with age. Third, even when rates of heavy drinking are reasonably comparable, lesbians and gay men tend to report more alcohol-related problems.

There is also evidence to suggest that, on the whole, drinking may be declining among lesbians and gay men (Crosby, Stall, Paul, & Barrett, 1998; Heffernan, 1998; Hughes, 2003; Hughes & Wilsnack, 1997; Remien et al., 1995). Possible reasons for this include greater awareness and concern about health and more moderate drinking among women and men in the general population, increased visibility and lessening of the social stigma and oppression of lesbians and gay men, and changing norms associated with drinking in some lesbian and gay communities. Nevertheless, because sexual minorities appear to be at heightened risk for heavy drinking and drinking-related problems, it is important to gain a better understanding of factors that influence this risk.

THEORETICAL FRAMEWORK OF RISK AND PROTECTIVE FACTORS

The conceptual model in Figure 9.1 is adapted from the work of Sharon and Richard Wilsnack (Wilsnack, Klassen, Sher, & Wilsnack, 1991; Wilsnack & Wilsnack, 1995; Wilsnack, Wilsnack, & Hiller-Sturmhofel, 1994), who have been engaged in a national longitudinal study of women's drinking since 1980.

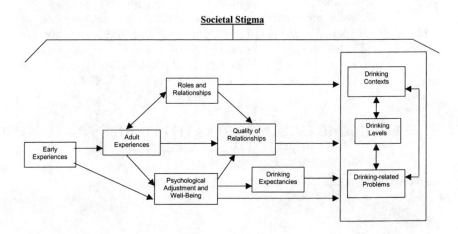

FIGURE 9.1 Conceptual model of drinking and drinking related problems among lesbians and gay men.[3]

Source: Adapted from Sharon C. Wilsnack unpublished Conceptual Model.

This model consists of six broad sets of influencing factors: early life experiences, adult life experiences, current roles and relationships, psychological adjustment and well-being, quality of current roles and relationships, and expectancies about the effects of alcohol. The six sets of factors are believed to directly or indirectly influence drinking contexts, drinking levels, and drinking-related problems.

Although variables within the Wilsnacks' model are relevant to drinking in both heterosexual and sexual minority populations, there are additional factors within each of the six categories that are specific to the lives of lesbians and gay men. Examples include stress associated with sexual identity development and "coming out" as lesbian or gay, level of sexual identity disclosure or "outness," lower or absent social support of family of origin, internalized homophobia (fear, shame, or self-hatred associated with being lesbian or gay), and high rates of mental health services utilization. Societal stigma is considered to be an overarching influence that affects each of these factors to varying degrees and leads to different risks or levels of risk for heterosexual and sexual minority women and men.

Using the six broad categories in Figure 9.1 as an organizing framework, the sections below summarize empirical findings related to drinking and drinking-related problems among lesbians and gay men. Emphasized are factors that may pose higher risk for lesbians and gay men, particularly those that stem from environmental or cultural influences, rather than genetic or biological factors, given that the latter two are assumed to be shared equally with their heterosexual counterparts. Although the terms *risk factor* and *protective factor* are used to suggest potential causal relationships, only a few longitudinal studies have been conducted. Thus, the predictive value of many of the factors discussed has not yet been evaluated. In the context of this chapter, risk and protective factors are variables found or hypothesized to be positively (risk) or negatively (protective) associated with heavy drinking or drinking-related problems. As used here, the term *protective factor* is similar to, but not synonymous with, *resilience*.

EMPIRICAL EVIDENCE RELATED TO RISK AND PROTECTIVE FACTORS

Early Experiences

Childhood Sexual Abuse (CSA)

Reported rates of CSA among women vary substantially but most often fall between 20% and 38% in community samples. Variations in rates are likely attributable to different definitions of sexual abuse and differences in age ranges and other characteristics of samples surveyed. Some previous studies that have assessed CSA among lesbians have found rates similar to those of heterosexual women (Descamps, Rothblum, Bradford, & Ryan, 2000; Neisen & Sandall, 1990). Two recent studies, however, found higher rates of CSA among lesbians than among demographically matched comparison groups of heterosexual women (Hughes & Johnson, 2003; Hughes, Johnson, & Wilsnack, 2001). It is possible that the higher rates of CSA among lesbians may be the result of reporting bias. Women who seek help for mental health problems—such as relationship problems, depression, and anxiety—may be more likely to recall and report CSA through their efforts to better understand their present difficulties (Kendler et al., 2000). This may be particularly true for lesbians, given the high number who report mental health counseling (see later section on mental health service use).

Literature on CSA among men is newer; but anecdotal, clinical, and research reports suggest that gay men are more likely than heterosexual men to have histories of sexual abuse, which, like reports of CSA by lesbians, can be partially accounted for by greater willingness to acknowledge such experiences. However, because the majority of CSA perpetrators are male, and given the historically rigid gender roles for men and myths that male-to-male sex is always gay sex, boys and young men who are sexually abused are likely to feel such shame that they may be unwilling to talk about the abuse or to seek professional help.

Not surprisingly, much of the focus of research on CSA among gay men is on adult sexual practices and the risk for sexually transmitted diseases. Two community-based studies—one with gay/bisexual men, another with men who have sex with men—found rates of reported childhood sexual coercion ranging from 21% to 28% (Jinich et al., 1998; Paul, Catania, Pollack, & Stall, 2001). Although empirical studies of CSA prevalence among sexual minority men are uncommon, the *Journal of Gay and Lesbian Social Services* devoted a volume to research and clinical practice with gay men who are survivors of CSA (Cassese, 2000), reflecting the growing awareness and interest in this health topic.

Clinicians and researchers increasingly recognize a link between CSA and substance abuse, especially in women (Clay, Olsheski, & Clay, 2000; Kendler et al., 2000; Langeland & Hartgers, 1998; Widom & Hiller-Sturmhofel, 2001). However, it is not clear whether substance abuse resulting from CSA is a factor in the development of other consequences, such as depression, or if depression comes first and alcohol or other drug abuse is used to cope. Much of what is known about the sequelae of CSA comes from reports of women in treatment for substance abuse or psychiatric problems. In one of the few studies to explore the relationship between CSA and alcohol abuse among women in the general population, Wilsnack, Vogeltanz, Klassen, and Harris (1997), found that CSA was strongly related to most drinking measures used in their survey, including alcohol use in the past 30 days, intoxication, and number of problem conse-quences and alcohol dependence symptoms in the past 12 months. In addition, CSA continued to have effects on drinking in 1991 (predicting increased drinking and alcohol dependence symptoms over a 10-year period), controlling for 1981 drinking levels (Wilsnack, Wilsnack, Kristjanson, & Harris, 1998).

Only five studies were found that examined the association of CSA and alcohol use or abuse in lesbians or gay men (Bartholow et al., 1994; Descamps et al., 2000; Hughes & Johnson, 2003; Hughes et al., 2001; Neisen & Sandall, 1990). Findings from these studies suggest that lesbians and gay men who were sexually abused as children are at greater risk than those without CSA histories for heavy drinking and drinking-related problems.

Sexual Identity Development

The development of a sexual minority identity is a lengthy process that can take many years (Troiden, 1993). Although the first awareness of sexual orientation often occurs at quite young ages (D'Augelli & Hershberger, 1993; Parks & Hughes, in press; Pattatucci & Hamer, 1995), such awareness can occur at any age. Developing a positive sexual identity is a normal part of adolescence, but it can be particularly difficult for lesbian and gay adolescents because of societal stigma and lack of readily identifiable role models. Lesbians and gay men who are members of racial/ethnic minority groups have the challenge of integrating two major devalued aspects of their identity (Espin, 1993; Greene, 1994, 1997). Further, because the stigma associated with homosexuality is believed to be greater in communities of color, fear of sexual orientation disclosure and the resulting social and emotional isolation (e.g., from community, family, and peers) may complicate the sexual identity development of racial/ethnic minority lesbians and gay men. The reluctance of racial/ethnic minorities to use mental health services, including therapy or counseling, may further increase the risk for negative psychological outcomes (Greene, 1997) and the associated risk of heavy drinking.

Psychological Adjustment and Well-being

Psychological Distress, "Coming Out," and Internalized Homophobia

Beginning with Hooker's work (1957), nearly a half century of research has shown that lesbians and gay men do not differ significantly from heterosexual women and men in overall psychological adjustment (McKirnan & Peterson, 1989b; Ross, Paulsen, & Stalstrom, 1988; Rothblum & Factor, 2001). Nevertheless, some studies suggest that lesbians and gay men may have higher rates of current depression (Ayala & Coleman, 2000; Cochran & Mays, 1994; Gilman et al., 2001; Oetjen & Rothblum, 2000; Valanis et al., 2000) and lifetime depression (Hughes & Johnson, 2003; Hughes et al., in press; Sandfort et al., 2001).

Members of sexual minority groups must contend with the psychological consequences of stigma throughout their lives. Beginning with their first awareness of same-gender attraction, lesbians and gay men learn from society to hate themselves—to internalize society's homonegativity. Internalized homophobia has been positively associated with depression and anxiety symptoms, substance abuse, and suicidal ideation (DiPlacido, 1998a,b; Meyer, 1995; Meyer & Dean, 1998). Disclosure of sexual orientation is believed to be negatively associated with internalized homophobia and positively associated with mental health (DiPlacido, 1998a,b; Jordan & Deluty, 1998; Morris, Waldo, & Rothblum, 2001; Schmitt & Kurdek, 1987). For example, in a study of 2,401 lesbian and bisexual women, sexual orientation disclosure was found to predict lower psychological distress, which in turn predicted lower suicidality (Morris et al., 2001). However, increased stress related to sexual minority status can be a cost of such disclosure. Lesbians and gay men who disclose their sexual orientation risk alienation from their families, discrimination at work, loss of child custody, verbal harassment, and physical assault (DiPlacido, 1998a; Herek, 1991; Purcell & Hicks, 1996). Moreover, the costs of "coming out" are not the same for all groups. Racial/ethnic minorities appear to be at even greater risk for psychological distress associated with coming out because they are often subjected to multiple forms of discrimination, including intense homophobia within their cultural group and racism within lesbian/gay communities (Cochran & Mays, 1994; Greene, 1994, 1997; Mays, Cochran, & Rhue, 1993; Morris et al., 2001; Savin-Williams, 1996).

Limited time-ordered data from studies conducted in the general population suggest that depression can be both an antecedent and a consequence of alcohol abuse (Dixit & Crum, 2000; Gilman & Abraham, 2001; Hesselbrock & Hesselbrock, 1997). Some studies have found that depression is more likely to precede alcohol abuse in women than in men (Gilman & Abraham, 2001; Moscato et al., 1997), and others have found the risk of secondary depression is higher among women with alcohol dependency than is the risk for depressed women to become alcohol dependent (Gilman & Abraham, 2001). Wilsnack et al. (1991) found that depression was a more consistent predictor of chronic problem drinking among women already experiencing alcohol-related problems than it was of onset of problem drinking.

A few studies have examined the relationship between psychological distress and alcohol abuse in lesbians and gay men. Hughes and Johnson (2003) examined lifetime and past year predictors of psychological distress in a diverse sample of 450 self-identified lesbians in Chicago. In this study, CSA, along with childhood physical abuse and age at first sexual intercourse, predicted lifetime psychological distress (but not psychological distress in the past year). In a longitudinal study of the relationship between substance abuse and psychological distress, 39 gay, lesbian, and bisexual college students were compared with a matched control group of 156 heterosexual students (DeBord, Wood, Sher, & Good, 1998).

Stronger associations were found between psychological distress and alcohol dependence in lesbian, gay, and bisexual college students than in heterosexual students. In contrast to the strength of the prospective design, this study was limited by the small number of sexual minority participants. In a much larger community-based study conducted by McKirnan and Peterson (1989b), lesbians and gay men had relatively low rates of depression, alienation, and general stress. However, 13% of the lesbians and 22% of the gay men reported that they used alcohol "half of the time" or more when coping with personal stress. Hence, although there is evidence of heightened risk of both psychological distress and alcohol abuse among lesbians and gay men, the manner and extent to which the two are linked remain unclear.

Adult Experiences

Age and Social Roles

Younger age is among the most robust predictors of heavy drinking in the general population. Women and men are more likely to drink heavily in early adulthood; for the majority of the population, both quantity and frequency of use decrease with age (Kandel, Warner, & Kessler, 1998; U.S. Department of Health and Human Services [USDHHS], 2000a). Problems related to drinking also tend to be highest in early adulthood, and then decrease with age, although age-related risk varies by racial/ethnic group (USDHHS, 2000a). In the 1991 National Study of Health and Life Experiences of Women (NSHLEW), 26% of the 21- to 30-year-old women reported at least one drinking problem in the past 12 months, compared with rates ranging from 2% to 17% in older age groups (Wilsnack et al., 1994). One reason younger adults have higher rates of alcohol-related problems is their greater tendency to engage in heavy episodic (binge) drinking (Wechsler & Issac, 1992; Wilsnack, 1996).

Role socialization theory (Yamaguchi & Kandel, 1985) argues that age-related decline in alcohol and other drug use is the result of assuming adult social roles and relationships, such as full-time employment, marriage, and parenting. Results from the NSHLEW suggest that women's drinking and drinking-related problems are more variable than men's and that the greatest changes occur among women 21 to 34 years old (Wilsnack et al., 1994). These fluctuations appear to be influenced by changes in drinking contexts and drinking partners and in social roles such as employment and marriage, common changes among this age group. Further, using data from the National Longitudinal Alcohol Epidemiologic Study, investigators found that the probability of current drinking and heavy drinking was higher among the never married, separated, and divorced than among married men and women (Dawson, Grant, Chou, & Pickering, 1995).

Relatively few studies have directly examined age-specific patterns of drinking among lesbians and gay men. Available data suggests that, compared with heterosexuals, rates of drinking and/or drinking-related problems decline less with age and that fewer older lesbians and gay men are abstainers (Bergmark, 1999; Bradford & Ryan, 1987; McKirnan & Peterson, 1989a; Skinner & Otis, 1996; Stall & Wiley, 1988; Valanis et al., 2000). For example, in the National Lesbian Health Care Survey (NLHCS), daily drinking was reported by 3% of lesbians 34 years old and younger, 7% of those 35 to 44 years old, 10% of those 45 to 54 years old, and 21% of those 55 years or older (Bradford & Ryan, 1987). McKirnan and Peterson (1989a) found that rates of alcohol problems among lesbians in all age groups were higher than those of women in the general population (rates for gay men were higher only in the 31–40 and 41–60 age groups). Lesbians in the three oldest age groups (26–30, 31–40, and 41–60) were 3 times as likely to report alcohol problems as women in comparable age groups in the general population.

There are two possible cohort-related explanations for smaller declines in age-related drinking patterns and problems. First, older cohorts of lesbians and gay men may be continuing patterns of drinking developed when they were younger and gay bars were among the few places to socialize and meet potential partners. It is also possible that younger lesbians and gay men may drink less than their older counterparts did at the same age. Recent changes in societal attitudes and institutional policies toward homosexuality have created a substantially different environmental context for young women and men now coming to terms with a sexual minority identity. Such changes may lessen the stigma, alienation, and isolation experienced by many lesbians and gay men and may contribute to decline in use of alcohol and other drugs as coping strategies. Nevertheless, it appears that older age confers less protection against drinking-related problems in lesbians and gay men than in heterosexual women and men.

Marriage and Parenting

Social roles such as marriage and parenting appear to be protective against drinking problems in heterosexual women and men (Chilcoat & Breslau, 1996). Reasons include social support gained from family, increased responsibilities, and greater social monitoring and feedback that may discourage excessive drinking (Wilsnack & Wilsnack, 1995). However, social roles differ substantially for lesbians and gay men. First, fewer have children (Hughes et al., 2000; Patterson, 1998). Until recently, lesbians and gay men in the United States have been unable to legally marry their partners, and even same-gender couples in stable, long-term relationships generally receive less sanction and support for their relationships than do unmarried heterosexual cohabiting couples. Thus, fewer lesbians and gay men engage in traditional roles (e.g., marriage, childbearing, and child rearing), or have responsibilities associated with combinations of social roles believed to limit substance use among women and men in the general population. For lesbians and gay men who do have children, the stresses associated with parenting may be exacerbated. Lesbian and gay parents must often deal with the realistic fear of child custody loss, homophobic remarks made to the children, partners' roles in child rearing, and revealing their sexual orientation to the children (Falk, 1993; Greene, 1994; Purcell & Hicks, 1996). On the one hand, these stressors may contribute to heavier drinking in some lesbians and gay men. On the other, several studies have documented that same-gender relationships tend to be characterized by more equitable distribution of responsibilities than are heterosexual relationships (Green, Bettinger, & Zacks, 1996; Matthews, Tataro, & Hughes, 2003; Schneider, 1986). Thus, for lesbians and gay parents who are in relationships, the stress of parenting (and the potential risk for heavy drinking) may be buffered to some degree.

Paid Employment

Employed persons' greater economic resources and social opportunities to drink have also been used to explain the relationship between alcohol consumption and paid employment, especially among women. Such a link may be particularly salient to lesbians' risk because they, more often than heterosexual women, work outside the home (Morgan & Brown, 1993). Furthermore, lesbians may not be as restricted as heterosexual women by gender-role socialization and thus may more likely choose jobs that are nontraditional (i.e., male dominated), a factor also found in several studies to be associated with greater alcohol consumption among women in the general population (LaRosa, 1990; Wilsnack & Wright, 1991).

The psychological difficulties for lesbians and gay men that are created by managing disclosure of sexual orientation on the job are well documented (Croteau, 1996; Morgan & Brown, 1993; Sorensen & Roberts, 1997). Hiding one's sexual orientation, vigilance around coworkers, having to listen to antigay jokes and comments, anxiety, and fear are not uncommon among employed lesbians and gay men. In a rare study of the relationship between workplace harassment and drinking among lesbians and gay men, Nawyn, Richman, Rospenda, and Hughes (2000) found that, although rates of sexual harassment did not differ between lesbian/bisexual and heterosexual women, the relationship between workplace harassment and alcohol-related outcomes was stronger for lesbians and bisexual women. Gay and bisexual men experienced significantly more sexual harassment than heterosexual men, but they did not report a corresponding increase in alcohol use or abuse. Findings such as these suggest that employment and work-related factors may have a greater influence on lesbians' drinking than on gay men's.

Quality of Relationships

Relationship Status and Satisfaction

Compared with persons who do not have an intimate relationship, those in relationships report greater well-being (Kurdek, 1994; Taylor, 1995; Wayment & Peplau, 1995; Wood, Rhodes, & Whelan, 1989). Further, the dissolution of an important relationship is one of life's most stressful events (Dohrenwend, Krasnoff, Askenasy, & Dohrenwend, 1978; Hope, Rodgers, & Power, 1999; Horwitz, White, & Howell-White, 1996; Kurdek, 1991). In comparing relationship satisfaction of lesbian/gay and heterosexual couples, one finds few differences (Duffy & Rusbult, 1986; Kurdek & Schmitt, 1986; Matthews et al., 2003; Peplau, Cochran, & Mays, 1997; Zak & McDonald, 1997). However, because lesbians' and gay men's relationships develop without the support of social institutions and often without the support of family of origin (Kurdek, 1994), they may be more vulnerable to disruption and dissolution. Relationship dissolution has been found to be an important risk factor for psychological distress (Hope et al., 1999; Horwitz et al., 1996) and for drinking-related problems (Chilcoat & Breslau, 1996; Power, Rodgers, & Hope, 1999), especially among women (Fillmore et al., 1997; Horwitz et al., 1996; Neff & Mantz, 1998). Although no studies have examined the association between relationship status or satisfaction and alcohol use among lesbians and gay men, relationship dissolution is believed to be an important reason for lesbians' depression (Kurdek, 1997; Rothblum, 1994), which, in turn, may increase risk of heavier drinking. In addition, lesbians and gay men without partners may be more likely than those with partners to frequent gay bars or other social settings where heavy drinking is normative (Heffernan, 1998; Parks, 1999b).

Relationship Distress

The reluctance to acknowledge intimate partner violence (IPV) in same-gender relationships, by society at large and by lesbian and gay communities, has resulted in limited attention to this problem (Coleman, 1994; Leventhal & Lundy, 1999). Most existing research has focused on IPV in lesbian relationships; only a few of these studies explored the relationship between same-gender partner violence and the use of alcohol (Renzetti, 1992, 1994; Schilit, Lie, & Montagne, 1990), and findings are inconsistent. Although the majority (64%) of women in Schilit et al.'s study (1990) reported that both they and their partners used alcohol or other drugs (AODs) during or prior to the incidents of IPV, only 35% of Renzetti's respondents (1992) reported that their partners were under the influence of AODs at the time IPV occurred (28% reported that both they and their partners were under the influence). A number of respondents reported that both they and their partner were near-abstainers.

Although less well documented than in lesbian couples, several studies have also found evidence of IPV in gay relationships. For example, in a survey of gay men in Minneapolis–St. Paul, 17% of the respondents indicated that they had been in a physically violent relationship with another man (Elliott, 1996). Using findings from a study conducted in San Francisco, Lettelier (1996) estimated that one in five men in same-gender relationships experienced violence. No studies were found that explored the relationships between IPV and AOD use/abuse among gay or bisexual men.

The issues related to IPV in same-gender relationships are arguably more complex than those in heterosexual relationships. For lesbians and gay men in violent relationships, isolation associated with being a member of a marginalized population group and society's tendency to view IPV through the lens of gender inequality and male dominance make it exceedingly difficult for them to seek help. Such isolation and stigmatization may induce or increase alcohol use in lesbians and gay men, and alcohol use may increase vulnerability to further violence in the relationship. Because of societal attitudes and gender-role norms, men who are battered are even less likely than battered women to seek help. Gay men who attempt to seek help are likely to find that women's shelters are not equipped to serve them and have staffs who do not understand their experiences.

Social Support

Research findings suggest that social support moderates the effects of stress. Individuals who experience high levels of stress but receive adequate social support are less likely to become ill than those who experience similar levels of stress but do not receive adequate social support (Cohen & Hoberman, 1983; Cohen & Willis, 1985). Research with lesbians and gay men suggest that social support of family and friends is associated with psychological well-being (Ayala & Coleman, 2000; Jordan & Deluty, 1998; Mays, Beckman, Oranchak, & Harper, 1994; Oetjen & Rothblum, 2000; Wayment & Peplau, 1995), but studies often find that lesbians and gay men report substantially lower levels of support from family than from friends (e.g., Fobair et al., 2001; Vincke & Bolton, 1994). The relationship between social support and drinking behaviors is complex, and findings vary substantially based on the social support measure used. For example, some types of social support, such as attachment support, which is supplied primarily by close and committed relationships (e.g., close friend or partner), are generally found to buffer psychological distress, which may reduce the risk of heavy drinking. Other measures of social support, such as number of friends, may tap into a broader construct in which greater social support is associated with more opportunities to drink.

Drinking Expectancies

Preconceived beliefs about the effects of alcohol appear to play an important role in moderating the relationship between psychological distress and drinking

(Cooper, Russell, Skinner, Frone, & Mudar, 1992; Williams & Clark, 1998); in particular, the expectancy of tension reduction has been shown to predict heavier alcohol use. McKirnan and Peterson (1989b) tested the hypothesis that the expectancy that drinking alcoholic beverages reduces tension (attitudinal vulnerability) and bar orientation (cultural vulnerability) were important predictors of alcohol abuse among lesbians and gay men. As hypothesized, tension reduction expectancies and bar orientation were strongly related to drinking, frequency of intoxication, and drinking-related problems in both lesbians and gay men. In analyses comparing high- and low-vulnerability groups, both social and stress-related drinking had substantially stronger correlations with alcohol-related problems among high—compared with low—vulnerability respondents (no gender differences were found). The authors argue that lesbians' and gay men's alcohol-related problems are not predicted by alcohol-use behaviors or level of consumption alone, but by psychological factors such as alcohol expectancies and social orientation toward bars.

Leigh (1990) found that lesbians and gay men hold stronger alcohol expectancies for decreased nervousness and increased sexual risk taking than heterosexual women and men. Such expectancies may be more salient for individuals who have identified as lesbian or gay more recently or who are conflicted about their sexual orientation (Ghindia & Kola, 1996).

Drinking Contexts and Drinking Norms

Drinking behavior is governed to a large extent by social structures (rules, role expectations, norms, and values) of the individual's cultural group and by the drinking behavior of peers (Brenan & Moos, 1996; Clark, 1991; Greenfield & Room, 1997). For example, Herd (1993) found that alcohol-related problems were strongly related to drinking norms in both African American and White women, and that African American women's drinking norms were less permissive than those of White women. In terms of peer networks, a recent longitudinal study of young married couples found that peer networks characterized by higher levels of alcohol involvement were strongly related to heavier drinking in both women and men, and that this relationship was independent of the partner's drinking (Leonard & Mudar, 2000). Weinberg (1994) found evidence for both partner and peer influence on gay men's drinking. In this study, alcohol consumption was higher among gay men whose partners were heavy drinkers, and partner's drinking was a strong predictor of alcohol-related problems. Weinberg also found that gay men whose social lives revolved around bar settings were likely to have friends who were heavier drinkers. Socializing in bars was associated with both availability of alcohol and peer pressure to drink.

A frequently noted characteristic of women's drinking is that alcohol consumption patterns often parallel those of significant others (Wilsnack, 1996). Whether this affects lesbians' drinking is yet to be explored. On the one hand, lesbians could be at lower risk of having a heavy-drinking partner because women, in general, are less likely than men to drink or to drink heavily. On the other hand, some studies have found that lesbians' drinking patterns and drinking-related problems are similar to those of gay men (Bergmark, 1999; McKirnan & Peterson, 1989a; Skinner, 1994). In the context of other cultural factors, such as more opportunities to drink and fewer traditional role restrictions and social prohibitions against drinking (Hughes & Wilsnack, 1997), and because lesbian relationships are characterized by greater intimacy and shared activities (Hurl-bert & Apt, 1993; Vargo, 1987), the influence of problem-drinking partners may be stronger on lesbians' than on heterosexual women's or gay men's drinking. Although gay and lesbian communities are generally characterized as having permissive drinking norms, this assumption has not been empirically tested. This and many other questions remain about the influence of drinking contexts on lesbians' and gay men's drinking.

Mental Health Service Use

Research suggests that lesbians and gay men use some mental health services, particularly therapy/counseling, at high rates (Bell & Weinberg, 1978; Bradford & Ryan, 1987; Cochran & Mays, 2000; Hughes et al., 2000, in press; Jones & Gabriel, 1999; Liddle, 1997; McDermott, Tyndall, & Lichtenberg, 1989; Morgan, 1992; Sorensen & Roberts, 1997). For example, in a study of women in the Midwest, Morgan (1992) found that 78% of lesbians compared with 29% of heterosexual women reported having been in therapy at some time in their lives. Rates in Morgan's study (1982) are similar to Bradford and Ryan's finding (1987) that 73% of the lesbians in the NLHCS had been in therapy at some point in their lives and to Hughes et al.'s findings (2000) that 78% of lesbians (compared with 56% of heterosexual women) in the Multi-site Women's Health Study (MWHS) had been in therapy. In the NLHCS and the MWHS, problems with partners and feeling sad, depressed, or anxious were among the most common reasons for seeking help. However, AOD problems were also commonly reported reasons; 13% of lesbians in the MWHS and 16% of lesbians in the NLHCS reported AOD problems as a reason for seeking help.

As in the general population, sexual minority men appear to be less likely than their female counterparts to seek mental health counseling. The only study located for this review that reported rates of mental health service use among adult gay men found that 56% of gay men compared with 27% of the heterosexual comparison group had consulted with a professional about emotional problems at some point in their lives (Bell & Weinberg, 1978).

Are lesbians and gay men more likely to seek mental health services because they experience more mental health problems associated with their sexual orientation, or because therapy/counseling is more normative and acceptable in gay and lesbian communities? Recent study results suggest that both are true. Meyer

(2003) conducted a meta-analysis of 10 studies that reported prevalence of diagnosed psychiatric disorders and compared lesbians, gay men, and/or bisexuals (variously defined) with heterosexual women and men. He examined the prevalence of any psychiatric disorder and the prevalence of general subclasses of disorders, including mood, anxiety, and substance use disorders. Comparisons of sexual minority and heterosexual women and men suggested a clear trend: Whenever significant differences were found, sexual minority groups had a higher prevalence. For example, in the five studies providing data on any lifetime mental disorders, lesbians and gay men were about 2.5 times more likely than their heterosexual counterparts to have had a mental disorder in their lifetime. Both lesbians and gay men had higher prevalence rates on most lifetime and current disorders; gay men, however, did not differ significantly from heterosexual men in terms of substance use disorders, and prevalence rates of these disorders were lower for gay men than for lesbians.

Conflict about sexual orientation, which often arises from internalized homophobia, has been found to be associated with psychological distress (DiPlacido, 1998a; Meyer, 1995) and substance use (Cabaj, 1996, 2000; Glaus, 1989; Kus, 1995) in lesbians and gay men. It seems reasonable, then, that use of therapy may moderate the relationship between distress associated with sexual orientation and drinking among some lesbians and gay men. For example, therapy may reduce the risk of heavy drinking by challenging the use of alcohol to self-medicate distress, or by increasing awareness of drinking behavior and the consequences of heavy drinking. Studies using more complex models and more sophisticated data analytic techniques are needed to permit more accurate assessment of whether the use of therapy is a consequence of dysfunctional drinking, a buffer against stress that helps to reduce heavy drinking, or both. Further, because young White women and men are more likely than their racial/ethnic minority and older counterparts to use mental health services, especially psychological counseling (Hasin & Link, 1988; Matthews & Hughes, 2001; Padgett, Harman, Burns, & Schlesinger, 1998), the effect of therapy on the relationship between psychological distress and drinking may be more salient for White than for racial/ethnic minority and for younger than older lesbians and gay men.

Summary of Risk and Protective Factors

Risks of heavy drinking or drinking-related problems are not associated with sexual orientation per se, but are a consequence of cultural and environmental factors associated with stigma and marginalization. Lesbians and gay men suffer from discrimination in housing, employment, and basic civil rights. In addition, they frequently feel uncomfortable with or rejected by their families of origin and often lose traditional social support when they disclose their sexual identity (Strommen, 1993; Vincke, Bolton, Mak, & Blank, 1993). In part because of societal stigma and discrimination, most lesbians and gay men do not bear or raise children (Patterson, 1998); lesbians, in particular, are less likely to assume many of the other traditional roles and responsibilities that are believed to limit drinking among heterosexual women (Hughes & Wilsnack, 1997). Until recently gay bars were among the few places lesbians and gay men could safely socialize and meet prospective partners.

Even in the presence of these risk factors, the majority of lesbians and gay men do not drink excessively or experience alcohol-related problems. This suggests that many lesbians and gay men have developed adaptive coping skills and resiliency that serve to protect them from heavy drinking. Understanding how resiliency develops in members of sexual minority groups could greatly enhance the effectiveness of prevention, early intervention, and treatment.

ASSESSMENT AND TREATMENT ISSUES

Although journal articles about sexual minority health that do not specifically include substance use/abuse among the top concerns are rare, there is a surprising dearth of empirical studies on assessment and treatment of alcohol problems in this population.

Assessment

The most effective means of outreach to lesbians and gay men who have problems related to their use of alcohol would be the routine inclusion of questions about sexual orientation in all health assessments, including those used to evaluate the severity of alcohol-related problems. Such questions can be readily integrated as part of the assessment of family, important relationships, social support, and sexual history.

Although the importance of considering gender and cultural differences in alcohol assessments and interventions is now well recognized (Bradley, Boyd-Wickizer, Powell, & Burman, 1998; O'Hare & Tran, 1997), little empirical work has been done to address the psychometric properties of standard screening or assessment instruments when used with sexual minorities. If, as suggested by McKirnan and Peterson (1989a), lesbians and gay men are more likely than heterosexual women and men to report alcohol-related problems, even at comparable levels of consumption, quantity–frequency measures alone might fail to identify individuals at risk in this population. Two studies were found that examined the reliability and validity of the CAGE alcohol screening tool with lesbians and gay men (Johnson & Hughes, in press; Knowlton, McCusker, Stoddard, Zapka, & Mayer, 1994). Results of these studies suggest that the CAGE has adequate validity and reliability in lesbians (Johnson & Hughes, in press) and in homosexually active men (Knowlton et al., 1994). No other studies were found that focused on screening or assessment of alcohol-related problems in sexual minority populations.

Treatment

In an early report about alcohol treatment for lesbians, Weathers (1980) described three major types of negative interactions between alcohol dependent lesbians and treatment providers. These included refusal of services if the woman's sexual orientation is known or suspected; provision of services on a limited basis, or with attitudes not conducive to support, growth, self-disclosure, or the maintenance of sobriety; and provision of services directed toward isolating and "curing" lesbianism as the primary problem, with little or no attention to the alcohol dependency itself (p. 146). Although the treatment options for lesbians and other sexual minorities are now greater and treatment providers' attitudes appear to be less negative, finding affirmative or sensitive treatment remains difficult (Eliason, 2000).

Pride Institute, founded in 1986, was the first, and remains one of the few, lesbian- and gay-affirmative inpatient treatment programs in the United States Pride's programs—now in five U.S. cities—actively promote self-acceptance of sexual minority identity as a central component of recovery and work to dispel myths and stereotypes about sexual minorities. The treatment philosophy is one that overtly affirms lesbians, gays, and bisexuals, their sexual orientation, and their families of choice (Pride Institute, www.pride-institute.com). In addition, although still relatively scarce, a growing number of treatment programs are lesbian- and gay-sensitive. Providers in these programs are knowledgeable about and sensitive to the unique concerns of sexual minorities and the difficulties and challenges that face them in recovery. These programs generally have a separate treatment "track" that includes education and therapy groups that are specific to sexual minorities.

Treatment Models

Current treatment models for sexual minority groups described in the literature are similar to traditional, mainstream treatment models; that is, they are based on the medical or disease perspective of addiction, generally provide education and therapy groups, incorporate the 12-step recovery system (e.g., Alcoholics Anonymous [AA], Narcotics Anonymous [NA]), and take into account other addictions or problems that may interfere with a client's ability to achieve and maintain sobriety. "Gay" AA groups now exist in all major cities and in many smaller suburbs and towns. However, because AA is commonly viewed as linked to religion and because many religious institutions denounce or condemn homosexuality, members of sexual minority groups may be resistant to treatment models that rely heavily on AA. This may be particularly true for lesbians, because many of them view AA as a male institution that has little consideration for them as women—and especially as lesbians—or because of the emphasis on powerlessness, which they feel emphasizes their status as victims (SAMHSA, 2001). In addition to awareness of potential difficulties with mainstream treatment philosophies such as AA, affirmative or sensitive alcohol-treatment programs and providers must demonstrate understanding of heterosexism as a form of cultural victimization and societal oppression (Neisen, 1997; Ratner, 1988).

Other recommendations for improving effectiveness of treatment services for sexual minorities include developing outreach programs and strategies specific to sexual minority clients, collecting data on sexual orientation at intake in order to track the use of services by these clients, increasing sexual minority oriented in-service training for staff, and including partners and families of choice in the treatment plan and process (Paul, Stall, & Bloomfield, 1991; Underhill & Wolverton, 1993). Such recommendations for improved quality of care for sexual minorities are actually recommendations for culturally competent practice (SAMHSA, 2001). Thus, assessment of cultural competency provides the basis for evaluations of quality of care.

Knowledge and Attitudes of Health Care Providers

As suggested above, knowledge and attitudes of health care providers are critical components in the treatment of sexual minority clients. The counselor–client relationship is a microcosm of the larger American social structure. It reflects the beliefs, stratifications, tensions, and injustices that exist in American society. Like race/ethnicity, sexual orientation may increase the complexity of the counselor–client relationship and the likelihood of misunderstandings between counselors and clients. Cultural misunderstandings may lead to difficulties in communication, obscure expectations, affect quality of care, and dramatically alter the lesbian's or gay client's willingness or ability to continue with treatment and adhere to treatment recommendations.

Aside from HIV/AIDS, much of the literature on health care for sexual minorities has focused primarily on lesbians. This literature reveals that many lesbians deeply distrust health care providers and that this mistrust is often well founded. In a comprehensive review of research related to health care providers' attitudes toward lesbians and to lesbians' experiences in health care encounters, Stevens (1992) documented blatantly homophobic attitudes of many providers. In the studies reviewed by Stevens, lesbians frequently interpreted providers' behavior as hostile and rejecting, and often feared for their safety in health care interactions.

Although the literature focusing on alcohol treatment suggests that attitudes of providers have improved over the past several decades, surveys of these providers indicate that they have limited knowledge about how to assess and treat lesbian, gay, or bisexual clients and that they often do not discuss sexual orientation with their clients, even when they consider it important to do so (Eliason, 2000; Hellman, Stanton, Tytun, & Vachon, 1989).

Do Gender and Sexual Orientation of Treatment Providers Matter?

Studies of mental health services use have typically focused on either racial/ ethnic or gender differences (Padgett et al., 1998), and generally find that White women are most likely to use these services. The few studies that have examined the influence of sexual orientation on mental health service use suggest that lesbians and gay men are among the most active—but least acknowledged— consumers of mental health counseling (Bell & Weinberg, 1978; Bradford, Ryan, & Rothblum, 1994; Hughes et al., 2000; Jones & Gabriel, 1999; Liddle, 1997; Morgan, 1992; Sorensen & Roberts, 1997). Although not focused on alcohol treatment, there has been a fair amount of speculation in the literature about whether sexual minority women and men who seek treatment need counselors who share their group membership. In an early article on homophobia among psychologists, Gartrell (1984) argued that lesbian therapists have access to life experiences in common with lesbian clients, and thus have a deeper understanding of what it means to be lesbian and of cultural influences that are important to this group. In general, the literature on the preferences of lesbians and gay clients suggests that, although counselors' sexual orientation is important (McDermott, Tyndall, & Lichtenberg, 1989), it is less important than gender (Hughes et al., 2000; Jones & Gabriel, 1999; Matthews & Hughes, 2001; Modrcin & Wyers, 1990). This is particularly true for lesbians. In most of the studies reviewed, the vast majority of lesbians preferred a female counselor or therapist. Little is known about how lesbians and gay men find or choose mental health service providers, or about their satisfaction with the services they receive (Razzano, Matthews, & Hughes, 2002).

Are Lesbian/Gay-Specific Treatment Programs or Approaches Necessary?

The argument about whether lesbians and gay men who have alcohol-related problems need specialized treatment is similar to an older and ongoing debate about whether women do better in single or mixed-gender treatment. In a review of the literature on women in treatment, Hodgins, El-Guebaly, and Addington (1997) argue that women need gender-specific treatment approaches because they differ from men in their substance use histories, victimization histories, and gender-role expectations and conflicts. Similarly, as described earlier in this section, the experiences of lesbians and gay men differ from those of their heterosexual counterparts in ways that impact their treatment needs (Finnegan & McNally, 2002; Hughes & Wilsnack, 1997). However, whether these differences influence treatment outcomes is unknown, and this question will remain unanswered until well-designed clinical trials and other evaluation studies of lesbians and gay men treated for alcohol problems are conducted.

Treatment Evaluation

Currently, there are no evidence-based practice guidelines (and no data to support the development of such guidelines) to assist alcohol treatment providers in program development and service delivery for sexual minorities. Accrediting bodies such as the Joint Commission on Accreditation of Healthcare Organizations (JCAHO), the National Committee on Quality Assurance (NCQA), and the Commission on the Accreditation of Rehabilitation Facilities (CARF) have established standards for the key components and functions of health care organizations, including substance abuse treatment facilities. In addition, the American Psychological Association (APA) provides recommendations for professional development and practice related to psychotherapy with lesbian, gay, and bisexual clients (APA, Division 44, 2000). These standards and guidelines provide a framework that can be used to guide the development or improvement of services for sexual minorities (SAMHSA, 2001).

Although no published evaluations of the effectiveness of alcohol treatment for sexual minorities were found, Pride Institute's Web site states that an independent outcome study found that Pride's graduates were more likely to remain chemically free than lesbian/gay graduates of mainstream programs (www.prideinstitute.com). An unpublished evaluation study compared 14-month treatment outcomes of patients treated at Pride Institute with 6-month outcomes of patients treated in five similar, lesbian/gay sensitive, but not lesbian/gay affirmative, treatment programs. Results suggest that Pride graduates did substantially better on almost all outcome measures (Ratner, Kosten, & McLellan, 1991).

Well-controlled clinical trials are needed to determine whether outcomes of programs tailored for sexual minority clients produce better treatment outcomes and to evaluate the cost–benefit ratio of such programs. The absence of evaluation data severely limits understanding of the effectiveness of programs or services and inhibits the development of effective assessment and treatment strategies for sexual minority population groups.

METHODOLOGICAL ISSUES

There is a growing body of research focusing on sexual minority health, including alcohol-related problems. This research, however, is characterized by a plethora of methodological problems. The most important methodological issues in re-search with lesbians and gay men—whether the focus is on alcohol use/abuse or other health concerns—include biases related to sampling methods and the samples studied, use of inconsistent and nonstandard measures, and the almost complete lack of prospective or longitudinal studies.

Study Samples and Research Designs

Until recently, the vast majority of studies conducted with sexual minorities have used cross-sectional research designs conducted with nonprobability samples. Although data collected at one point in time from a convenience sample can provide greater depth of understanding of the people and topics examined, the extent to which the information is generalizable remains an important issue.

Random samples are very difficult to obtain because very large numbers of persons must be screened to identify a sufficient sampling frame of lesbians and/ or gay men for a given study. Currently, many researchers attempt to limit biases inherent in convenience samples by using multiple sources and multiple methods of recruiting lesbian and gay participants. A few researchers have employed innovative sampling strategies that include combinations of data from census tracts, reports of HIV/AIDS infection rates, and gay organizations' mailing lists to obtain probability samples from areas believed to be more densely populated by gay men (Binson et al., 1996; Blair, 1999). These methods are useful in urban areas with densely populated and well-defined "gay" neighborhoods but are much less effective in sampling lesbians (Meyer, Rossano, Ellis, & Bradford, 2002) or sexual minority persons in rural areas or small towns because these groups are less likely to cluster in defined geographic locations. Further, this sampling strategy remains prohibitively expensive for the majority of researchers.

One of the most efficient and cost-effective means of obtaining representa-tive samples would be the inclusion of questions about sexual orientation in ongoing population-based studies that include a focus on substance use and abuse. Although political constraints have limited advances in this area, some progress has been made, including, for example, the inclusion of questions about sexual orientation in the National Health and Nutrition Examination Survey, the Youth Risk Behavior Surveillance System, the National Comorbidity Study, the 1996 National Household Survey on Drug Abuse, and the Women's Health Initiative. Unfortunately, when such questions are included, they typically ask about sexual behavior only. Regardless of the questions asked, given the relatively low base rate of homosexuality (or willingness to report it), these studies identify few lesbians and gay men. However, if questions about sexual orientation were asked as routinely as questions about other sociodemographic characteristics, samples from multiple years of the same study, or from several studies conducted within the same year, could be combined to form much larger probability samples.

Even with the best sampling methods, lesbians and gay men who are most "closeted" are likely to be excluded. Those willing to participate in research studies may be quite different from those who are unwilling to identify themselves as lesbian or gay (Morris & Rothblum, 1999). Judging from existing demographic profiles of study samples, lesbians and gay men who participate in research are more highly educated and more likely to be White and middle class than are women and men in general population surveys. This, of course, makes it difficult to compare findings from studies of lesbians and gay men with general population norms.

To date, only a handful of longitudinal studies have been conducted with sexual minority populations. All of these studies have focused on HIV-risk behaviors among men who have sex with men (e.g., Chesney, Barrett, & Stall, 1998; Jinich et al., 1998; Ostrow et al., 1993; Woody et al., 1999).[4] Although cross-sectional studies provide important information about the health risks and health needs of sexual minority groups, such studies are unable to assess changes in alcohol-use patterns and problems over time and cannot determine the temporal order of risk factors and indicators of alcohol-related problems.

Measures of Sexual Orientation

There is growing consensus that full assessment of sexual orientation requires measurement of multiple dimensions, including behavior, identity, and attraction or desire (Brogan, Frank, Elon, & O'Hanlan, 2001; Laumann et al., 1994; Meyer, Silenzio, Wolfe, & Dunn, 2000; Sell & Becker, 2001; Solarz, 1999). Currently, there is little consistency in how this construct is defined and measured. The terms *sexual orientation* and *sexual identity* are often used interchangeably, and *same-gender behavior* is frequently used as a proxy for *sexual identity* in studies of lesbians and gay men. The lack of standard terms and definitions greatly complicates efforts to estimate the number of lesbian, gay, and bisexual persons within the overall population and the prevalence of various health conditions within these sexual minority groups (Meyer et al., 2000). Until researchers explicitly and consistently describe how sexual orientation is operationally defined, comparisons across studies will be tentative at best.

Characteristics of the Researcher

A less recognized methodological "issue" relates to characteristics of researchers who wish to conduct studies related to sexual minority health. This concern is most salient for heterosexual investigators and for those who are new to sexual minority research. Only recently have questions been raised about whether heterosexual or "straight" researchers can conduct sensitive and meaningful research with groups oppressed because of their sexual minority status. This question looms largest in research that aims to gather sensitive information such as data about violence, victimization, sexuality, and substance use/abuse. Researchers who are not themselves members of the group they wish to study face the challenge of gaining access to the community and securing the ongoing cooperation of its members. Heterosexual researchers are often suspected of using sexual minority groups to enhance their own careers—rather than generating information to reduce social myths and improve health care practices—and must adopt culturally sensitive strategies that enable them to be considered more than an intrusive outsider. McClennan (2003), a heterosexual woman who studies same-gender intimate partner violence, wrote about the difficulties she encountered as an "outsider" researcher. In addition to gaining access to sexual minority communities and the trust of community members, she emphasized the need for outsider researchers to be aware of heterosexist biases that may negatively influence the formulation of research questions and the interpretation of results. She acknowledged that insider researchers may formulate questions that might not occur to outsiders, have greater knowledge about where and how to reach their samples, and have greater ease in gaining entry into settings where study participants can be recruited. She rightly noted that being an insider does not, however, guarantee a productive, working relationship between the researcher and community or group of interest. Trust must also be gained by lesbian, gay, and bisexual investigators who study the groups to which they belong. Further, insider researchers who are new to sexual minority research may not understand the importance of precise definitions of sexual orientation or the need for community involvement in formulating research questions and hypotheses and in choosing or developing culturally sensitive research questions.

RECOMMENDATIONS FOR FUTURE RESEARCH

This literature review points to numerous gaps and issues in the research focusing on alcohol use among sexual minority groups, including the general need for more research and for research with bisexuals, older sexual minority group members, and racial/ethnic sexual minority group members in particular. In addition, there is a clear need for clinical trials and other studies of treatment effectiveness, as well as a need for greater methodological rigor in research with sexual minorities.

Understanding the differential distribution of risk factors and negative outcomes related to alcohol use/abuse within sexual minority population groups and between sexual minorities and heterosexuals requires greater attention to how historical, social, economic, political, and cultural contexts shape health-damaging and health-enhancing variables that are typically measured at the individual level. For example, are older individuals who came out before the gay rights movement of the 1960s, when gay bars were among the few places to socialize and meet other lesbians/gay people, at greater risk for drinking-related problems than their age-matched counterparts who came out later? Are bisexual women at greater risk than lesbians? If so, does heavy drinking stem from the potentially greater stress associated with having an identity that is largely invisible—both in the general society and in gay and lesbian communities? Is same-gender behavior, in the absence of a sexual minority identity, simply one of a cluster of high-risk behaviors shared by a segment of the population? What are the individual and environmental factors most predictive of resilience in sexual minority women and men? Alcohol studies of same-gender twins or other sibling pairs in which one sibling is homosexual and the other heterosexual, such as those focusing on self-esteem and mental health in female siblings (Rothblum & Factor, 2001) and suicidality in male twins (Herrell et al., 1999), would be particularly informative.

Many research questions appear more amenable to qualitative than quantitative research designs. Much of the qualitative work on alcohol use and abuse in sexual minority groups has been conducted with lesbians, and the largest focus of this research has been on the recovery process among lesbians (Hall, 1993, 1994; McNally & Finnegan, 1992). A notable exception is Parks' work (1999a, 1999b) that examines the relationships between alcohol use and the developmental process of "coming out" in three generational age cohorts of lesbians. More qualitative work, particularly studies that more fully examine the life experiences of lesbians and gay men and the meaning of alcohol in their lives, would provide valuable information to inform the development of more theoretically sound research and clinical practice.

Very little is known about the health behavior and health concerns of lesbians and gay men (or bisexual women and men) across the life span. Sexual behaviors, economic status, and relationship patterns differ substantially across different age groups and between women and men. Life-course or life-span research that focuses on various age cohorts to help more clearly identify age- and gender-specific factors associated with risk vulnerability is needed. Longitudinal studies of a cohort or generation of lesbians, gays, and bisexual women and men would provide an even more powerful tool for risk-factor identification. More sophisticated research designs and data analytic strategies that permit examination of complex explanatory models such as those containing mediating and moderating variables would greatly expand our understanding of sexual minority health. Also important are studies that include larger samples of persons of color to better understand whether or how race/ethnicity interacts with sexual orientation to influence alcohol-abuse risk at various stages of development.

In addition to the need for more rigorously designed studies on risk factors for alcohol abuse in sexual minority populations, balanced attention must be given to protective factors and resilience. For example, although many lesbians and gay men have experienced abuse or violence in childhood or adulthood, and all members of sexual minority groups are exposed to myriad stressors associated with their nonheterosexual behavior or identity, most of them do not drink excessively. Focusing on resilient groups, by far the majority, can inform the development of prevention and intervention strategies by highlighting effective coping and problem-solving skills. Further, focusing on strengths and resilience might help to lessen the tendency of health care providers and others to view sexual minorities through a pathological lens and would send a much more positive message to sexual minority individuals. This would help boost self-esteem and encourage greater attention to their health and to the use of preventive health care services.

PROGRESS IN THE FIELD

Although a number of gaps remain and greater methodological rigor is needed, an impressive amount of progress has been made, especially given the short history of alcohol research among lesbians and gay men and the barriers faced by researchers in this field. Until the mid-1980s, researchers obtained very little federal money for research on sexual orientation. Since then, considerably more funding has been available for research related to substance abuse and sexual orientation, but this funding has largely focused on HIV/AIDS-related research. Silvestre (1999) reviewed reports of research funded by the National Institutes of Health (NIH) between 1974 and 1992 that listed homosexuality as a primary or secondary focus. Only 13% of grants dealt with non-HIV-related issues. Research projects on homosexuality unrelated to HIV averaged only $532,000 per year (excluding funds for building facilities) compared with about $20 million per year since 1982 for HIV-related projects. Research on HIV/AIDS has substantially improved understanding of the relationship between alcohol abuse and unsafe sexual behavior in MSMs, and this information has informed interventions that have substantially reduced the risk of HIV/AIDS among this sexual minority group. There is no question about the importance of this research; however, the interest and attention devoted to HIV/AIDS has inevitably diverted attention and funding from other health problems, including non-HIV/AIDS-related AOD use/abuse. Further, the linking of homosexuality with unsafe sex practices, AOD abuse, and the HIV/AIDS epidemic continues to fuel socially conservative lawmakers' efforts to block or reverse gains made in understanding sexual minority health and in the civil rights of sexual minority groups. The recent threat that funding for studies of sexual minorities (or studies that focus on sexuality in any population group) might be withdrawn is a real concern and could discourage investigators or students who wish to study health concerns of these population groups (Chronicle of Higher Education, 2003).

Despite multiple barriers to research with sexual minority populations, including attempts by socially conservative groups to monitor and restrict funding for research focusing on health concerns of sexual minorities, progress continues to be made. Examples of recent initiatives aimed at improving understanding of sexual minority health are the Institute of Medicine's report *Lesbian Health: Current Assessment and Directions for the Future* (Solarz, 1999), funded by the NIH Office of Research on Women's Health and the Centers for Disease Control and Prevention's (CDC) Office of Women's Health; the Removing the Barriers project (Scout, Bradford, & Fields, 2001), funded by the CDC; the inclusion of sexual orientation in Healthy People 2010 as one of six population groups for which health disparities exist (USDHHS, 2000b); and the *Healthy People 2010 Companion Document for Lesbian, Gay, Bisexual, and Transgender Health* (GLMA & LGBT Experts, 2001). In addition, the Substance Abuse and Mental Health Services Administration released *A Provider's Introduction to Substance Abuse Treatment for Lesbian, Gay, Bisexual, and Transgender Individuals* (SAMHSA, 2001), and the *American Journal of Public Health* (2001) published a special issue on sexual minority health. Such initiatives, in combination with greater funding opportunities for health-related studies, should help to stimulate further research, prevention, and treatment efforts aimed at improving the health and lives of lesbians and gay men as well as other sexual minority groups.

NOTES

[1]Because sexual identity is much less stable in children and adolescents, and because the issues related to alcohol use and abuse varies greatly among lesbian, gay, and bisexual (LGB) youth and adults, this review is limited to studies of adult LGB populations.

[2]Bisexual women and men are included in this review to the extent possible. However, because the samples of the research studies reviewed differ (e.g., some include only lesbians, some only lesbians and gay men, and some combined samples of lesbian/gay/bisexual participants), the terms used to describe the specific samples will be used. It should also be noted that many samples described as "lesbian" or "gay" likely include some bisexual women or men.

[3]The conceptual model is an adaptation of a model from Sharon and Richard Wilsnack's national longitudinal study of women's drinking. It has been modified slightly for simplicity and for closer fit with the literature related to lesbians' and gay men's drinking.

[4]The author is currently collecting the second wave of data in a longitudinal study that focuses on risk and protective factors for heavy drinking and drinking-related problems among lesbians.

ACKNOWLEDGMENTS

Development of this chapter was supported by funding from the National Institute on Alcohol Abuse and Alcoholism (K01 #AA0026 and R01 #AA13328). The author wishes to acknowledge her colleague Cheryl Parks and members of her research staff (Frances Aranda, Wendy Bostwick, Aimee Callanan, Kristin Jacobson, and Kelly Martin), who assisted with preparation of the paper. In addition, the author is especially grateful to Sharon Wilsnack—mentor, colleague, and friend—whose work provides the basis for the conceptual model included in this review and for the author's research on risk and protective factors for heavy drinking and drinking-related problems among lesbians.

REFERENCES

American Psychological Association (APA), Division 44. (2000). Guidelines for psychotherapy with lesbian, gay, and bisexual clients. *American Psychologist, 55*(12), 1440–1451.

American Public Health Association. (1999, September). The need for acknowledging transgender individuals within research and clinical practice. *The Nation's Health,* 46–48.

Ayala, J., & Coleman, H. (2000). Predictors of depression among lesbian women. *Journal of Lesbian Studies, 4*(3), 71–86.

Bartholow, B. N., Doll, L. S., Joy, D., Douglas, J. M., Bolan, G., Harrison, J. S., et al. (1994). Emotional, behavioral and HIV risks associated with sexual abuse among adult homosexual and bisexual men. *Child Abuse and Neglect, 18,* 747–761.

Bell, A. P., & Weinberg, M. S. (1978). *Homosexualities: A study of diversity among men and women.* New York: Simon & Schuster.

Bell, A. P., Weinberg, M. S., & Hammersmith, S. K. (1981). *Sexual preference: Its development in men and women.* Bloomington: Indiana University Press.

Bergmark, K. H. (1999). Drinking in the Swedish gay and lesbian community. *Drug and Alcohol Dependence, 56,* 133–143.

Binson, D., Moskowitz, J., Mills, T., Anderson, K., Paul, J., Stall, R., et al. (1996). Sampling men who have sex with men: Strategies for a telephone survey in urban areas in the United States. *Proceedings of the American Statistical Association, 1,* 68–72.

Blair, J. (1999). A probability sample of gay urban males: The use of two-phase adaptive sampling. *Journal of Sex Research, 36*(1), 39–44.

Bloomfield, K. A. (1993). A comparison of alcohol consumption between lesbians and heterosexual women in an urban population. *Drug and Alcohol Dependence, 33,* 257–269.

Bradford, J., & Ryan, C. (1987). *The National Lesbian Health Care Survey: Final report.* Washington, DC: National Lesbian and Gay Health Foundation.

Bradford, J., Ryan, C., & Rothblum, E. D. (1994). National lesbian health care survey: Implications for mental health care. *Journal of Consulting and Clinical Psychology, 62*(2), 228–242.

Bradley, K. A., Boyd-Wickizer, J., Powell, S. H., & Burman, M. L. (1998). Alcohol screening questionnaires in women: A critical review. *Journal of the American Medical Association, 280*(2), 166–171.

Brenan, P. L., & Moos, R. H. (1996). Late-life problem drinking: Personal and environmental risk factors for 4-year functioning outcomes and treatment seeking. *Journal of Substance Abuse, 8*(2), 167–180.

Brogan, D., Frank, E., Elon, L., & O'Hanlan, K. (2001). Methodologic concerns in defining lesbian for health research. *Epidemiology, 12*(1), 109–113.

Cabaj, R. P. (1996). Substance abuse in gay men, lesbians, and bisexuals. In R. P. Cabaj & T. S. Stein (Eds.), *Textbook of homosexuality and mental health* (pp. 783–799). Washington, DC: American Psychiatric Press.

———. (2000). Substance abuse, internalized homophobia, and gay men and lesbians: Psychodynamic issues and clinical implications. *Journal of Gay and Lesbian Psychotherapy, 3*(3–4), 5–24.

Caldwell, M. A., & Peplau, L. A. (1984). The balance of power in lesbian relationships. *Sex Roles, 10,* 587–599.

Cass, V. (1984). Homosexual identity: A concept in need of a definition. *Journal of Homosexuality, 9,* 105–126.

Cassese, J. (Ed.). (2000). Gay men and childhood sexual trauma: Integrating the shattered self. *Journal of Gay and Lesbian Social Services, 12*(1–2), 1–17.

Chesney, M. A., Barrett, D. C., & Stall, R. (1998). Histories of alcohol use and risk behavior: Precursors to HIV seroconversion in homosexual men. *American Journal of Public Health, 88*(1), 113–116.

Chilcoat, H. D., & Breslau, N. (1996). Alcohol disorders in young adulthood: Effects of transitions into adult roles. *Journal of Health and Social Behavior, 37,* 339–349.

Chng, C. L., & Geliga-Vargas, J. (2000). Ethnic identity, gay identity, sexual sensation seeking and HIV risk taking among multiethnic men who have sex with men. *AIDS Education and Prevention, 12*(4), 326–339.

Chronicle of Higher Education. (2003, October 27). Congress asks NIH to justify more than 160 research projects. Retrieved October 27, 2003, from http://chronicle.com/daily/2003/10/2003102701n.htm

Clark, W. B. (1991). Introduction to drinking contexts. In W. B. Clark & M. E. Hilton (Eds.), *Alcohol in America: Drinking practices and problems* (pp. 249–255). Albany: State University of New York Press.

Clay, K. M., Olsheski, J. A., & Clay, S. W. (2000). Alcohol use disorders in female survivors of childhood sexual abuse. *Alcoholism Treatment Quarterly, 19*(4), 19–29.

Cochran, S. D., Keenan, C., Schober, C., & Mays, V. M. (2000). Estimates of alcohol use and clinical treatment needs among homosexually active men and women in the US population. *Journal of Consulting and Clinical Psychology, 68*(6), 1062–1071.

Cochran, S., & Mays, V. (1994). Depressive distress among homosexually active African American men and women. *American Journal of Psychiatry, 151*(4), 524–529.

———. (2000). Relation between psychiatric syndromes and behaviorally defined sexual orientation in a sample of the US populations. *American Journal of Epidemiology, 151*(5), 516–523.

Cohen, S., & Hoberman, H. M. (1983). Positive life events and social supports as buffers of life change stress. *Journal of Applied Social Psychology, 13,* 99–125.

Cohen, S., & Willis, T. A. (1985). Stress, social support, and the buffering hypothesis. *Psychology Bulletin, 98,* 310–357.

Coleman, V. E. (1994). Lesbian battering: The relationship between personality and the perpetration of violence. *Violence and Victims, 9*(2), 139–152.

Cooper, M. L., Russell, M., Skinner, J. B., Frone, M. R., & Mudar, P. (1992). Stress and alcohol abuse: Moderating effects of gender, coping, and alcohol expectancies. *Journal of Abnormal Psychology, 101,* 139–152.

Crosby, G. M., Stall, R. D., Paul, J. P., & Barrett, D. C. (1998). Alcohol and drug use patterns have declined between generations of younger gay-bisexual men in San Francisco. *Drug and Alcohol Dependence, 52*, 177–182.

Croteau, J. M. (1996). Research on the work experience of lesbian, gay, and bisexual people: An integrative review of methodology and findings. *Journal of Vocational Behavior, 48*, 195–209.

D'Augelli, A. R., & Hershberger, S. L. (1993). Lesbian, gay, and bisexual youth in community settings: Personal challenges and mental health problems. *American Journal of Community Psychology, 21*(4), 421–448.

Dawson, D. A., Grant, B. F., Chou, S. P., & Pickering, R. P. (1995). Subgroup variation in U. S. drinking patterns: Results of the 1992 National Longitudinal Alcohol Epidemiologic Study. *Journal of Substance Abuse, 7*, 331–334.

DeBord, K. A., Wood, P. K., Sher, K. J., & Good, G. E. (1998). The relevance of sexual orientation to substance abuse and psychological distress among college students. *Journal of College Student Development, 39*(2), 157–168.

Descamps, M. J., Rothblum, E., Bradford, J., & Ryan, C. (2000). Mental health impact of child sexual abuse, rape, intimate partner violence and hate crimes in the National Lesbian Health Care Survey. *Journal of Gay and Lesbian Social Services, 11*(1), 27–55.

Diamond, L. M. (2000). Sexual identity, attractions, and behavior among young sexual minority women over a 2-year period. *Developmental Psychology, 36*(2), 241–250.

DiPlacido, J. (1998a, August). *Minority stress and well-being among lesbians and bisexual women.* Presented at the American Psychological Association Conference, San Francisco.

———. (1998b). Minority stress among lesbians, gay men, and bisexuals. A consequence of heterosexism, homophobia, and stigmatization. In G. M. Herek (Ed.), *Stigma and sexual orientation: Psychological perspectives on lesbian and gay issues* (Vol. 4, pp. 138–159). Thousand Oaks, CA: Sage.

Dixit, A. R., & Crum, R. M. (2000). Prospective study of depression and the risk of heavy alcohol use in women. *American Journal of Psychiatry, 157*(5), 751–758.

Dohrenwend, B. S., Krasnoff, L., Askenasy, A. R., & Dohrenwend, B. P. (1978). Exemplification of a method for scaling life events: The PERI Life Events Scale. *Journal of Health and Social Behavior, 19*, 205–229.

Duffy, S. M., & Rusbult, C. E. (1986). Satisfaction and commitment in homosexual and heterosexual relationships. *Journal of Homosexuality, 12*, 1–23.

Eliason, M. (2000). Substance abuse counselors' attitudes regarding lesbian, gay, and bisexual and transgender clients. *Journal of Substance Abuse, 12*, 311–328.

Eliason, M., & Hughes, T. (2004). Treatment counselor's attitudes about lesbian, gay, bisexual, and transgendered clients: Urban vs. rural settings. *Substance Use and Misuse, 39*(4), 625–644.

Elliott, P. (1996). Shattering illusions: Same-sex domestic violence. *Journal of Gay and Lesbian Social Services, 4*(1), 1–8.

Espin, O. (1993). Issues of identity in the psychology of Latina lesbians. In L. D. Garnets & D. C. Kimmel (Eds.), *Psychological perspectives on lesbian and gay male experience* (pp. 348–363). New York: Columbia University Press.

Falk, P. (1993). Lesbian mothers: Psychosocial assumptions and family law. In L. D. Garnets & D. C. Kimmel (Eds.), *Psychological perspectives on lesbian and gay male experience* (pp. 420–436). New York: Columbia University Press.

Fifield, L. H., Latham, J. D., & Phillips, C. (1977). *Alcoholism in the gay community: The price of alienation, isolation, and oppression*. Los Angeles: Gay Community Services Center.

Fillmore, K. M., Golding, J. M., Leino, E. V., Motoyoshi, M., Shoemaker, C., Terry, H., Ager, C. R., et al. (1997). Patterns and trends in women's and men's drinking. In R. W. Wilsnack & S. C. Wilsnack (Eds.), *Gender and alcohol: Individual and social perspectives* (pp. 21–48). New Brunswick, NJ: Rutgers Center of Alcohol Studies.

Finnegan, D. G., & McNally, E. B. (2002). *Counseling lesbian, gay, bisexual, and transgender substance abusers*. New York: Haworth Press.

Firestein, B. A. (1996). *Bisexuality: The psychology and politics of an invisible minority*. Thousand Oaks, CA: Sage.

Fobair, P., O'Hanlan, K., Koopman, C., Classen, C., Dimiceli, S., Drooker, N., et al. (2001). Comparison of lesbian and heterosexual women's response to newly diagnosed breast cancer. *Psycho-Oncology, 10*, 40–51.

Gartrell, N. (1984). Combating homophobia in psychologists. *Women and Therapy, 3*, 13–29.

Gay and Lesbian Medical Association (GLMA) & LGBT Experts. (2001). *Healthy People 2010: Companion document for lesbian, gay, bisexual, and transgender (LGBT) health*. Retrieved Oct. 27, 2003, from www.glma.org

Ghindia, D. J., & Kola, L. A. (1996). Co-factors affecting alcohol abuse among homosexual men: An investigation within a Midwestern gay community. *Drug and Alcohol Dependence, 41*, 167–177.

Gilbert, J. M., & Collins, R. L. (1997). Ethnic variation in women's and men's drinking. In R. W. Wilsnack & S. C. Wilsnack (Eds.), *Gender and alcohol* (pp. 357–378). New Brunswick, NJ: Rutgers Center of Alcohol Studies.

Gilman, S. E., & Abraham, H. D. (2001). A longitudinal study of the order of onset of alcohol dependence and major depression. *Drug and Alcohol Dependence, 63*(3), 277–286.

Gilman, S. E., Cochran, S. D., Mays, V. M., Hughes, M., Ostrow, D., & Kessler, R. C. (2001). Risk of psychiatric disorders among individuals reporting same-sex sexual partners in the National Comorbidity Study. *American Journal of Public Health, 91*(6), 933–939.

Glaus, K. O. (1989). Alcoholism, chemical dependency and the lesbian client. *Women and Therapy, 8*(1–2), 131–144.

Gomez, C. A., Garcia, D. R., Kegebein, V. J., Shade, S. B., & Hernandez, S. R. (1996). Sexual identity versus sexual behavior: Implications for HIV prevention strategies for women who have sex with women. *Women's Health: Research on Gender, Behavior, and Policy, 2*(1–2), 91–109.

Green, R. J., Bettinger, M., & Zacks, E. (1996). Are lesbian couples fused and gay male couples disengaged? Questioning gender straightjackets. In J. Laird & R. J. Green (Eds.), *Lesbians and gays in couples and families: A handbook for therapists* (pp. 185–230). San Francisco: Jossey-Bass.

Greene, B. (1994). Lesbian and gay sexual orientations. In B. Greene & G. M. Herek (Eds.), *Lesbian and gay psychology: Theory, research, and clinical applications* (Vol. 1, pp. 1–24). Thousand Oaks, CA: Sage.

———. (1997). Ethnic minority lesbians and gay men. Mental health and treatment issues. In B. Greene (Ed.), *Ethnic and cultural diversity among lesbians and gay men* (pp. 216–239). Thousand Oaks, CA: Sage.

Greenfield, T. K., & Room, R. (1997). Situational norms for drinking and drunkenness: Trends in the U.S. adult population, 1979–1990. *Addiction, 92*(1), 33–47.

Gruskin, E. P., Hart, S., Gordon, N., & Ackerson, L. (2001). Patterns of cigarette smoking and alcohol use among lesbians and bisexual women enrolled in a large health maintenance organization. *American Journal of Public Health, 91*(6), 976–979.

Hall, J. M. (1993). Lesbians and alcohol: Patterns and paradoxes in medical notions and lesbian beliefs. *Journal of Psychoactive Drugs, 25*(2), 109–122.

———. (1994). How lesbians recognize and respond to alcohol problems: A theoretical model of problematization. *Advances in Nursing Science, 16*(3), 46–63.

Hasin, D. S., & Link, B. (1988). Age and recognition of depression: Implications for a cohort effect in major depression. *Psychological Medicine, 18,* 683–688.

Heffernan, K. (1998). Nature and predictors of substance use among lesbians. *Addictive Behaviors: An International Journal, 23*(4), 517–528.

Hellman, R. E., Stanton, M., Lee, J., Tytun, A., & Vachon, R. (1989). Treatment of homosexual alcoholics in government-funded agencies: Provider training and attitudes. *Hospital and Community Psychiatry, 40*(11), 1163–1168.

Herd, D. (1993). An analysis of alcohol-related problems in black and white women drinkers. *Addiction Research, 1*(3), 181–198.

Herek, G. M. (1991). Stigma, prejudice, and violence against lesbians and gay men. In J. C. Gonsiorek & J. D. Weinrich (Eds.), *Homosexuality: Research implications for public policy* (pp. 60–80). Newbury Park, CA: Sage.

Herrell, R., Goldberg, J., True, W. R., Ramakrishman, V., Lyons, M., Eisen, S., et al. (1999). Sexual orientation and suicidality. *Archives of General Psychiatry, 56,* 867–874.

Hesselbrock, M. N., & Hesselbrock, V. M. (1997). Gender, alcoholism, and psychiatric comorbidity. In R. W. Wilsnack & S. C. Wilsnack (Eds.), *Gender and alcohol: Individual and social perspectives* (pp. 49–71). New Brunswick, NJ: Rutgers Center of Alcohol Studies.

Hodgins, D. C., El-Guebaly, N., & Addington, J. (1997). Treatment of substance abusers: Single or mixed gender programs? *Addiction, 92,* 805–812.

Hooker, E. (1957). The adjustment of the male overt homosexual. *Journal Projective Techniques, 21,* 18–31.

Hope, S., Rodgers, B., & Power, C. (1999). Marital status transitions and psychological distress: Longitudinal evidence from a national population sample. *Psychological Medicine, 29,* 381–389.

Horwitz, A. V., White, H. R., & Howell-White, S. (1996). The use of multiple outcomes in stress research: A case study of gender differences in response to marital dissolution. *Journal of Health and Social Behavior, 37,* 278–291.

Hughes, T. L. (2003). Lesbians' drinking patterns: Beyond the data. *Substance Use and Misuse, 38,* 1739–1758.

Hughes, T. L., Haas, A. P., & Avery, L. (1997). Lesbians and mental health: Preliminary results from the Chicago Women's Health Survey. *Journal of the Gay and Lesbian Medical Association, 1*(3), 133–144.

Hughes, T. L., Haas, A. P., Razzano, L., Cassidy, R., & Matthews, A. K. (2000). Comparing lesbians' and heterosexual women's mental health: Findings from a multi-site study. *Journal of Gay and Lesbian Social Services, 11*(1), 57–76.

Hughes, T. L., & Johnson, T. (2003, June). *Risk factors for drinking-related problems among adult lesbians.* Paper presented at the 26th Annual Scientific Meeting of the Research Society on Alcoholism, Fort Lauderdale, FL.

Hughes, T. L., Johnson, T. P., & Wilsnack, S. C. (2001). Sexual assault and alcohol abuse: A comparison of lesbians and heterosexual women. *Journal of Alcohol Abuse, 13*, 515–532.

Hughes, T. L., Matthews, A. K., Razzano, L., & Aranda, F. (2003). Psychological distress in African American lesbians and heterosexual women. *Journal of Lesbian Studies, 7*(1), 51–68.

Hughes, T. L., & Wilsnack, S. C. (1997). Use of alcohol among lesbians: Research and clinical implications. *American Journal of Orthopsychiatry, 66*(1), 20–36.

Hughes, T. L., Wilsnack, S. C., & Johnson, T. (in press). Investigating lesbians' mental health and alcohol use: What is an appropriate comparison group? In A. Omoto & H. Kurtzman (Eds.), *Recent research on sexual orientation, mental health, and substance use.* Washington, DC: APA Books.

Hurlburt, D., & Apt, C. (1993). Female sexuality: A comparative study between women in homosexual and heterosexual relationships. *Journal of Sex and Marital Therapy, 19*, 315–327.

Israelstam, S., & Lambert, S. (1983). Homosexuality as a cause of alcoholism: A historical review. *International Journal of the Addictions, 18*(8), 1085–1107.

Jinich, S., Paul, J. P., Stall, R., Acree, M., Kegeles, S., Hoff, C., et al. (1998). Childhood sexual abuse and HIV risk-taking behavior among gay and bisexual men. *AIDS and Behavior, 2*(1), 41–51.

Johnson, T., & Hughes, T. L. (in press). The reliability and concurrent validity of the CAGE screening questions: A comparison of lesbian and heterosexual women. *Journal of Substance Use and Misuse.*

Jones, M., & Gabriel, M. A. (1999). Utilization of psychotherapy by lesbians, gay men, and bisexuals: Findings from a nationwide survey. *American Journal of Orthopsychiatry, 69*(2), 209–219.

Jordan, K. M., & Deluty, R. H. (1998). Coming out for lesbian women: Its relation to anxiety, positive affectivity, self-esteem, and social support. *Journal of Homosexuality, 35*(2), 41–63.

Jorm, A. F., Dear, K. B. G., Rodgers, B., & Christensen, H. (2003). Cohort differences in sexual orientation: Results from a large age-stratified population sample. *Gerontology, 49*, 392–395.

Jorm, A. F., Korten, A. E., Rodgers, B., Jacomb, P. A., & Christensen, H. (2002). Sexual orientation and mental health: Results from a community survey of young and middle-aged adults. *British Journal of Psychiatry, 180*, 423–427.

Kandel, D. B., Warner, L. A., & Kessler, D. (1998). The epidemiology of substance use and dependence among women. In C. L. Weatherington & A. Roman (Eds.), *Drug addiction research and the health of women* (NIH Pub. No. 98-4290, pp. 105–130). Rockville, MD: National Institute on Drug Abuse.

Kendler, K. S., Bulik, C. M., Silberg, J., Hettema, J. M., Myers, J., & Prescott, C. A. (2000). Childhood sexual abuse and adult psychiatric and substance use disorders in women: An epidemiological and co-twin control analysis. *Archives of General Psychiatry, 57*(10), 953–959.

Kinsey, A. C., Pomeroy, W. B., & Martin, C. E. (1948). *Sexual behavior in the human male.* Philadelphia: W. B. Saunders.

Kinsey, A. C., Pomeroy, W. B., Martin, C. E., & Gebhard, P. H. (1953). *Sexual behavior in the human female.* Philadelphia: W. B. Saunders.

Kitzinger, C., & Wilkinson, S. (1995). Transition from heterosexuality to lesbianism: The discursive production of lesbian identities. *Developmental Psychology, 31*, 95–104.

Knowlton, R., McCusker, J., Stoddard, A., Zapka, J., & Mayer, K. (1994). The use of the CAGE questionnaire in a cohort of homosexually active men. *Journal of Studies on Alcohol, 55*, 692–694.

Kurdek, L. A. (1991). The dissolution of gay and lesbian couples. *Journal of Personal and Social Relationships, 8*, 265–278.

———. (1994). The nature and correlates of relationship quality in gay, lesbian, and heterosexual cohabiting couples. In B. Greene & G. Herek (Eds.), *Lesbian and gay psychology: Theory, research, and clinical applications* (pp. 133–155). Thousand Oaks, CA: Sage.

———. (1997). Adjustment to relationship dissolution in gay, lesbian, and heterosexual partners. *Personal Relationships, 4*(2), 145–161.

Kurdek, L. A., & Schmitt, J. P. (1986). Relationship quality of partners in heterosexual married, heterosexual cohabiting, and gay and lesbian relationships. *Journal of Personality and Social Psychology, 51*, 711–720.

Kus, R. J. (Ed.). (1995). *Addiction and recovery in gay and lesbian persons.* Binghamton, NY: Harrington Park Press.

Langeland, W., & Hartgers, C. (1998). Child sexual and physical abuse and alcoholism. *Journal of Studies on Alcohol, 59*, 336–348.

LaRosa, J. H. (1990). Executive women and health: Perceptions and practices. *American Journal of Public Health, 80*, 1450–1454.

Laumann, E. O., Gagnon, J. H., Michael, R. T., & Michaels, S. (1994). *The social organization of sexuality: Sexual practices in the United States.* Chicago: University of Chicago Press.

Leigh, B. C. (1990). The relationship of sex-related alcohol expectancies to alcohol consumption and sexual behavior. *British Journal of Addictions, 85*, 919–928.

Leonard, K. E., & Mudar, P. J. (2000). Alcohol use in the year before marriage: Alcohol expectancies and peer drinking as proximal influences on husband and wife alcohol involvement. *Alcoholism: Clinical and Experimental Research, 24*(11), 1666–1679.

Lettelier, P. (1996). Twin epidemics: Domestic violence and HIV infection among gay and bisexual men. *Journal of Gay and Lesbian Social Services, 4*(1), 69–82.

Leventhal, B., & Lundy, S. E. (Eds.). (1999). *Same-sex domestic violence.* Thousand Oaks, CA: Sage.

Liddle, B. J. (1997). Gay and lesbian clients' selection of therapists and utilization of therapy. *Psychotherapy, 34*(1), 11–18.

Lohrenz, L., Connely, J., Coyne, L., & Spare, L. (1978). Alcohol problems in several Midwest homosexual populations. *Journal of Studies on Alcohol, 39*, 1959–1963.

Markovic, N., Aaron, D. J., & Danielson, M. E. (2001, June). *Using sexual identity vs. behavior among lesbian and bisexual women to assess health status.* Paper presented at the National Lesbian Health Conference, San Francisco.

Matthews, A. K., & Hughes, T. L. (2001). Mental health service use by African American women: Exploration of subpopulation differences. *Cultural Diversity and Ethnic Minority Psychology, 7*(1), 75–87.

Matthews, A. K., Tataro, J., & Hughes, T. L. (2003). A comparative study of lesbian and heterosexual women in committed relationships. In T. L. Hughes, C. Smith, &

A. J. Dan (Eds.), *Mental health issues for sexual minority women* (pp. 101–114). New York: Haworth Press.

Mays, V. M., Beckman, L. J., Oranchak, E., & Harper, B. (1994). Perceived social support for help-seeking behaviors of Black heterosexual and homosexually active women alcoholics. *Psychology of Addictive Behaviors, 8*, 235–242.

Mays, V. M., & Cochran, S. D. (2001). Mental health correlates of perceived discrimination among lesbians, gay, and bisexual adults in the United States. *American Journal of Public Health, 91*(6), 1869–1876.

Mays, V. M., Cochran, S. D., & Rhue, S. (1993). The impact of perceived discrimination on the intimate relationships of Black lesbians. *Journal of Homosexuality, 25*(4), 1–14.

McClennan, J. C. (2003). Researching gay and lesbian domestic violence: The journey of a non-LGBT researcher. *Journal of Gay and Lesbian Social Services, 15*(1–2), 31–45.

McDermott, D., Tyndall, L., & Lichtenberg, J. W. (1989). Factors related to counselor preference among gays and lesbians. *Journal of Counseling and Development, 68*, 31–35.

McKirnan, D. J., & Peterson, P. L. (1988). Stress, expectancies, and vulnerability to alcohol abuse: A test of a model among homosexual men. *Journal of Abnormal Psychology, 97*(4), 461–466.

———. (1989a). Alcohol and drug use among homosexual men and women: Epidemiology and population characteristics. *Addictive Behaviors, 14*, 545–553.

———. (1989b). Psychosocial and cultural factors in alcohol and drug abuse: An analysis of a homosexual community. *Addictive Behaviors, 14*, 555–563.

McNally, E. B., & Finnegan, D. G. (1992). Lesbian recovering alcoholics: A qualitative study of identity transformation—A report on research and applications to treatment. *Journal of Chemical Dependency, 5*(1), 93–103.

Meyer, I. H. (1995). Minority stress and mental health in gay men. *Journal of Health and Social Behavior, 7*, 9–25.

———. (Ed.). (2001). Lesbian, gay, bisexual and transgender public health [Special issue]. *American Journal of Public Health, 91*(6), 856–991.

———. (2003). Prejudice, social stress, and mental health in lesbian, gay, and bisexual populations: Conceptual issues and research evidence. *Psychological Bulletin, 129*(5), 674–697.

Meyer, I. H., & Dean, L. (1998). Internalized homophobia, intimacy and sexual behavior among gay and bisexual men. In G. M. Herek (Ed.), *Stigma and sexual orientation: Understanding prejudice against lesbians, gay men, and bisexuals* (pp. 160–186). Thousand Oaks, CA: Sage.

Meyer, I. H., Rossano, L., Ellis, J. M., & Bradford, J. (2002). A brief telephone interview to identify lesbian and bisexual women in random digit dialing sampling. *Journal of Sex Research, 39*(2), 139–144.

Meyer, I., Silenzio, V., Wolfe, D., & Dunn, P. (2000). Introduction and background. In L. Dean, I. H. Meyer, K. Robinson, R. L. Sell, et al. (Eds.), *Lesbian, gay, bisexual, and transgender health: Findings and concerns* (pp. 4–5). New York: Center for Lesbian, Gay, Bisexual and Transgender Health.

Modrcin, M. J., & Wyers, N. L. (1990). Lesbian and gay couples: Where they turn when help is needed. *Journal of Gay and Lesbian Psychotherapy, 1*(3), 89–104.

Money, J. (1988). *Gay, straight, and in-between: The sexology of erotic orientation.* New York: Oxford University Press.

Morales, E. S., & Graves, M. A. (1983). *Substance abuse: Patterns and barriers to treatment for gay men and lesbians in San Francisco.* San Francisco: Department of Public Health.

Morgan, K. S. (1992). Caucasian lesbians' use of psychotherapy: A matter of attitude. *Psychology of Women Quarterly, 16,* 127–130.

Morgan, K. S., & Brown, L. S. (1993). Lesbian career development, work behavior, and vocational counseling. In L. D. Garnets & D. C. Kimmel (Eds.), *Psychological perspectives on lesbian and gay male experience* (pp. 267–286). New York: Columbia University Press.

Morris, J. R., & Rothblum, E. D. (1999). Who fills out a "lesbian" questionnaire? *Psychology of Women Quarterly, 23,* 537–547.

Morris, J. F., Waldo, C. R., & Rothblum, E. D. (2001). A model of predictors and outcomes of outness among lesbian and bisexual women. *American Journal of Orthopsychiatry, 71*(1), 61–71.

Moscato, B. S., Russell, M., Zielezny, M., Bromet, E., Egri, G., Mudar, P., et al. (1997). Gender differences in the relation between depressive symptoms and alcohol problems: A longitudinal perspective. *American Journal of Epidemiology, 146*(11), 966–974.

Nawyn, S. J., Richman, J. A., Rospenda, K. M., & Hughes, T. L. (2000). Sexual identity and alcohol-related outcomes: Contributions of workplace harassment. *Journal of Substance Abuse, 11*(3), 289–304.

Neff, J. A., & Mantz, R. J. (1998). Marital status transition, alcohol consumption, and number of sex partners over time in a tri-ethnic sample. *Journal of Divorce and Remarriage, 29*(1–2), 19–42.

Neisen, J. H. (1997). An inpatient psychoeducational group model for gay men and lesbians with alcohol and drug abuse problems. In L. D. McVinney (Ed.), *Chemical dependency treatment: Innovative group approaches* (pp. 37–51). New York: Haworth Press.

Neisen, J. H., & Sandall, H. (1990). Alcohol and other drug abuse in gay/lesbian populations: Related to victimization? *Journal of Psychology and Human Sexuality, 3*(1), 151–168.

Oetjen, H., & Rothblum, E. (2000). When lesbians aren't gay: Factors affecting depression among lesbians. *Journal of Homosexuality, 39,* 49–73.

O'Hare, T., & Tran, T. V. (1997). Predicting problem drinking in college students: Gender differences and the CAGE questionnaire. *Addictive Behaviors, 22*(1), 13–21.

Ostrow, D. G., Beltran, E. D., Joseph, J. G., DiFrancesco, W., Wesch, J., & Chmiel, J. S. (1993). Recreational drugs and sexual behavior in the Chicago MACS/CCS cohort of homosexually active men. *Journal of Alcohol Abuse, 5*(4), 311–325.

Padgett, D. K., Harman, C. P., Burns, B. J., & Schlesinger, H. J. (1998). Women and outpatient mental health services. In B. L. Levin, A. K. Blanch, & A. Jennings (Eds.), *Women's mental health services* (pp. 34–54). Thousand Oaks, CA: Sage.

Parks, C. (1999a). Bicultural competence: A mediating factor affecting alcohol use practices and problems among lesbian social drinkers. *Journal of Drug Issues, 29*(1), 135–154.

———. (1999b). Lesbian identity development: An examination of differences across generations. *American Journal of Orthopsychiatry, 69*(3), 347–361.

Parks, C. A., & Hughes, T. L. (in press). Age differences in lesbian identity development and drinking. *Journal of Substance Use and Misuse.*

Pattatucci, A. M., & Hamer, D. H. (1995). Development and familiarity of sexual orientation in females. *Behavior Genetics, 25*(5), 407–420.

Patterson, C. J. (1998, May). *Sexual orientation and fertility.* Paper presented at Infertility in the Modern World conference, Cambridge Biosocial Society. Cambridge, England.

Paul, J. P., Catania, J., Pollack, L., & Stall, R. (2001). Understanding childhood sexual abuse as a predictor of sexual risk-taking among men who have sex with men: The Urban Men's Health Study. *Child Abuse and Neglect, 25,* 557–684.

Paul, J. P., Stall, R., & Bloomfield, K. A. (1991). Gay and alcoholic: Epidemiologic and clinical issues. *Alcohol Health and Research World, 15*(2), 151–160.

Peplau, L. A., Cochran, S. D., & Mays, V. (1997). A national survey of the intimate relationships of African American lesbians and gay men. In B. Greene (Ed.), *Ethnic and cultural diversity among lesbians and gay men* (pp. 11–38). Thousand Oaks, CA: Sage.

Power, C., Rodgers, B., & Hope, S. (1999). Heavy alcohol consumption and marital status: Disentangling the relationship in a national study of young adults. *Addiction, 94*(10), 1477–1487.

Purcell, D. W., & Hicks, D. W. (1996). Institutional discrimination against lesbians, gay men, and bisexuals: The courts, legislature, and the military. In R. P. Cabaj & T. S. Stein (Eds.), *Textbook of homosexuality and mental health* (pp. 763–782). Washington, DC: American Psychiatric Press.

Ratner, E. (1988). A model for treatment of lesbian and gays alcohol abusers. *Alcoholism Treatment Quarterly, 5*(1–2), 25–43.

Ratner, E. F., Kosten, T., McLellan, A. T., Roiblatt, M. A., Demston, K., & Magnan, R. (1991). Treatment outcome of Pride Institute patients: First wave—Patients admitted from September 1988 through February 1989. Unpublished outcome report. Eden Prairie, MN: Pride Institute.

Razzano, L. A., Matthews, A., & Hughes, T. L. (2002). Utilization of mental health services: A comparison of lesbian and heterosexual women. *Journal of Gay and Lesbian Social Services, 14*(1), 51–66.

Remien, R. H., Goetz, R., Rabkin, J. G., Williams, J. B., Bradbury, M., Ehrhardt, A. A., et al. (1995). Remission of substance use disorders: Gay men in the first decade of AIDS. *Journal of Studies on Alcohol, 56,* 226–232.

Renzetti, C. M. (1992). *Violent betrayal: Partner abuse in lesbian relationships.* Newbury Park, CA: Sage.

———. (1994). Understanding and responding to violence in lesbian relationships: Part III. *Treating Abuse Today, 4*(1), 20–24.

Roberts, S. J., & Sorensen, L. (1999). Prevalence of childhood sexual abuse and related sequelae in a lesbian population. *Journal of the Gay and Lesbian Medical Association, 3*(1), 11–19.

Ross, M. W., Paulsen, J. A., & Stalstrom, O. W. (1988). Homosexuality and mental health: A cross-cultural review. *Journal of Homosexuality, 15,* 131–152.

Rothblum, E. D. (1994). I only read about myself on bathroom walls: The need for research on the mental health of lesbians and gay men. *Journal of Counseling and Clinical Psychology, 62*(2), 213–220.

Rothblum, E. D., & Factor, R. (2001). Lesbians and their sisters as a control group: Demographic and mental health factors. *Journal of Psychological Science, 12,* 63–69.

Rust, P. (1993). Coming out in the age of social constructionism: Sexual identity formation among lesbians and bisexual women. *Gender and Society, 7,* 50–77.

Saghir, M. T., & Robins, E. (1973). *Male and female homosexuality: A comprehensive investigation.* Baltimore: Williams & Wilkins.

Sandfort, T. G. M., Graaf, R. D., Bijl, R. V., & Schnabel, P. (2001). Same-sex sexual behavior and psychiatric disorders. *Archives of General Psychiatry, 58*(1), 85.

Savin-Williams, R. C. (1996). Self-labeling and disclosure among gay, lesbian, and bisexual youth. In J. Laird & R. J. Green (Eds.), *Lesbians and gays in couples and families: A handbook for therapists* (pp. 153–182). San Francisco: Jossey-Bass.

Scheer, S., Parks, C. A., McFarland, W., Page-Shafer, K. P., Delgado, V., & Ruiz, J. D., et al. (2003). Self-reported sexual identity, sexual behaviors and health risks: Examples from a population-based survey of young women. *Journal of Lesbian Studies, 7*(1), 69–84.

Schilit, R., Lie, G., & Montagne, M. (1990). Alcohol abuse as a correlate of violence in intimate lesbian relationships. *Journal of Homosexuality, 19*(3), 51–65.

Schmitt, J. P., & Kurket, L. A. (1987). Personality correlates of positive identity and relationship involvement in gay men. *Journal of Homosexuality, 13,* 101–109.

Schneider, M. S. (1986). The relationships of cohabiting lesbian and heterosexual couples: A comparison. *Psychology of Women Quarterly, 10,* 234–239.

Scout, Bradford, J., & Fields, C. (2001). Removing the barriers: Improving practitioners' skills in providing health care to lesbians and women who partner with women [Research letter]. *American Journal of Public Health, 91,* 989.

Sell, R. L., & Becker, J. B. (2001). Sexual orientation data collection and progress toward Healthy People 2010. *American Journal of Public Health, 91*(6), 876–882.

Silvestre, A. J. (1999). Gay male, lesbian and bisexual health-related research funded by the National Institutes of Health between 1974 and 1992. *Journal of Homosexuality, 37*(1), 81–94.

Skinner, W. F. (1994). The prevalence and demographic predictors of illicit and licit drug use among lesbians and gay men. *American Journal of Public Health, 84*(8), 1307–1310.

Skinner, W. F., & Otis, M. D. (1996). Drug and alcohol use among lesbian and gay people in a Southern US sample: Epidemiological, comparative, and methodological findings from the trilogy project. *Journal of Homosexuality, 30*(3), 59–91.

Solarz, A. L. (Ed.). (1999). *Lesbian health: Current assessment and directions for the future.* Washington, DC: National Academy Press.

Sorensen, L., & Roberts, S. J. (1997). Lesbian uses of and satisfaction with mental health services: Results from the Boston Lesbian Health Project. *Journal of Homosexuality, 33*(1), 35–49.

Stall, R., Paul, J. P., Greenwood, G., Pollack, L. M., Bein, E., Crosby, G. M., et al. (2001). Alcohol use, drug use and alcohol-related problems among men who have sex with men: The Urban Men's Health Study. *Addiction, 96,* 1589–1601.

Stall, R., & Wiley, J. (1988). A comparison of alcohol and drug use patterns of homosexual and heterosexual men: The San Francisco Men's Health Study. *Drug and Alcohol Dependence, 22,* 63–73.

Stevens, P. (1992). Lesbian health care research: A review of the literature from 1970 to 1990. *Health Care for Women International, 13*(2), 91–120.

Strommen, E. F. (1993). "You're a what?" Family member reactions to the disclosure of homosexuality. In L. D. Garnets & D. C. Kimmel (Eds.), *Psychological perspectives on lesbian and gay male experiences* (pp. 248–266). New York: Columbia University Press.

Substance Abuse and Mental Health Services Administration (SAMHSA). (2001). *A provider's introduction to substance abuse treatment for lesbian, gay, bisexual, and transgender individuals* (DHHS Pub. No. SMA 01-3498). Rockville, MD: Author.

Taylor, S. E. (1995). *Health psychology* (3rd ed.). New York: Random House.

Troiden, R. R. (1993). The formation of homosexual identities. In L. D. Garnets & D. C. Kimmel (Eds.), *Psychological perspectives on lesbian and gay male experience* (pp. 192–217). New York: Columbia University Press.

Underhill, B. L., & Wolverton, T. (1993). *Creating visibility: Providing lesbian-sensitive and lesbian-specific alcoholism recovery services*. Los Angeles: Alcoholism Center for Women.

U.S. Department of Health and Human Services (USDHHS). (2000a). *10th special report to the U.S. Congress on alcohol and health* (pp. 28–53). Washington, DC: Author.

———. (2000b). *Healthy People 2010: Understanding and improving health*. Washington, DC: Office of Disease Prevention and Health Promotion.

Valanis, B. G., Bowen, D. J., Bassford, T., Whitlock, E., Charney, P., & Carter, R. A. (2000). Sexual orientation and health. *Archives of Family Medicine, 9*(9), 843.

Vargo, S. (1987). The effect of women's socialization on lesbian couples. In Boston Lesbian Psychologies Collective (Eds.), *Lesbian psychologies* (pp. 161–173). Chicago: University of Illinois Press.

Vincke, J., & Bolton, R. (1994). Social support, depression, and self-acceptance among gay men. *Human Relations, 49*(9), 1049–1062.

Vincke, J., Bolton, R., Mak, R., & Blank, S. (1993). Coming out and AIDS-related high-risk sexual behavior. *Archives of Sexual Behavior, 22*(6), 559–586.

Wayment, H. A., & Peplau, L. A. (1995). Social support and well being among lesbian and heterosexual women: A structural modeling approach. *Personality and Social Psychology Bulletin, 21*(11), 1189–1199.

Weathers, B. (1980). Alcoholism and the lesbian community. In C. C. Eddy & J. L. Fords (Eds.), *Alcoholism in women* (pp. 142–149). Dubuque, IA: Kendall/Hunt Publishing.

Wechsler, H., & Issac, N. (1992). "Binge" drinking at Massachusetts's colleges: Prevalence, drinking styles, time trends and associated problems. *Journal of the American Medical Association, 267*, 2929–2931.

Weinberg, T. S. (1994). *Gay men, drinking, and alcoholism*. Carbondale: Southern Illinois University Press.

Weinberg, M. S., Williams, C. J., & Prior, D. W. (1994). *Dual attraction: Understanding bisexuality*. New York: Oxford University Press.

Welch, S., Howden-Chapman, P., & Collings, S. C. D. (1998). Survey of drug and alcohol use by lesbian women in New Zealand. *Addictive Behaviors: An International Journal, 23*(4), 543–548.

Widom, C. S., & Hiller-Sturmhofel, S. (2001). Alcohol abuse as a risk factor for and consequence of child abuse. *Alcohol Research and Health, 25*(1), 52–57.

Williams, A., & Clark, D. (1998). Alcohol consumption in university students: The role of reasons for drinking, coping strategies, expectancies, and personality traits. *Addictive Behaviors, 23*(3), 371–378.

Wilsnack, R. W., Wilsnack, S. C., Kristjanson, A. F., & Harris, T. R. (1998). Ten-year prediction of women's drinking behavior in a nationally representative sample. *Women's Health: Research on Gender, Behavior and Policy, 4*, 199–230.

Wilsnack, R. W., & Wright, S. L. (1991, August). *Women in predominately male occupations: Relationships to problem drinking*. Paper presented at the annual meeting of the Society for the Study of Social Problems, Cincinnati.

Wilsnack, S. C. (1995). Alcohol use and alcohol problems in women. In A. L. Stanton & S. J. Gallant (Eds.), *The psychology of women's health: Progress and challenges in research and application* (pp. 381–443). Washington, DC: American Psychological Association.

———. (1996). Patterns and trends in women's drinking: Recent findings and some implications for prevention. In J. M. Howard, S. E. Martin, P. D. Mail, M. E. Hilton, &

E. D. Taylor (Eds.), *Women and alcohol: Issues for prevention research* (pp. 19–63, National Institute on Alcohol Abuse and Alcoholism Research Monograph Series). Washington, DC: U.S. Government Printing Office.

Wilsnack, S. C., Klassen, A. D., Sher, B. E., & Wilsnack, R. W. (1991). Predicting onset and chronicity of women's problem drinking: A five-year longitudinal analysis. *American Journal of Public Health, 81*, 305–318.

Wilsnack, S. C., Vogeltanz, N. D., Klassen, A. D., & Harris, T. R. (1997). Childhood sexual abuse and women's alcohol abuse: National survey findings. *Journal of Studies on Alcohol, 58*, 264–271.

Wilsnack, S. C., & Wilsnack, R. W. (1995). Drinking and problem drinking in US women: Patterns and recent trends. In M. Galanter, et al. (Eds.), *Recent developments in alcoholism: Alcoholism and women* (Vol. 12, pp. 29–60). New York: Plenum.

Wilsnack, S. C., Wilsnack, R. W., & Hiller-Sturmhofel, S. (1994). How women drink: Epidemiology of women's drinking and problem drinking. *Alcohol Health and Research World, 18*(3), 173–181.

Wood, W., Rhodes, N., & Whelan, M. (1989). Sex differences in positive well being: A consideration of emotional style and marital status. *Psychological Bulletin, 106*, 249–264.

Woody, G. E., Donnell, D., Seage, G. R., Metzger, D., Marmor, M., Koblin, B. A., et al. (1999). Non-injection substance use correlates with risky sex among men having sex with men: Data from HIVNET. *Drug and Alcohol Dependence, 53*(3), 197–205.

Yamaguchi, K., & Kandel, D. B. (1985). On the resolution of role incompatibility: A life event history analysis of family roles and marijuana use. *American Journal of Sociology, 90*, 1284–1325.

Zak, A., & McDonald, C. (1997). Satisfaction and trust in intimate relationships: Do lesbians and heterosexual women differ? *Psychological Reports, 80*(3), 904–906.

Chapter 10

Alcohol and Risky Behaviors

Colleen M. Corte and Marilyn Sawyer Sommers

ABSTRACT

The purpose of this chapter is to review and critique the literature on risky drinking, driving, and sexual behaviors. To complete this review, electronic searches using databases from the disciplines of nursing, medicine, and psychology were used with keywords alcohol and risky behavior, risky drinking, risky driving, risky sex, and sexual aggression, as well as other relevant terms.

The basic tenets of contemporary theoretical models of risky behaviors are used as a framework for reviewing the literature. Most relevant to the discussion are the relationships among the behaviors, risk and protective factors, and major unresolved theoretical and methodological issues. In the literature, sensation seeking was differentially associated with risky drinking, driving, and sex, but causal assertions are premature.

Important conceptual and physiological issues are clarified. First, unconventionality contributes to risky drinking, risky driving, and, among adolescents, risky sex. Second, the pharmacologic effects of alcohol on cognitive processing contribute to risky sex, but only among persons who feel conflicted about risky sex (e.g., condom use). This perception may be particularly true for men who have a belief that alcohol will enhance sex. Third, sexual aggression appears to stem from a variety of factors, including the pharmacologic effects of alcohol on aggression and stereotypes about drinking women.

Exploration of risk and protective factors adds breadth and depth to the discussion of risk taking. Risk factors include (1) high tolerance for deviance, (2) unconventional attitudes and behaviors such as early alcohol use and precocious sex, (3) peer norms for deviance, (4) high sensation seeking, and, to a lesser extent, (5) disturbed risk perception and positive beliefs about alcohol. Protective factors appear to mitigate risk and include (1) conventional attitudes and behaviors and (2) having peers that model conventional attitudes and behaviors. Although empirical evidence suggests that risky behaviors tend to covary, most intervention trials to date have focused on single behaviors, and often are based on clinical information rather than existing theoretical and empirical knowledge.

Keywords: risky drinking, risky driving, risky sex, risk taking

Risky drinking, driving, and sexual behaviors are sources of considerable morbidity and mortality, particularly among young people. Compared with the rest of the life span, mortality rates rise most sharply during adolescence, with three fourths of all deaths among teens being due to preventable causes (Centers for Disease Control and Prevention [CDC], 1999). Motor vehicle crashes are the most common cause of death in young adults (National Center for Injury Prevention and Control [NCIPC], 2000). More than one third of all traffic fatalities in the United States are alcohol-related, and 75% of these fatalities involve people between 16 and 44 years of age (CDC, 2004d; Yi, Williams, & Dufour, 2003). Yet one in three college students engages in risky behavior involving alcohol at least once per month (National Institute for Alcohol Abuse and Alcoholism [NIAAA], 2000). In addition, young people under age 25 account for nearly two thirds of sexually transmitted infections in the United States (CDC, 1999), and 4.9% of teens between the ages of 15 and 19 gave birth in 2000 (Moore et al., 2001). Recent data also show that high school students are increasingly drinking alcohol prior to sexual intercourse, motivating a call for alcohol-related interventions aimed at decreasing the percentage of sexually active high school students with sexually transmitted diseases and unwanted pregnancies (CDC, 2002). Risky drinking, particularly in combination with driving and risky sex, clearly escalates the potential for adverse events.

A clear understanding of factors that contribute to as well as protect against risky behaviors is essential for the development of effective interventions. Although the goal of any intervention program is to reduce the enactment of risky behaviors, interventions aimed at changing behavior without reducing risk factors and/or enhancing protective factors are not likely to have long-term success. Behavioral change has long been an important focus of nursing intervention. As such, the systematic investigation of risk and protective factors for risky behaviors is of considerable relevance to nursing science. Nurse-researchers are well positioned to lead the effort to develop theoretically based and empirically derived interventions to reduce risky behaviors.

In this chapter, the diverse body of literature on risky behaviors is synthesized to identify important risk and protective factors for enacting these behaviors, as well as the mechanisms through which they exert their influences. Although much is known about the prevalence of these behaviors, less is known about the underlying mechanisms driving these behaviors. Three questions guided our review. First, what are the relationships among the different risky behaviors? There is considerable evidence that risky behaviors tend to covary (Donovan & Jessor, 1985), and many of the antecedents may be similar (Igra & Irwin, 1996). Yet much of the literature has focused on single behaviors such as risky driving or risky sex. Second, what factors contribute to and protect against risky behaviors? And third, what further research is needed to advance knowledge about risky behaviors?

METHODS

The search was limited to articles published between 1999 through 2004, except when other search methods led to seminal or other important earlier works. Using the keywords *risk taking* and *alcohol*, the searches of the following computerized databases elicited 150 articles from the Cumulative Index of Nursing and Allied Health Literature (CINAHL), 459 articles from Medline, 56 articles from Psychology and Behavioral Sciences Collection, and 199 articles from PsycINFO. Searches were also completed on keywords and phrases including *alcohol and risky behavior, risky drinking, risky driving, risky sex,* and *interventions or programs for risky behavior.*

Articles were then classified into the following categories for review: theoretical models, epidemiology, risky drinking and driving behaviors, and risky drinking and sexual behaviors. Research focusing on persons with alcohol dependence was deemed outside the scope of this review. In addition, the authors used their own compilation of relevant articles, and reviewed the reference lists of relevant articles from all databases to locate other articles of interest and benchmark studies. Relevant reviews and meta-analyses from the general literature and the Cochrane database were used to explore the scientific evidence and discuss relevance to nursing practice. Electronic searches were also completed on the Web sites of the NIAAA, the Substance Abuse and Mental Health Services Administration (SAMHSA), and the CDC.

Two national agencies collect and report data on risky behaviors that were useful for this review. The CDC supports ongoing risk surveillance in the United States. The Youth Risk Behavior Surveillance System (CDC, 2004e; YRBSS http://www.cdc.gov/HealthyYouth/yrbs/index.htm) allows scientists to monitor six priority areas that cause health risks among youth and young adults 10 to 24 years of age. These behaviors include (1) unintentional injuries and violence; (2) tobacco use; (3) alcohol and other drug use; (4) sexual behaviors that contribute to pregnancy and sexually transmitted diseases (STDs), including human immunodeficiency virus (HIV) infection; (5) unhealthy dietary behaviors; and (6) and physical inactivity/overweight (Grunbaum et al., 2004). The Youth Risk Behavior Survey (YRBS), conducted as part of the surveillance system, is a national school-based survey conducted by the CDC in collaboration with states and local educational health agencies. Reports are released each year and published in the *Morbidity and Mortality Weekly Report*. In the 2004 national survey, 15,240 questionnaires were completed in 158 schools (Grunbaum et al., 2004). Finally, the Behavioral Risk Factor Surveillance System (CDC, 2004b; BRFSS; available at http://www.cdc.gov/BRFSS) allows scientists to monitor risk behaviors for chronic disease so that health education and intervention programs can be initiated. It is an ongoing, state-based telephone survey of the U.S. civilian, noninstitutionalized population older than 18 years of age. The questions relate to health status, health care access, exercise, eating patterns, asthma, diabetes, oral health, vaccination, tobacco and alcohol use, seatbelt use, family planning, use of firearms, women's health, cancer screening, and HIV infection. The sample size in 2002 was 247,964 (Balluz et al., 2004).

The sequence of this chapter is (1) definition of the terms *risky drinking, risky driving,* and *risky sexual behavior* for this review; (2) discussion of the theoretical models used to examine risky behaviors; (3) review of the relevant research highlighting relationships among the behaviors, risks, and protective factors, together with major unresolved theoretical and methodological issues; (4) description of recent and ongoing intervention studies aimed at reducing risky behaviors; and (5) recommendations for future research.

DEFINITION OF RISKY BEHAVIORS

Risky behaviors are potentially destructive behaviors, engaged in voluntarily, with or without understanding of possible adverse consequences (Byrnes, 1998; Igra & Millstein, 1991). There is considerable variability in the types of behaviors that may fall into the broad category of risky behaviors (Byrnes, 1998). One way to conceptualize risky behaviors is on a continuum, with one pole representing hazardous variants of normative behaviors (e.g., maladaptive drinking, reckless driving, precocious sex), and the other pole representing more extreme, atypical behaviors that may be considered hazardous or dangerous (e.g., bungee jumping, skydiving). This chapter is focused on relationships among three risky behaviors that are hazardous variants of normative behaviors that have been linked with

serious health consequences—risky drinking, risky driving, and risky sexual behaviors. Although sexual aggression is not deemed a hazardous variant of a
"normative" behavior, it is included because of the documented relationship
between alcohol and sexual aggression.

Risky drinking is defined as patterns of alcohol use associated with increased
odds of adverse health effects and/or alcohol dependence (Allen, Litten, Fertig, &
Babor, 1997). Risky drinking is often problem drinking, which occurs when
people drink above the recommended limits of alcohol use (see chapter 2,
Table 2.1, for definitions of risky drinking, problem drinking, and recommended
drinking limits). Another example of risky drinking is underage drinking. Adolescent drinking has the potential to harm because, compared to the adult brain, the
adolescent brain is more vulnerable to the effects of alcohol (Kelley, Schochet, &
Landry, 2004; Spear, 2004). In addition, early drinking onset is a very strong
predictor of later alcohol dependence (Brown & Tapert, 2004).

Risky driving is defined as operating a motor vehicle illegally or dangerously
so as to endanger others physically and/or psychologically (Dula & Geller, 2003;
Iverson & Rundmo, 2004). Risky driving includes speeding, illegal passing, lane
and right-of-way violations, turn and control signal violations, failure to wear a
safety restraint, and (more recently noted in the literature) road rage and lapses
of attention such that occurs during cellular phone use. Interestingly, drinking
and driving has also been considered a risky "driving" practice, yet research has
shown that it is only moderately correlated with other types of risky driving
(Bingham & Shope, 2004; Donovan, 1993; Jessor, Turbin, & Costa, 1997),
suggesting that these behaviors are independent factors. Consequently, we distinguish risky driving from drinking/driving.

Risky sex is defined as activities that increase the odds of developing a
sexually transmitted infection or an unwanted pregnancy. Risky sexual behaviors
include precocious sex (initiation of sexual intercourse before age 15), unprotected sex, and having two or more sexual partners in the previous 3 months
(Kalichman, Cain, Zweben, & Swain, 2003; Santelli, Brener, Lowry, Bhatt, &
Zabin, 1998; Santelli et al., 2004). Sexual aggression is defined as coercing or
forcing a sex act on an unwilling partner (Abbey, Zawacki, Buck, Clinton, &
McAuslin, 2001; Testa, 2002). The present review is limited to sexual assaults
involving male perpetrators and female victims because the majority of sexual
assaults involve such dyads (George & Stoner, 2000).

THEORETICAL CONSIDERATIONS

The majority of research on risky behaviors has been conducted with adolescent
and young adult samples. This is not surprising, given that risky behaviors tend
to peak in late adolescence/early adulthood (Arnett, 1999; Jonah, 1997; Lejuez

et al. 2002). Although risky behaviors show considerable stability across adolescence and young adulthood (Lane & Cherek, 2002), they do sometimes persist beyond early adulthood (Iversen & Rundmo, 2004). It is not clear, however, whether the underlying mechanisms driving these behaviors in middle and older adults are the same or different than they are for adolescents and young adults.

Although the epidemiology of these behaviors and of their co-occurrence is well defined, the underlying mechanisms driving these behaviors are less clear. Increasing evidence suggests that risky behaviors stem from the interaction of multiple causal factors from biological, psychological, and social domains. This complexity might explain the dearth of studies testing interventions to reduce risk and adverse events. Intervention studies to date have tended to focus on single risky behaviors (underage drinking, teen pregnancy, drinking and driving) rather than on multiple co-occurring risky behaviors.

The current state of the science contributes to difficulties understanding the causal mechanisms of risky behaviors. Alcohol is sometimes conceptualized as a risky behavioral outcome of risky driving and risky sex, and other times as a contributor to risky driving and risky sex. Some investigators have focused on single risky behaviors, whereas others have focused on relationships among behaviors. To complicate matters further, diverse theoretical orientations have been used, although sometimes implicitly. Although multiple theories can be useful, they can also be confusing when a multitude of interacting underlying mechanisms may exist.

Theoretical Approaches Used to Examine Risky Drinking and Risky Driving

Risky drinking, risky driving, and the relationship between alcohol and risky driving have been primarily examined using models that focus on individual differences to explain why certain individuals are more inclined to take risks than other individuals. One model focuses on individual differences in sensation seeking, one on individual differences in risk perception, and one on individual differences in the degree of unconventionality (see Figure 10.1, in which risky drinking is an outcome in each model).

Sensation Seeking/Impulsivity

The perception that high sensation seeking contributes to risky behaviors is widely held. Sensation seeking is characterized by the propensity to search for novel and varied experiences, as well as willingness to take risks for such experiences (Zuckerman, 1991). Sensation seeking represents a broad personality dimension that is comprised of different aspects including disinhibition/impulsivity (inability to control impulses resulting in behavior without forethought), experi-

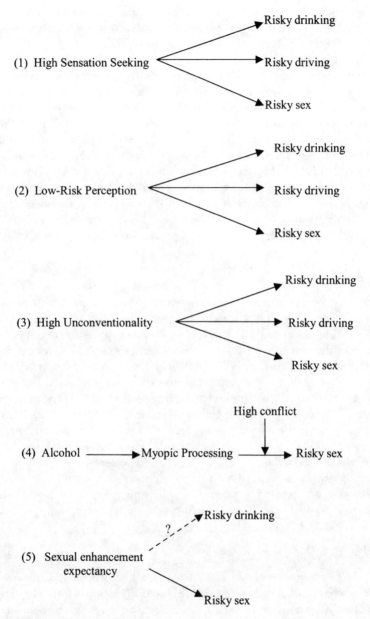

FIGURE 10.1 Theoretical models of risky behaviors: (1) sensation-seeking model, (2) risk perception model, (3) problem behavior model, (4) alcohol myopia model, (5) sexual expectancy model.

ence seeking (desire for novel experiences), thrill and adventure seeking, and boredom sensitivity. Although the different aspects of sensation seeking are correlated, they appear to be differentially related to risky behaviors (Greene, Kremar, Walters, Rubin, & Hale, 2000; Jonah, 1997).

According to this theoretical perspective, risky behaviors are viewed as behavioral expressions of underlying high impulsivity (or the broader dimension of sensation seeking). Because sensation seeking reflects a stable personality disposition, it is not easily amenable to change. Impulsivity has been conceptualized as having both direct effects on risky behaviors (Cherpitel, 1999; Sayette, Kirchner, Moreland, Levine, & Travis, 2004) as well as indirect effects that are mediated by more proximal mechanisms such as perceived risk (Jonah, 1997) or beliefs about alcohol (Kalichman, Tannenbaum, & Nachimson, 1998). Impulsivity and risky behaviors have similar gender differences and developmental trajectories—both tend to be higher in males compared with females (Igra & Irwin, 1996; Irwin & Millstein, 1991; Jonah, 1997; Stanford et al., 1996), and both tend to peak during adolescence (Arnett, 1999; Igra & Irwin, 1996).

Risk Perception

Risk perception involves an assessment of perceived costs and benefits of behavior. This model posits that persons who engage in risky behavior either underestimate the risks associated with the behaviors and/or overestimate the perceived benefits of the behavior, with the net result being that the behavior is deemed "worth the risk" (Weinstein, 1984, 1989). The perception of risk may be "adjusted downward" over time if the person fails to experience adverse consequences of risky behaviors such as getting arrested for drunk driving or becoming pregnant after unprotected sex (Goldberg, Halpern-Felsher, & Millstein, 2002). If involvement in one type of risky behavior does not lead to negative outcomes, the downward adjustment in perception of risk may generalize to other forms of risky behavior (Goldberg et al., 2002). For adolescents, there may be many perceived benefits associated with risky behavior, such as autonomy, defiance of authority, and peer recognition. Risky drinking, risky driving, and risky sex would thus be direct outcomes of disturbances in risk perception.

Problem Behavior Theory

According to another individual difference model, risky behaviors are not single, isolated behaviors, but rather are an organized constellation of interrelated behaviors. These behaviors stem from unconventionality across several domains (personality, social environment, and behavior) that lead to transgression of social norms (Donovan & Jessor, 1983; Jessor, Donovan, & Costa, 1991; Jessor & Jessor, 1977). This complex biopsychosocial model can be explained by factors from multiple domains. The social environment (e.g., parental monitoring, peer influences), personality (e.g., tolerance of deviance), behavioral system (e.g., problem behaviors [alcohol and drug use] vs. conventional behaviors [commitment to academic achievement, involvement with church]), and biology (e.g., genetic predisposition to alcoholism) interact to form a "web of causation" (MacMahon, Pugh, & Ipsen, 1960). According to the model, overall psychosocial proneness to risky behavior is conceptualized as a balance between risk and protective factors from these multiple domains.

Self-Concept in Risky Behaviors

The self-concept may be an important focus for future research on risky behaviors. With the exception of a few studies (Corte & Stein, 2003; Stein, Roeser, & Markus, 1998), the role of the self-concept in risky behaviors has been largely unexplored. Disturbances of the self-concept, however, are briefly mentioned in the discussion sections of papers as a possible factor in the enactment of risky behaviors. Irwin and Millstein (1991) suggested that self-perceptions may be an important distal influence on the development of risk perception. Other investigators have noted that risky behaviors are indicators of poor self-regulation (Lipsitt & Mitnick, 1991; Raffaelli & Crockett, 2003). Steinberg (2004) argued that by inducing more rapid maturation of the brain in areas that govern self-regulation, scientists might be able to affect risky behaviors. Consequently, the self-concept may be an important mediator of the onset and persistence of risky behaviors, as well as a viable target of interventions designed to reduce and/or prevent risky behaviors.

RISKY DRINKING

Data from the Monitoring the Future study, an ongoing national survey that follows individuals from high school into adulthood, show that young adults have the highest incidence of risky drinking (Johnston, O'Malley, Bachman, & Schulenberg, 2004). The 2-week prevalence of consuming 5+ drinking (see Table 2.1, chapter 2) is approximately 40% for young adults between the ages of 21 and 24, but by age 40 it decreases to 20%. Risky drinking patterns can ultimately lead to alcohol dependence, a major mental disorder as defined by the *Diagnostic and Statistical Manual of Mental Disorder* (4th ed., *DSM-IV*) that spans adolescence through older adulthood.

   Research findings support the hypothesis that disinhibition/impulsivity contributes to risky drinking. A cross-sectional study by Greene et al. (2000) examined the relationship between different aspects of sensation seeking and risky behaviors in adolescents and young adults. Alcohol consumption was positively correlated with the disinhibition aspect of sensation seeking ($r = 0.69$), as well as with the experience seeking ($r = 0.36$), boredom sensitivity ($r = 0.35$), and thrill seeking ($r = 0.34$) aspects of sensation seeking. One longitudinal study used a person-centered approach to group adolescents based on personality profiles and drinking behavior (Colder, Campbell, Ruel, Richardson, & Flay, 2002). Risk-taking scores distinguished groups of adolescents who differed in terms of their drinking profiles. Adolescents who had high risk-taking dispositions had more escalating and heavy drinking patterns compared with those who had low risk-taking dispositions. A study using a behavioral measure of impulsivity in women without alcohol problems showed that those who had their first drink prior to age 18 had higher impulsivity as compared with those who had their first drink at 21 years or later (Dougherty, Mathias, Tester, & Marsh, 2004). Taken together, these studies suggest that individual differences in disinhibition/impulsivity are associated with earlier drinking onset and heavier drinking over time.

The perceived benefits of drinking may loom larger than the perceived risks of drinking, particularly for adolescents. From an evolutionary perspective, risky behaviors in adolescence have adaptive benefit—moving toward independence (Lejuez et al., 2002). A cross-sectional study of adults showed that although higher perceived risk of addiction was associated with lower intentions to drink, higher perceived benefit of drinking was associated with greater intention to drink (Goldberg & Fischhoff, 2000). In a sample of adolescents, Goldberg and colleagues (2002) found that perceived benefits of drinking significantly predicted drinking behaviors 6 months later, and that, over time, the benefits of drinking were perceived to be more likely and the risks of drinking were perceived to be less likely. The majority of adolescents who drank did not experience negative consequences, and over 6 months, the self-generated number of positive outcomes increased, whereas the self-generated number of negative outcomes did not. These results suggest that interventions need to go beyond assessing risks for alcohol problems to consider perceived benefits and ways to counter them.

RISKY DRIVING

Risky driving can be classified into aggressive and nonaggressive practices. Aggressive driving practices (speeding, illegal passing, unsafe lane changes, following too closely, running stop signs or red lights) and road rage have alarming prevalence rates and serious consequences. Aggressive driving was involved in 59.5% of fatal crashes, 54.7% of crashes leading to injury, and 50.3% of all vehicular crashes in the United States in 2001 (National Safety Council [NSC], 2003). Road rage is defined as aggressive behavior by the operator or passenger of one motor vehicle toward the operator or passenger of another motor vehicle on the roadway (Miller, Azrael, Hemenway, & Solop, 2002). In a large cross-sectional telephone survey of adults ages 18 and older, one third of the respondents (34%)

admitted to shouting, cursing, or making rude gestures at another driver, and 44% reported that they were shouted at, cursed at, or had rude gestures directed at them in the past year (Miller et al., 2003).

Nonaggressive risky driving practices such as lack of safety belt compliance and driver inattention are also associated with adverse consequences. When lap and shoulder safety belts are used, they reduce the risk to fatal injury to front-seat passengers by 45% and reduce the risk of moderate to critical injury by 50% (NSC, 2003). The National Safety Council (2003) estimated that in 2001, safety belts saved more than 12,000 lives. Overall, belt use among Americans has risen to 79% (Glassbrenner, 2004), but there are systematic age, gender, socioeconomic, and ethnic differences in safety belt use. The lowest rate of use (72%) occurs in males between 16 and 24 years of age. When age and geographic region are considered, in the southern part of the United States children 8 to 15 years of age have a compliance rate of 49%, and individuals older than 70 years have a compliance rate of 33% (Glassbrenner, 2004). Drivers in rural areas, drivers with poor driving records, low-income persons, and African Americans are more likely to have poor safety belt compliance (Lerner et al., 2001; Reinfurt et al., 1996).

In a national study of unsafe driving acts, the National Highway Traffic Safety Administration (NHTSA, 1999) found that driver inattention was the leading cause of vehicular crashes in the United States. Driver inattention caused 22.7% of traffic crashes, as compared with excessive speeding (18.7%), alcohol impairment (18.2%), perceptual errors (15.1%), decision errors (10.1%), and incapacitation (falling asleep, 6.4%). Driver inattention results from factors inside and outside the vehicle. Observing passing scenery, eating or drinking, attending to the radio or sound system, or talking on a cellular phone can all serve as driver distractions (Utter, 2001).

A recent observational survey study showed that drivers who frequently use cellular phones in their vehicles have a higher risk of collision than drivers who use them infrequently or not at all while driving, a finding that was particularly strong for females (Wilson, Fang, Wiggins, & Cooper, 2003). Driving records revealed that persons who used cellular phones while driving had higher counts of aggressive driving violations and alcohol violations over the previous 4 years (Wilson et al., 2003). It is not clear from existing research whether cell phone users while driving have more violations because of distraction, or whether cell phone usage while driving is itself an indicator of high risk taking, nor is it clear that the other factors involved in driver inattention are related to risk taking.

Risky Driving in Adolescents and Young Adults

Risky driving is more prevalent among young drivers compared with older drivers. Young drivers are more likely than older drivers to speed, run red lights, make illegal turns, ride with an intoxicated or a drinking driver, and drive after drinking alcohol (CDC, 1999; Hingson & Howland, 1993). Interestingly, although most risky drivers are young people, they are not new drivers. The highest incidence of risky driving is seen in males between the ages of 20 and 28 years (Department of Licensing, State of Washington, 2002), followed by a linear decline (Jessor et al., 1997). This trend suggests that driver inexperience alone does not account for risky driving behaviors. According to the NIAAA (1996), lack of driving experience, combined with a penchant for risky driving behaviors, a tendency to underestimate the dangerous consequences of such behaviors, and a tendency to overestimate driving skill, contributes to the high crash rate among young drivers.

Evidence also suggests that risky driving persists beyond young adulthood. Although the fatal crash involvement rate for 16-year-olds is the highest across all national drivers (94 per 100,000), approximately 75% of all crashes occur with drivers over the age of 25 (NSC, 2003). Risky and aggressive driving is not only the purview of the young. Miller et al. (2002) found that 26% of respondents between ages 35 and 59 and 11% of respondents who were 60 or older admitted to engaging in road rage.

Sensation Seeking and Risky Driving

Empirical support was found for the hypothesis that high sensation seeking (thrill and adventure seeking in particular) is associated with risky driving, but causal evidence is limited. In Jonah's (1997) comprehensive review examining the relationship between sensation seeking and risky driving, positive relationships between sensation seeking and risky driving were found across all 15 studies. Risky driving behaviors (i.e., speeding, passing in no passing zones, and lack of compliance with seatbelt use) were more strongly associated with the thrill- and adventure-seeking aspect of sensation seeking than other aspects of sensation seeking. More recently, a survey study showed that adults (mean age 45) with high sensation seeking reported risky driving more frequently than those with low sensation seeking (Iversen & Rundmo, 2004).

A similar relationship has also been found in high school adolescents using a person-centered approach to classify individuals into groups based on personality profiles and risky driving attitudes and behaviors (Ulleberg, 2002). A survey study of early and middle adolescents showed that sensation seeking was also related to risky driving attitudes (Harre, Brandt, & Dawe, 2000). Furthermore, boys had riskier attitudes about driving behaviors compared with girls, and middle adolescents had riskier attitudes about driving compared with early adolescents. Both of these patterns are consistent with the known developmental trajectory of impulsivity. Although theoretically it makes sense that high sensation seeking would contribute to risky driving, causal evidence for this claim is lacking.

Risky Driving as Part of a Cluster of Behaviors

The evidence for risky driving being part of a larger cluster of problem behavior is mixed. From this perspective, risky driving is part of a general lifestyle of unconventionality that covaries with other risky behavioral outcomes. In a three-wave longitudinal study of young adults, Jessor et al. (1997) found that when controlling for drinking and driving, risky driving behaviors (e.g., speeding, running red lights) were predicted by unconventionality. Among the riskiest drivers in the sample, adopting more conventional social roles was negatively associated with risky driving (controlling for drinking and driving). These investigators concluded that risky driving is another type of problem behavior.

Conversely, Bingham and Shope (2004) found that unconventionality during adolescence did not predict risky driving behaviors (speeding, passing, following, lane usage, right of way, turn and control signal violations) 8 years later. One possible reason for the discrepancy between these two studies is that there may be only a modest relationship between unconventionality and risky driving that held over a 2-year period in the Jessor study but not over an 8-year period in the Bingham study. Another possibility is that after 8 years, when participants were in their mid-20s, individuals in the Bingham study had adopted more conventional adult roles, such as securing employment, getting married, and having children, a factor that has been shown to be associated with a decline in risky drinking (Chassin, Presson, Sherman, & Edwards, 1992; Merline, O'Malley, Schulenberg, Bachman, & Johnston, 2004).

Risky Drinking and Risky Driving

The first question addressed in this chapter is, what are the relationships among the different risky behaviors? Examining patterns of association in co-occurring maladaptive behaviors is a useful strategy that informs both research and practice. Data consistently show that risky driving is frequently associated with alcohol use. Alcohol-impaired drivers account for 41% of all traffic deaths (CDC, 2004d) and 7% of all traffic crashes in general at an estimated cost of $34.1 billion each year (NSC, 2003). In addition to traffic crashes, alcohol is associated with road rage perpetration and victimization (Mann, Smart, Stoduto, Adlaf, & Ialometeanu, 2004).

The relationship between alcohol and risky driving is multifaceted. There is little experimental evidence to suggest that alcohol induces persons to engage in risky driving behaviors (Leigh, 1999), but the pharmacologic effects of alcohol are what make the driving risky. Alcohol interferes with the processing of information, decision making, and reaction times (Schweizer, Jolicoeur, Vogel-Sprott, & Dixon, 2004), thus heightening the risk associated with potentially dangerous behaviors that require full concentration, sharp psychomotor skills, and fast reaction times (e.g., driving).

Drinking/driving is consistently associated with sensation seeking, and perhaps disinhibition/impulsivity in particular. Arnett, Offer, and Fine (1997) found a positive relationship between sensation seeking and drinking/driving. Arnett (1990) found that high school students who reported drunk driving had higher scores on the disinhibition/impulsivity, thrill and adventure seeking, and boredom sensitivity aspects of sensation seeking compared with students who reported that they did not engage in drunk driving. Jonah (1997) found that drinking/driving was most strongly associated with the disinhibition/impulsivity aspect of sensation seeking across 18 studies, as compared with his finding that risky driving behaviors such as speeding were most strongly associated with the thrill-and adventure-seeking aspect of sensation seeking. Although it is certainly consistent with theoretical predictions that high sensation seeking would lead to drinking/driving, causal evidence to support this claim is limited. Further work is needed to clarify the relationships between the different aspects of sensation seeking and drinking/driving. These studies indicate that careful interpretation is warranted for studies that use various indicators of personality traits.

Disturbances in risk perception may mediate the effects of sensation seeking on drinking/driving, as it apparently does with other risky driving behaviors, such as speeding. Evidence suggests that adolescents who are high in sensation seeking and engage in drunk driving report lower perceived risk of having a traffic crash and receiving a traffic citation compared with students who do not engage in drunk driving (Arnett, 1990). This finding is consistent with that of Irwin and Millstein (1991), who argued that risk perception may be a proximal factor that mediates other, more distal causes of risky behaviors.

The evidence that drinking/driving is part of a cluster of problem behaviors is stronger than the evidence that other risky driving behaviors are part of a cluster of problem behaviors. In the longitudinal study by Bingham and Shope (2004), unconventionality during adolescence predicted drinking/driving behaviors 8 years later, though it did not predict other types of risky driving behaviors, such as speeding. This suggests a strong relationship between unconventionality and drinking/driving that persists into the mid-20s, a time when more conventional roles, such as employment and marriage, are usually adopted (Merline et al., 2004). Bingham and Shope argue that drinking/driving is a much more deviant behavior, whereas risky driving behaviors, such as speeding, are more normative. In any case, the evidence suggests that drinking/driving is different than other aggressive risky driving behaviors (speeding, passing in no passing zones) and nonaggressive behaviors (driver inattention, lack of safety restraint), and these behaviors should be distinguished in future research.

Summary and Critique

A variety of mechanisms play a role in risky drinking and risky driving. Existing studies suggest that both high sensation seeking (particularly disinhibition/impulsivity) and high unconventionality contribute to risky drinking. Sensation seeking is also associated with risky driving and with drinking/driving, and may be mediated by disturbances in risk perception for men. Unconventionality also contributes to risky driving, and especially drinking/driving. Making distinctions among different risky driving behaviors is critical because evidence suggests that behaviors such as speeding are not the same as drinking/driving. It is not clear from existing research whether nonaggressive driving behaviors (safety belt use and driver inattention) share the same antecedents as aggressive driving behaviors (speeding, running red lights).

Data from the risk surveillance systems clearly dictate a "call to arms" against risky behaviors. Given that the federal government maintains annual risk surveillance systems, scientists ought to shift the focus from epidemiological studies and instead expend efforts in two directions. First, additional studies are needed to explore the causal mechanisms underlying risky behaviors. Second, theoretically derived interventions need to be developed and tested.

Although research on risk taking is fairly extensive, few studies have explored factors related to risky driving behaviors beyond young adulthood. Risky driving behaviors are clearly an issue for adults in middle and older age groups, but studies of this population are almost entirely missing from the literature. In fact, the Behavioral Risk Factor Surveillance System (BRFSS) asks only one question on safety belt use and no questions on risky driving behaviors and alcohol-related driving (CDC, 2004b). Further work is required in these populations to determine whether antecedents are the same across all age groups.

Important methodological issues also complicate this research. Among adolescents, most risky behaviors are enacted in the context of a group setting (Sayette et al., 2004) and under conditions of high emotional arousal (Steinberg, 2004). Yet these factors are difficult to replicate in a research setting. Participants usually respond to questionnaires or participate in laboratory studies individually and efforts are made to minimize emotional influences. Finally, although there are a wide variety of existing measures of sensation seeking, different measures tap different aspects of sensation seeking, such as disinhibition/impulsivity versus thrill and adventure seeking. Investigators sometimes use these terms interchangeably—a practice that contributes to conceptual and methodological blurring.

THEORETICAL APPROACHES USED TO EXAMINE RISKY DRINKING AND RISKY SEX

Risky sex and the role of alcohol in risky sex have been examined in a number of ways. One model focuses on contextual factors to explain why environmental circumstances promote risky behaviors (alcohol myopia), and a second model focuses on both individual difference and social context variables to explain why certain individuals in certain situations tend to engage in risky behaviors (alcohol expectancy); individual difference models described earlier have also been used. Although risky drinking is an outcome in four of the models, alcohol consumption is a precursor to risky sexual outcomes in the alcohol myopia model (see Figure 10.1).

Alcohol Myopia Theory

Both the pharmacologic properties of alcohol and circumstances in the social context (a high conflict situation) explain risky behaviors (Steele & Josephs, 1990). According to the model, alcohol intoxication leads to a narrowing of perception by limiting attention to the most salient cues. As a result of this "myopic" processing, attention to other stimuli such as worries and concerns is reduced. In a situation in which the person is feeling conflicted about a decision, such as whether or not to use a condom, the model suggests that alcohol interferes with cognitive processing of more distal information (the risk of pregnancy or a sexually transmitted infection), and enables only cognitive processing of cues in the immediate environment, such as feelings associated with the current sexual experience. These factors may lead to risky sexual behavior, such as the decision not to use a condom.

Alcohol Outcome Expectancy

This model focuses on the social context to explain why certain individuals in certain situations engage in risky behaviors. Alcohol expectancy is a belief that alcohol will have a beneficial effect in a specific affective (reducing tension) or behavioral (enhancing sex) domain (Brown, Christiansen, & Goldman, 1987). The basic tenet of the expectancy model is that a person with a belief that alcohol will enhance sex will be more inclined to drink in situations where sex is a possible outcome. Although such a belief may lead to risky drinking behaviors, the expectancy effect itself is indicated by a direct relationship between the belief that alcohol will enhance sex and the risky sexual outcome.

Two types of methods have been used to examine the effects of alcohol expectancies on sexual behavior. Descriptive studies have used self-report questionnaires, such as the Alcohol Expectancy Questionnaire (Brown et al., 1987), to examine the presence or absence of alcohol outcome expectancies. Experimental studies have used the balanced placebo design to study the effects of alcohol outcome expectancy on sexual behavior in the laboratory. The balanced placebo design enables investigators to control two properties of drinking: actual alcohol content (pharmacologic effect) and the perceived alcohol content (expectancy), in order to disentangle the pharmacologic properties of alcohol from beliefs about the effects of alcohol. The design includes four randomly assigned groups:

expect alcohol/receive alcohol, expect alcohol/receive placebo, expect no alcohol/receive alcohol, and expect no alcohol/receive placebo. Positive expectancy effects are indicated by persons in the "expect alcohol" groups when they have a stronger response to the experimental manipulation than the "expect no alcohol" groups regardless of actual alcohol consumption.

RISKY SEX

Three issues point out the health consequences of the seriousness of risky sex: sexual precociousness, sexually transmitted infections, and violence against women. Data from the Youth Risk Behavior Survey (Grunbaum et al., 2002) show that more than one third of 9th graders have had sexual intercourse, and by the 12th grade, nearly one fourth of students reported having multiple sex partners. Despite the current emphasis on safe sex and increasing awareness about sexual risk, two out of five sexually active students (42%) reported that they did not use a condom at their last intercourse, which places them at high risk for sexually transmitted infections and pregnancy.

Human immunodeficiency virus (HIV) and the resulting acquired immunodeficiency syndrome (AIDS) is on the rise in the United States. Recent preliminary data show a 2.2% increase in new AIDS diagnoses (CDC, 2004c), and since 1994, the number of persons who had a newly diagnosed HIV infection increased 14% among homosexual men and 10% among heterosexuals. In addition, recent syphilis outbreaks among HIV-positive homosexual men suggest that sexual risk taking is increasing in homosexual men (CDC, 2004c).

Violence against women is epidemic. The National Violence Against Women (NVAW) survey found that of 8,000 women surveyed, 18% had experienced an attempted or completed rape at some time in their lives. In the year prior to the survey, 2% of the participants reported being raped, physically assaulted, or both. Considering the number of women who experienced multiple assaults per year, an estimated 876,000 rapes are perpetrated against U.S. women annually (Tjaden & Thoennes, 1998).

Some evidence suggests a modest relationship between high sensation seeking and risky sex, but there is little support for causality. In a review of the sensation-seeking literature, Zuckerman (1991) found that individuals who were high in sensation seeking had a greater number of sexual partners and more varied sexual experiences compared with individuals who were low in sensation seeking. More recently, Kalichman et al. (1998) found a correlation of $r = 0.30$ between sensation seeking and the number of male sex partners in a cross-sectional survey study of gay and bisexual men. Data from the National Longitudinal Survey of Youth showed that, among adolescents, attraction to risk taking was not a significant predictor of risky sex (unprotected sex and multiple sex partners) 4 years later (Raffaelli & Crockett, 2003).

There is empirical evidence that psychosocial unconventionality contributes to precocious sex. Because studies using the problem behavior model to examine risky sex typically focus on risky sex together with other risky behaviors, they will be discussed in the next section on the relationship between risky drinking and risky sex.

Relationship between Risky Drinking and Risky Sex

Descriptive studies demonstrate that alcohol is associated with sexual risk taking in adolescents and adults (Abbey, McAuslin, & Ross, 1998; George & Stoner, 2000; Santelli et al., 2004). YRBS data from 8,450 adolescents and young adults between the ages of 14 and 22 show that alcohol and illicit drug use were associated with initiation of sexual intercourse, and these findings were particularly strong for males and African Americans. Alcohol use was also associated with multiple sexual partners for both males and females. As the number of alcohol-related behaviors increased, the adjusted proportion of respondents who had multiple partners rose from 8% to 48% among females and from 23% to 61% among males (Santelli et al., 1998).

A strong relationship was also found between alcohol and early sexual experiences among pregnant and parenting adolescents (Kellogg, Hoffman, & Taylor, 1999), and between alcohol and risky sex (precocious sex and multiple sex partners) among alcohol-abusing adolescents (Bailey, Pollock, Martin, & Lynch, 1999). A review of research on alcohol use and risky sex in adolescents showed that alcohol was associated with lack of condom use, but primarily for first-time sexual intercourse events rather than ongoing sexual relationships (Halpern-Fisher, Millstein, & Ellen, 1996). In adult samples, alcohol use was found to be associated with unprotected sex with casual or one-time partners in inner-city men (Kalichman et al., 2003) and inconsistent condom use among women (Wingood & DiClemente, 1998).

The relationship between drinking and risky sex may be much stronger than what has been reported in the literature. Methodological reviews suggest that assessment of sensitive topics such as sexual behavior is difficult (Weinhardt, Forsyth, Carey, Jaworski, & Durant, 1998). Because of the questionable validity of self-reports about sexual behavior, obtaining accurate accounts of the relationship between drinking and sexual behavior is challenging. To address this problem, LaBrie and Earleywine (2000) asked participants to indicate the number of items that were true in a series of random statements. Half the sample received a series with the item of interest, a 6-item series that included a statement about having sex without a condom after drinking, and half the sample received a 5-item series with no item about sex. Because the groups were randomly assigned, the difference in the mean score for the two groups reflected the estimated frequency of having sex without a condom after drinking. This method revealed a much higher frequency of having sex without a condom after drinking (65%) compared with a self-reported survey (36%).

Physiological Effects of Alcohol

The pharmacologic effects of alcohol have differential effects on physiological and subjective arousal. Experimental studies have demonstrated that alcohol decreases penile tumescence (Cooper, 1994) and vaginal blood volume (Wilson & Lawson, 1978), and increases latency to orgasm for both men and women (Malatesta, Pollack, Wilbanks, & Adams, 1979). However, alcohol may also interfere with the ability to control heightened subjective arousal in men. Wilson and Niaura (1984) found that men who received low doses of alcohol and were instructed to suppress arousal experienced earlier physiologic arousal compared with controls.

Alcohol Expectancies

A belief that alcohol will enhance sex increases both physiologic and subjective arousal in men (George & Marlatt, 1986; Wilson, Niaura, & Adler, 1985). After consuming placebo drinks, men with a sexual enhancement expectancy reported higher sexual arousal compared with men without sexual enhancement expectancy (George, Stoner, Norris, Lopez, & Lehman, 2000). Given the known effects of alcohol on physiologic arousal, however, George and Stoner (2000) argue that "a man's increased arousal after drinking is mostly a product of what he believes about alcohol" (p. 96). The effects for women have been mixed (Dermen & Cooper, 2000; Dermen, Cooper, & Agocha, 1998; Wilson & Lawson, 1978). Expectancy effects may be strongest in women who have high anxiety about sex (Leigh, 1999). Abbey et al. (2001) argue that the lack of expectancy effects in women is because drunken excess is considered less acceptable in women than men, and women are concerned about the label of promiscuity and their increased vulnerability to sexual and nonsexual aggression. "Consequently, women's expectancies about alcohol's sexual effects are less positive than men's expectancies, because the social costs associated with alcohol use and sexual behavior are greater for women" (p. 48).

Alcohol Myopia Model

There is evidence to support the alcohol myopia model. Alcohol interferes with cognitive processing and decision making (Fillmore & Vogel-Sprott, 1999; Schweitzer et al., 2004), which is relevant for persons who have a strong impulse to engage in risky sex and simultaneously have a strong awareness of potential adverse consequences. Logan, Cole, and Leukefeld (2002) argue that this is the primary reason that alcohol is associated with sexual risk taking. In a study of 407 men, MacDonald, Zanna, and Fong (1996) found that alcohol consumption decreased the likelihood of condom use. In subsequent experiments, they found that intoxicated participants were more likely than their sober counterparts to report intentions to engage in unprotected sex, but this finding did not hold when intoxicated participants were exposed to a strong inhibitory cue (McDonald, Zanna, Fong, & Martineau, 2000). Dermen and Cooper (2000) similarly found that the quantity of alcohol consumed was inversely related to condom use during first sexual intercourse among those college students who had a high degree of conflict about using condoms. George and Stoner's (2000) review of research on the acute effects of alcohol on sexual behavior across many nonexperimental and experimental studies led them to conclude that the myopia model convincingly explains risky sexual behavior.

Alcohol Expectancies versus Alcohol Myopia

Recently, investigators have pitted the expectancy model against the myopia model to further examine the relationship between alcohol and risky sex. Dermen and Cooper (2000) found support for both models in college students. After drinking, condom use was lower if persons had an alcohol expectancy about sex, internal conflict about condom use, or both. Morris and Albery (2001) argue that alcohol expectancies might moderate the relationship between alcohol-induced myopic processing and risky sex. They posit that after alcohol narrows the scope of attention and cognitive processing, alcohol expectancy may in fact be the salient cue that is attended to in a sexual situation. When considered together with the results of a meta-analysis of laboratory studies that showed that expectancy effects were strongest under conditions of high conflict (Steele & Southwick, 1985), studies based on an integration of these two theories may be particularly useful.

Role of Unconventionality

Alcohol and risky sex may both be outcomes stemming from high unconventionality in adolescents, as compared with the view that alcohol is a contributor to risky sex. Costa, Jessor, Donovan, and Fortenberry (1996) found that greater unconventionality predicted earlier first sexual intercourse in middle and high school students. Significant findings included (1) twice as many unconventional adolescents had intercourse by the end of high school as compared with conventional adolescents, and (2) nonvirgins were significantly more likely to be problem drinkers as compared to virgins. Santelli et al. (2004) found that indicators of unconventionality in early adolescence—alcohol and drug use and poor academic performance—predicted the initiation of sexual intercourse. Furthermore, indicators of conventionality—peer norms for refraining from sex—were protective against initiation of sexual intercourse.

Alcohol and Sexual Aggression

Sexual aggression frequently occurs in the context of alcohol-related social situations. Aggressive or coercive sex is often perpetrated by acquaintances and often occurs in bars, at fraternity parties, or on dates where alcohol is a central activity (Brecklin & Ullman, 2002; Buddie & Parks, 2003). Some investigators have hypothesized that women may find that the potential opportunity to establish a relationship outweighs the potential risks associated with such environments (Norris, Nurius, & Dimeff, 1996; Parks, Miller, Collins, & Zetes-Zanatta, 1998; Testa, Livingston, & Collins, 2000).

The majority of sexual assaults involve alcohol use by the perpetrator (Brecklin & Ullman, 2002; Testa, 2002). Drinking levels and rates of alcohol dependence are higher in perpetrators compared with nonperpetrators of sexual aggression (Abrecen, Looman, & Anderson, 2000; Borowsky, Hogan, & Ireland, 1997; McKeown, Jackson, & Valois, 1998; Ouimette, 1997). Abbey et al. (2001) suggested that heavy drinkers may use alcohol intoxication as an excuse for socially unacceptable behavior, including sexual assault. The use of alcohol may in fact be one strategy used to obtain sex by college men (Tyler, Hoyt, & Whitbeck, 1998).

Interestingly, many victims of sexual assault also report drinking at the time of sexual assault, although the mechanisms by which alcohol influences a woman's vulnerability to sexual aggression are not well understood. A review by Testa and Parks (1996) showed that women's alcohol consumption was positively associated with experiencing sexual aggression. A more recent epidemiologic study supports their findings. In a study of 23,980 at 199 colleges across the United States, 4.7% reported being raped, and 72% of the victims reportedly experienced being raped while they were intoxicated (Mohler-Kuo, Dowdall, Koss, & Wechsler, 2004). A possible mechanism is through alcohol's effect on risk perception. Testa et al. (2002) studied 59 women to determine the impact of women's alcohol consumption on their perceptions of risk and intended behaviors in a hypothetical situation that could lead to establishing a relationship but could also lead to sexual aggression. Compared to women in the no-alcohol condition, women in the alcohol condition rated the male character in the vignette more positively and anticipated less risk and more benefit from the interaction. Similar associations between alcohol and reduced risk perception were noted in a comprehensive review of the literature on women and HIV risk behaviors (Logan, Cole, & Leukefeld, 2002).

Role of Alcohol Expectancy

Although alcohol expectancy appears to play a role in risky sex, the pharmacologic effects of alcohol seem to have a more powerful effect on aggression. Ito, Miller, and Pollock (1996) found that alcohol increased aggressive behavior in subjects who consumed alcohol, but not in subjects who expected to consume alcohol but received a nonalcoholic beverage. The effects of alcohol on sexual aggression may be subtle. For example, intoxicated men have been shown to be less empathetic in their evaluation of a victim of sexual assault (Norris et al., 1999) and more likely to rate a woman as highly aroused (Gross, Bennett, Sloan, Marx, & Juergens, 2001). Marx, Gross, and Juergens (1997) found that intoxicated men were slower to stop sexual advances in a date rape situation as compared to sober men.

Based on a review of surveys and lab studies on alcohol and sexual assault, Abbey et al. (2001) posit that alcohol contributes to sexual assault through multiple pathways, including stereotypes about drinking women. A series of experimental studies have shown that men tend to rate drinking women as more sexually available than women who were not drinking (George, Cue, Lopez, Crowe, & Norris, 1995; George et al., 1997). Furthermore, both men and women assert less blame on a drinking rapist than a sober rapist (Richardson & Campbell, 1982), but assert more blame on a drinking victim than a sober victim (Barbaree & Marshall, 1991). Abbey and colleagues contend that complex interactions between such stereotypes, together with the pharmacologic effects of alcohol on impulse control, aggression and cognitive processing, and men's beliefs about the effect of alcohol on sex, all contribute to sexual aggression.

Summary and Critique

A variety of mechanisms appear to play a role in the relationship between risky sex and alcohol. The relationship between sensation seeking and risky sex appears to be much weaker than the relationship with risky drinking and risky driving behaviors. Unconventionality plays a causal role in risky sex, particularly in adolescents, and experimental studies support causal assertions about the role of alcohol in risky sexual behaviors. Alcohol contributes to sexual aggression through a variety of mechanisms, including the pharmacologic properties of alcohol on aggression and stereotypes about drinking women.

A troublesome trend exists in the body of work on risky sexual behaviors. Scientists have investigated sexual risk taking in populations that might be considered vulnerable, including minority women (Wingood & DiClemente, 1998), patients at inner-city clinics (Kalichman et al. 2003), inner-city middle school students (Santelli et al., 2004), pregnant adolescents (Kellogg et al., 1999), and adolescents with alcohol use disorders (Bailey et al., 1999). Although large-scale surveys exist in the college population, studies on inner-city and minority populations predominate in the literature (Logan et al., 2002). It seems difficult to justify scientifically that sexual risk taking is a phenomenon that exists primarily in vulnerable populations.

Methodological issues also complicate our understanding of contributing factors to risky drinking and risky sex. There is a big difference between responding to a hypothetical risky sexual situation on a questionnaire or in a laboratory setting, and actual behavioral responses in a situation that holds the potential for risky sex. Laboratory paradigms are artificial, and research participants know that their responses do not have real-life consequences. As illustrated by Steinberg (2004), it is much easier to use a condom in a hypothetical sexual encounter than it is to use a real one in the throes of passion of a real sexual encounter.

RISK AND PROTECTIVE FACTORS

The second major question addressed in this chapter is, what factors contribute to and protect against risky behaviors? There is a consistency about risk and protective factors across studies despite diverse theoretical approaches and methods. Risk factors such as male gender and being an adolescent or young adult are not malleable. A predisposition for sensation seeking and a high tolerance for deviance (manifested as unconventional attitudes and behaviors) may not be amenable to change.

Other risk factors, such as peer norms for deviance, lack of conventional involvements, perceived benefits of risky behavior, and expectancies about alcohol, may be more amenable to change. Peer norms for deviant behavior are critical because risky behaviors are enacted almost exclusively in the context of group settings (Sayette et al., 2004). In fact, peer norms are so important that in early adolescence they often are not distinguished from personal beliefs (Santelli et al., 2004), and they often carry a strong influence even into young adulthood (Steinberg, 2004). Lack of involvement with conventional institutions such as school, church, and community is another important risk factor. Given that self-concept and identity development is the central task of adolescence (Erikson, 1968), it is plausible that adolescents who fail to develop successful conventional involvements may use unconventional attitudes and behaviors as a way of establishing an identity.

Although it is not clear why some adolescents perceive more benefits than risks for behaviors such as drinking, challenging these perceived benefits may be an effective way to mitigate risk. Finally, beliefs about alcohol enhancing sex develop over time in the context of social experience. Challenging such beliefs about alcohol may be an effective means to prevent crystallization of a developing expectancy (Morris & Albery, 2001).

Traditionally, risk factors have received more attention than protective factors, but protective factors may moderate risk (Jessor et al., 1998) and potentiate other protective factors (Hawkins, Catalano, & Miller, 1992). Conventional involvements related to school, church, and community have been consistently found to be important factors in mitigating risk. Adolescents who are involved in a diverse collection of prosocial activities may have a more stable self-concept, and thus, be less likely to turn to unconventional behaviors as a way to define themselves. Finally, having a peer group that models conventional behavior is critical because peers have a great deal of influence from early adolescence into young adulthood.

INTERVENING TO REDUCE RISK

Motivational interviews may be successful for reducing drinking and driving (but not drinking alone) in adolescents, particularly when alcohol-related injury is salient. Monti et al. (1999) delivered a brief motivational interview to 94 adolescents (mean age 18.4 years) who were in the emergency department (ED) for an injury and either had a positive blood alcohol concentration or reported drinking prior to the injury. Although no differences in frequency and quantity of alcohol consumption were found between experimental and control subjects 6 months after the intervention, subjects in the experimental group reported fewer drinking and driving episodes and fewer alcohol-related injuries compared with the standard care cohort. This suggests that brief motivational interviews in adolescents immediately after an alcohol-related injury may have some sustained effectiveness for reducing drinking and driving and alcohol-related injuries.

An interactive, computerized intervention delivered in the ED after any type of acute injury was not successful in reducing the expected age-related increase in alcohol misuse among 14-18 year old adolescents, but did show promise for those who had experience with drinking and driving (Maio et al., 2005). The intervention was designed to provide informtion about alcohol and decrease intention to drive after drinking, but because the proportion of adolescents with drinking and driving experience in this study was small, further research is needed to determine its effectiveness in adolescents who drink and drive.

An ED intervention to reduce risky driving and problem drinking in young adults is being conducted by Marilyn Sommers. The aim of this study is to test the effectiveness of a brief intervention to limit risky driving behaviors (i.e., risky driving practices and lack of seatbelt compliance) and problem drinking. The intervention is a clinically based strategy that includes assessment and direct feedback, contracting and goal setting, behavior modification techniques, and the use of written materials that serve as a self-help manual (Fleming, Barry, Manwell, Johnson, & London, 1997). Participants are ED patients ages 18 to 44 who screen positive for both problem drinking and risky driving. At a 12-

month follow-up session, alcohol consumption, adverse events such as illnesses, injuries, traffic citations, and traffic crashes, and health care costs will be evaluated. Data collection will end in 2006 (CDC, 2004a).

There is a lack of interventions to reduce risky sexual behaviors that are linked with alcohol, although interventions have been developed to reduce risky sexual behaviors alone. Several investigators have developed programs to prevent sexually transmitted infections, pregnancy, HIV transmission, and sexual assault among adolescents (Jemmott, Jemmott, & Fong, 1992; 1998; Kirby & DiClemente, 1994; Talashek, Norr, & Dancy, 2003). These programs tend to be located in schools, hospitals and clinics, and residential treatment centers, or through outreach (locations in which young people congregate).

A review of 30 intervention studies illustrates the variety of strategies used to reduce risky sex in adolescents (Talashek et al., 2003). Some examples include increasing self-efficacy to use condoms (Jemmott, Jemmott, & Fong, 1998), improving decision-making skills (Kirby, Korpi, Adivi, & Weissman, 1997), developing assertiveness skills (Aarons et al., 2000), coping with emotions (Siegel, Aten, Roghmann, & Enaharo, 1998) and dealing with peer pressure (Goldfarb et al., 1999). Interventions focused on increasing condom use were more successful than those focused on delaying or refusing sexual intercourse. The interventions did not discuss the role of alcohol in HIV prevention or in the prevention of sexual risk taking. Talashek and colleagues (2003) refined a 13-week school-based intervention that focuses on social and cognitive mediating variables (e.g., behavioral skills related to condom use, self-esteem, communication, problem-solving skills) related to sexual initiation and unsafe sex practices rather than aiming to reduce the behaviors themselves.

A recent meta-analysis of 30 intervention studies to reduce risky sex in adults found a disappointingly small effect size ($d = 0.05$) (Logan et al., 2002). These investigators cited the large gap between existing theoretical and empirical knowledge and intervention strategies as the probable reason for such limited success. Interventions were critiqued in a *Psychological Bulletin* review paper in 1992 for tending to be based on practical experience instead of on existing theories of risky sex (Fisher & Fisher, 1992). The same critique was noted in review of interventions for risky sex nearly a decade later (Morris & Albery, 2001).

CONCLUSION AND FUTURE RESEARCH DIRECTIONS

The first question addressed in this chapter focused on relationships among risky behaviors. Despite consistent evidence that these behaviors are often related, a great deal of research and the majority of intervention studies tend to focus on individual risky behaviors. Sensation seeking is strongly associated with risky drinking, moderately associated with risky driving, and weakly associated with risky sex, but causal assertions are premature given existing data. Causal evidence exists that unconventionality contributes to risky drinking, risky driving, and, among adolescents, risky sex. In adults, there is consistent evidence that the pharmacologic properties of alcohol limit attention and perception, thereby enabling persons who are conflicted about risky sex to "temporarily forget" about their conflict and "give in" to risky sex. In men, this may be particularly true for those who have a belief that alcohol will enhance sex. Finally, sexual aggression appears to result from a variety of factors including the pharmacologic effects of alcohol on aggression and, possibly, stereotypes about drinking women.

The second question focused on risk and protective factors for risky behaviors. Risk factors such as male gender, being an adolescent or young adult, having unconventional attitudes and behaviors and a high tolerance for deviance, and having peers who have unconventional attitudes and behaviors are consistently seen across studies. Evidence that being impulsive, having disturbed risk perception (related to risky driving for males and risky sex for females), and having a belief that alcohol will enhance sex (for males) was documented but was less convincing. Protective factors, including being actively involved in a diverse collection of conventional activities and having peers that model conventional attitudes and behaviors, mitigate risk for engaging in risky drinking, risky driving, and risky sex.

The third question focused on future research directions to advance the knowledge base about risky behaviors. There is a need to go beyond epidemiologic work and move toward longitudinal testing of promising causal mechanisms that have been derived from existing theory and research findings. There is a need to develop interventions that are theoretically derived and empirically based and are focused on causes of multiple behaviors. Studies that test the efficacy of interventions across the life span and in diverse populations are needed, with particular attention to their long-term effectiveness. The existing potpourri of interventions for risky behaviors, some of which stem from clinical findings or practical experience rather than being based on scientific evidence, may be insufficient to move the science forward and prevent adverse health events. One of the most critical issues is that the focus of interventions needs to be shifted "upstream" to target root causes rather than the behaviors themselves being the targets of intervention. Although interventions are warranted to reduce risky behaviors, interventions also need to prevent risky behaviors. Nurse-scientists are particularly well positioned to implement intervention trials because of their interest in health promotion and prevention of adverse health events.

Given the current state of the science and promising theoretical models, there are clear and specific directions for intervention. For example, given that there is fairly strong evidence that high unconventionality contributes to all three risky behaviors in adolescents, efforts to foster involvements in school, church, and community-related activities will enhance conventionality. A second example relates to the role of expectancy in risky sex. Given beliefs about alcohol enhancing sex for men in particular, interventions aimed at challenging the formation of such beliefs in adolescents or challenging existing beliefs about the role of alcohol and sex would be effective. A third example has to do with the myopic processing view of the relationship between alcohol and risky sex in adults who feel conflicted about risky sex. Interventions should be aimed at decreasing the conflict about risky sex, thereby fostering certainty about the dangers of risky sex, promoting sexual health as a personal value, or decreasing alcohol consumption prior to sex.

Risky drinking, risky driving, and risky sexual behaviors lead to health-related consequences that can significantly decrease the health and well-being of the public. Although young people bear a disproportionate burden of the negative consequences of risky behaviors, individuals across the life span are also affected. The extent of the problem is clearly elucidated through epidemiologic studies; nurse-scientists have an opportunity to develop, refine, and test empirically derived nursing interventions to reduce risky behaviors. More importantly, with the health promotion focus of the discipline, nurse-scientists can ensure the health of our future generations by emphasizing preventive interventions.

ACKNOWLEDGMENT

This work was supported in part by the National Center for Injury Prevention and Control, Centers for Disease Control and Prevention, Grant R49/CCR-523225.

REFERENCES

Aarons, S., Jenkins, R., Raine, T., El-Khoratzy, M., Woddward, K., & Williams, R., et al. (2000). Postponing sexual intercourse among junior high school students: A randomized controlled evaluation. *Journal of Adolescent Health, 27,* 236–247.

Abbey, A., McAuslan, P., & Ross, L. T. (1998). Sexual assault perpetration by college men: The role of alcohol, misperception of sexual intent and sexual beliefs and experiences. *Journal of Social and Clinical Psychology, 17,* 167–195.

Abbey, A., Zawacki, T., Buck, P. O., Clinton, A. M., & McAuslan, P. (2001). Alcohol and sexual assault. *Alcohol Research and Health, 25,* 43–51.

Abrecen, J., Looman, J., & Anderson, D. (2000). Alcohol and drug abuse in sexual and nonsexual violent offenders. *Sexual Abuse: Journal of Research and Treatment, 12,* 263–274.

Allen, J. P., Litten, R. Z., Fertig, J. B., & Babor, T. F. (1997). A review of research on the Alcohol Use Disorders Identification Test (AUDIT). *Alcoholism: Clinical and Experimental Research, 21,* 613–619.

Arnett, J. (1990). Personality variables associated with traffic accidents. *Behavioural Research in Highway Safety, 1*, 3–18.

———. (1999). Adolescent storm and stress reconsidered. *American Psychologist, 54*, 317–326.

Arnett, J., Offer, D., & Fine, M. (1997). Reckless driving in adolescence: "State" and "trait" factors. *Accident Analysis and Prevention, 29*, 57–63.

Bailey, S. L., Pollock, N. K., Martin, C. S., & Lynch, K. G. (1999). Risky sexual behaviors among adolescents with alcohol use disorders. *Journal of Adolescent Health, 25*, 179–181.

Balluz, L., Ahluwalia, I. B., Murphy, W., Mokdad, A., Giles, W., & Harris, V. (2004). Surveillance for certain health behaviors among selected local areas: United States, Behavioral Risk Factor Surveillance System, 2002. *Mortality and Morbidity Weekly Report, 53*(SS-5), 1–100.

Barbaree, H., & Marshall, W. (1991). The role of male sexual arousal in rape: Six models. *Journal of Consulting and Clinical Psychology, 59*, 621–630.

Bingham, C. R., & Shope, J. (2004). Adolescent developmental antecedents of risky driving among young adults. *Journal of Studies on Alcohol, 65*, 84–94.

Borowsky, I. W., Hogan, M., & Ireland, M. (1997). Adolescent sexual aggression: Risk and protective factors. *Pediatrics, 100*, E7.

Brecklin, L. R., & Ullman, S. E. (2001). The role of offender alcohol use in rape attacks: An analysis of National Crime Victimization Survey data. *Journal of Interpersonal Violence, 16*, 3–21.

Brecklin, L. R., & Ullman, S. E. (2002). The role of victim and offender alcohol use in sexual assault: Results from the National Crime Victimization Survey data. *Journal of Studies on Alcohol, 63*, 57–63.

Brown, S., Christiansen, B., & Goldman, M. (1987. The Alcohol Expectancy Questionnaire: An instrument for the assessment and adult alcohol expectancies. *Journal of Studies on Alcohol, 48*, 483–491.

Brown, S. A., & Tapert, S. F. (2004). Adolescence and the trajectory of alcohol use: Basic to clinical studies. *Annals of the New York Academy of Sciences, 1021*, 234–244.

Buddie, A. M., & Parks, K. A. (2003). The role of the bar context and social behaviors on women's risk for aggression. *Journal of Interpersonal Violence, 18*, 1378–1393.

Centers for Disease Control and Prevention. (1999). Achievements in public health, 1900 to 1999. Motor-vehicle safety: A 20th century public health achievement. *Mortality and Morbidity Weekly Report, 48*, 369–374.

———. (2002). Trends in sexual risk behaviors among high school students–United States, 1991–2001. *Mortality and Morbidity Weekly Report, 51*, 856–859.

———. (2004a). Acute health care, rehabilitation and disability prevention research, National Center for Injury Prevention and Control. Retrieved September 15, 2004, from http://www.cdc.gov/ncipc/profiles/acutecare/default.htm

———. (2004b). Brief risk factor surveillance system. Retrieved September 15, 2004, from http://www.cdc.gov/brfss/

———. (2004c). CDC's new HIV initiative advancing HIV prevention: New strategies for a changing epidemic United States (National Center for HIV, STD and TB Prevention, Divisions of HIV/AIDS Prevention). Retrieved September 15, 2004, from http://www.cdc.gov/hiv/partners/question.htm

———. (2004d). Impaired driving facts. Retrieved September 15, 2004, from http://www.cdc.gov/ncipc/factsheets/drving.htm

————. (2004e). Youth Risk Behavior Surveillance System. Retrieved September 15, 2004, from http://www.cdc.gov/HealthyYouth/yrbs/index.htm

Chassin, L., Presson, C., Sherman, S., & Edwards, D. (1992). Parent educational attainment and adolescent cigarette smoking. *Journal of Substance Abuse, 4,* 219–234.

Cherpitel, C. J. (1999). Substance use, injury, and risk-taking dispositions in the general population. *Alcoholism Clinical and Experimental Research, 23,* 121–126.

Colder, C. R., Campbell, R. T., Ruel, E., Richardson, J. C., & Flay, B. R. (2002). A finite mixture model of growth trajectories of adolescent alcohol use: Predictors and consequences. *Journal of Consulting and Clinical Psychology, 70,* 976–985.

Cooper, A. (1994). The effects of intoxication levels of ethanol on nocturnal penile tumescence. *Journal of Sex and Marital Therapy, 20,* 14–23.

Corte, C., & Stein, K. (2003). *Role of the self in antisocial alcoholism: Content and structure of self-cognitions in antisocial alcohol dependence and recovery.* Paper presented at the annual meeting of the Midwest Nursing Research Society, Grand Rapids, MI.

Costa, F., Jessor, R., Fortenberry, D., & Donovan, J. (1996). Psychosocial conventionality, health orientation, and contraceptive use in adolescence. *Journal of Adolescent Health, 18,* 404–416.

Department of Licensing, State of Washington. (2002). *Road rage.* Retrieved September 15, 2004, from http://dol.wa.gov/ds/roadrage.htm.

Dermen, K., & Cooper, M. L. (2000). Inhibition conflict and alcohol expectancy as moderators of alcohol's relationship to condom use. *Experimental and Clinical Psychopharmacology, 8,* 198–206.

Dermen, K., Cooper, M. L., & Agocha, V. (1998). Sex-related alcohol expectancies as moderator of the relationship between alcohol use and risky sex in adolescents. *Journal of Studies on Alcohol, 59,* 71–77.

Donovan, J. E. (1993). Young adult drinking-driving: Behavioral and psychosocial correlates. *Journal of Studies on Alcohol, 54,* 600–613.

Donovan, J. E., & Jessor, R. (1983). Problem drinking and the dimension of involvement with drugs: A Guttman scalogram analysis of adolescent drug use. *American Journal of Public Health, 73,* 543–552.

————. (1985). Structure of problem behavior in adolescence and young adulthood. *Journal of Consulting and Clinical Psychology, 53,* 890–904.

Dougherty, D. M., Mathias, C. W., Tester, M., & Marsh, D. M. (2004) Age at first drink relates to behavioral measures of impulsivity: The immediate and delayed memory tasks. *Alcoholism Clinical and Experimental Research, 28,* 408–414.

Dula, C. S., & Geller, E. S. (2003). Risky, aggressive, or emotional driving: Addressing the need for consistent communication in research. *Journal of Safety Research, 34,* 559–566.

Erikson, E. (1968). *Identity: Youth and crisis.* New York: Norton.

Fillmore, M., & Vogel-Sprott, M. (1999). Response inhibition under alcohol: Effects of cognitive and motivational conflict. *Journal of Studies on Alcohol, 61,* 239–246.

Fleming, M. F., Barry, K. L., Manwell, L. B., Johnson, K., & London, R. (1997). Brief physician advice for problem alcohol drinkers: A randomized controlled trial in community-based primary care practices. *Journal of the American Medical Association, 277,* 1039–1045.

George, W., Cue, K., Lopez, P., Crowe, L., & Norris, J. (1995). Self-reported alcohol expectancies and postdrinking sexual inferences about women. *Journal of Applied Social Psychology, 25,* 164–186.

George, W., Lehman, G., Cue, K., Martinez, L., Lopez, P., & Norris, J. (1997). Postdrinking sexual inferences: Evidence for linear rather than curvilinear dosage effects. *Journal of Applied Social Psychology, 27,* 630–649.

George, W., & Marlatt, A., (1986). The effects of alcohol and anger on interest in violence, erotica, and deviance. *Journal of Abnormal Psychology, 95,* 150–158.

George, W. H., & Stoner, S. A. (2000). Understanding acute alcohol effects on sexual behavior. *Annual Review of Sex Research, 11,* 92–124.

George, W. H., Stoner, S. A., Norris, J., Lopez, P. A., & Lehman, G. L. (2000). Alcohol expectancies and sexuality: A self-fulfilling prophecy analysis of dyadic perceptions and behavior. *Journal of Studies on Alcohol, 61,* 168–176.

Glassbrenner, D. (2004). Safety belt use in 2003—demographic characteristics (National Center for Statistics and Analysis, Department of Transportation (DOT) Tech. Report HS 809 729). Retrieved September 15, 2004, from http://www.nhtsa.dot.gov/people/injury/airbags/809729.pdf

Goldberg, J., & Fischoff, B. (2000). The long-term risks in the short-term benefits: Perception of potentially addictive activities. *Health Psychology, 19,* 299–303.

Goldberg, J., Hapern-Felsher, B., & Millstein, S. (2002). Beyond invulnerability: The importance of the benefits in adolescents' decision to drink alcohol. *Health Psychology, 21,* 477–484.

Greene, K., Kremar, M., Walters, L., Rubin, D., Hale, J., & Hale, L. (2000). Targeting adolescent risk-taking behaviors: The contributors of egocentrism and sensation-seeking. *Journal of Adolescence, 23,* 439–461.

Gross, A. M., Bennett, T., Sloan, L., Marx, B. P., & Juergens, J. (2001). The impact of alcohol and alcohol expectancies on male perceptions of female sexual arousal in a date rape analog. *Experimental and Clinical Psychopharmacology, 9,* 380–388.

Grunbaum, J., Hann, L., Kinshen, S., Ross, J., Gowda, V., Collins, J., et al. (2002). Youth risk behavior surveillance: National Alternative High School Youth Risk Behavior Survey, Unites States, 1998. *Journal of School Health, 70,* 5–17.

Grunbaum, J. A., Kann, L., Kinchen, S., Ross, J., Hawkins, J., Lowry, R., et al. (2004). Youth risk behavior surveillance—United States 2003. *Morbidity and Mortality Weekly Report, 53*(SS02), 1–96.

Halpern-Felsher, B., Millstein, S., & Ellen, J. (1996). Relationship of alcohol use and risky sexual behavior: A review and analysis of findings. *Journal of Adolescent Health, 19,* 331–336.

Harre, N., Brandt, T., & Dawe, M. (2000). The development of risky driving in adolescence. *Journal of Safety Research, 31,* 185–194.

Hawkins, J., Catalano, R., & Miller, J. (1992). Risk and protective factors for alcohol and other drug problems in adolescence and early adulthood: Implications for substance abuse prevention. *Psychological Bulletin, 112,* 64–105.

Hingson, R., & Howland, J. (1993). Promoting safety in adolescents. In S. G. Millstein, A. C. Peterson, & E. O. Nightingale (Eds.), *Promoting the health of adolescents* (pp. 305–327). New York: Oxford University Press.

Igra, V., & Irwin, C. (1996). Theories of adolescent risk-taking behavior. In R. DiClemente, W. Hansen, & L. Ponton (Eds.), *Handbook of adolescent health risk behavior* (pp. 35–51). New York: Plenum Press.

Irwin, C. E., & Millstein, S. G. (1991). Correlates and predictors of risk-taking behavior during adolescence. In L. R. Lapsitt & L. L. Mitnick (Eds.), *Self-regulatory behavior and risk taking: Causes and consequences* (pp. 3–21). Norwood, NJ: Ablex.

Ito, T. A., Miller, N., & Pollock, V. E. (1996). Alcohol and aggression: A meta-analysis on the moderating effects of inhibitory cues, triggering events, and self-focused attention. *Psychological Bulletin, 120*, 60–82.

Iverson, H., & Rundmo, T. (2004). Attitudes toward traffic safety, driving behaviour and accident involvement among the Norwegian public. *Ergonomics, 47*, 555–572.

Jemmott, J. B., Jemmott, L. S., & Fong, G. T. (1992). Reductions in HIV risk-associated sexual behaviors among black male adolescents: Effects of an AIDS prevention intervention. *American Journal of Public Health, 82*, 372–377.

———. (1998). Abstinence and safer sex HIV risk-reduction interventions for African American adolescents: A randomized controlled trial. *Journal of the American Medical Association, 279*, 129–1536.

Jessor, R., Donovan, J., & Costa, F. (1991). *Beyond adolescence: Problem behavior and young adult development.* Cambridge: Cambridge University Press.

Jessor, R., & Jessor, S. (1977). *Problem behavior and psychosocial development: A longitudinal study of youth.* New York: Academic Press.

Jessor, R., Turbin, M. S., & Costa, F. M. (1997). Protective factors in adolescent health behavior. *Journal of Personality and Social Psychology, 75*, 788–800.

Johnston, L., O'Malley, P., Bachman, J., & Schulenberg, J. (2004). *Monitoring the future: National survey results on drug use, 1975–2003: Vol. 2. College Students and Adults Ages 19–45, 2003.* Bethesda, MD: U.S. Department of Health and Human Services, National Institute on Drug Abuse.

Jonah, B. (1997). Sensation seeking and risky driving: A review and synthesis of the literature. *Accident Analysis and Prevention, 29*, 651–665.

Kalichman, S., Cain, D., Zweben, A., & Swain, G. (2003). Sensation seeking, alcohol use and sexual risk behaviors among men receiving services at a clinic for sexually transmitted infections. *Journal of Studies on Alcohol, 64*, 564–569.

Kalichman, C., Tannebaum, L., & Nachimson, D. (1998). Personality and cognitive factors influencing substance use and sexual risk for HIV infection among gay and bisexual men. *Psychology of Addictive Behaviors, 12*, 262–271.

Kelley, A. E., Schochet, T., & Landry, C. F. (2004). Risk taking and novelty seeking in adolescence: Introduction to part I. *Annals of the New York Academy of Sciences, 1021*, 27–32.

Kellogg, N. D., Hoffman, T. J., & Taylor, E. R. (1999). Early sexual experiences among pregnant and parenting adolescents. *Adolescence, 34*, 293–303.

Kirby, D., & DiClemente, R. J. (1994). School-based interventions to prevent unprotected sex and HIV among adolescents. In R. J. DiClemente & J. L. Peterson (Eds.), *Preventing AIDS: Theories and methods of behavioral interventions* (pp. 117–139). New York: Plenum Press.

Kirby, D., Korpi, M., Adivi, C., & Weissman, J. (1997). An impact evaluation of project SNAPP: An AIDS and pregnancy prevention middle school program. *AIDS Education and Prevention, 9*(Suppl. A), 44–61.

Labrie, J., & Earlywine, M. (2000). Sexual risk behaviors and alcohol: Higher base rates revealed using the unmatched-count technique. *Journal of Sex Research, 37*, 321–326.

Lane, S., & Cherek, D. (2002). Risk taking by adolescents with maladaptive behavior histories. *Experimental and Clinical Psychopharmacology, 9*, 74–82.

Leigh, B. (1999). Peril, chance, adventure: Concepts of risk, alcohol use and risky behavior in young adults. *Addiction, 94*, 371–383.

Lipsitt, L., & Mitnick, L. (Eds.). (1991). *Self-regulatory behavior and risk taking: Causes and consequences.* Norwood, NJ: Ablex.

Logan, T., Cole, J., & Leukefeld, C. (2002). Women, sex, and HIV: Social and contextual factors, meta-analysis of published interventions, and implications for practice and research. *Psychological Bulletin, 128,* 851–885.

MacDonald, T. K., Zanna, M. P., & Fong, G. T. (1996). Why common sense goes out the window: The effects of alcohol on intentions to use condoms. *Personality and Social Psychology Bulletin, 22,* 763–775.

MacMahon, B., Pugh, T., & Ipsen, J. (1960). *Epidemiologic methods.* Boston: Little, Brown.

Malatesta, V., Pollack, R., Wilbanks, W., & Adams, H. (1979). Alcohol effects on the orgasmic-ejaculatory response in human males. *Journal of Sex Research, 15,* 101–107.

Mann, R., Smart, R., Stoduto, G., Adlaf, E., & Ialomiteanu, A. (2004). Alcohol consumption and problems among road rage victims and perpetrators. *Journal of Studies on Alcohol, 65,* 161–168.

Maio, R. F., Shope, J. T., Blow, F. C., Gregor, M. A., Zakrajsek, J. S., Weber, J. E. et al., (2005). A randomized controlled trial of an emergency department-based interactive computer program to prevent alcohol misuse among injured adolescents. *Annals of Emergency Medicine, 45,* 420–429.

Marx, B. P., Gross, A. M., & Juergens, J. P. (1997). The effects of alcohol consumption and expectancies in an experimental date rape analogue. *Journal of Psychopathology and Behavioral Assessment, 19,* 281–302.

McKeown, R. E., Jackson, K. L., & Valois, R. F. (1998). The frequency and correlates of violence behaviors in a statewide sample of high school students. *Family and Community Health, 20,* 38–53.

Merline, A., O'Malley, P., Schulenberg, J., Bachman, J., & Johnston, L. (2004). Substance use among adults 35 years of age: Prevalence, adulthood, predictors, and impact of adolescent substance use. *American Journal of Public Health, 94,* 96–102.

Miller, M., Azrael, D., Hemenway, D., & Solop, F. I. (2002). "Road rage" in Arizona: Armed and dangerous. *Accident Analysis and Prevention, 34,* 807–814.

Mohler-Kuo, M., Dowdall, G. W., Koss, M. P., & Wechsler, H. (2004). Correlates of rape while intoxicated in a national sample of college women. *Journal of Studies on Alcohol, 65,* 37–45.

Monti, P. M., Colby, S. M., Barnett, N. P., Spirito, A., Rohsenow, D. J., Myers, M., et al. (1999). Brief intervention for harm reduction with alcohol-positive older adolescents in a hospital emergency department. *Journal of Consulting and Clinical Psychology, 67,* 989 994.

Moore, K., Malove, J., Terry-Humen, E., Williams, S., Papillo, A., & Scarpa, J. (2001). *Child trends: Facts at a glance 2001.* Retrieved August, 16, 2004, from http://www.child trends.org/factlink.asp

Morris, A., & Albery, I. (2001). Alcohol consumption and HIV risk behaviours: Integrating the theories of alcohol myopia and outcome expectancies. *Addiction Research and Theory, 9,* 73–86.

National Center for Injury Prevention and Control (NCPIC). (2000). *Fact book for the year 2000: Working to prevent and control injury in the United States.* Atlanta: Author. Retrieved August 4, 2004, from http://www.cdc.gov/ncipc/pub-res/FactBook

National Highway Traffic Safety Administration (NHTSA). (1999). *Relative frequency of unsafe driving acts in serious traffic crashes: Summary of important findings.* Retrieved

October 25, 2004, from http://www.nhtsa.dot.gov/people/injury/research/UDAshort rpt/docum entation_page.html

National Institute on Alcohol Abuse and Alcoholism. (1996). Drinking and driving. *Alcohol Alert, 31*, 1–4.

National Safety Council. (2003). *Injury facts*. Itasca, IL: Author.

Norris, J., George, W. H., Davis, K. L., Cue, K. L., Martell, J., & Leonesio, R. J. (1999). Alcohol and hypermasculinity as determinants of men's emphatic responses to violent pornography. *Journal of Interpersonal Violence, 14*, 683–700.

Norris, J., Nurius, P. S., & Dimeff, L. A. (1996). Through her eyes: Factors affecting women's perceptions of and resistance to acquaintance sexual aggression threat. *Psychology of Women Quarterly, 20*, 123–145.

Ouimette, P. C. (1997). Psychopathology and sexual aggression in non-incarcerated men. *Violence and Victims, 12*, 389–395.

Parks, K. A., Miller, B. A., Collins, R. L., & Zetes-Zanatta, L. (1998). Women's descriptions of drinking in bars: Reasons and risks. *Sex Roles, 38*, 701–717.

Raffaelli, M., & Crockett, L. (2003). Sexual risk taking in adolescence: The role of self-regulation and attraction to risk. *Developmental Psychology, 39*, 1036–1046.

Richardson, D., & Campbell, J. (1982). Alcohol and rape: The effect of alcohol on attributions of blame for rape. *Personality and Social Psychology Bulletin, 8*, 468–476.

Reinfurt, D., Williams, J., Wells, J., & Rodgman, E. (1996). Characteristics of drivers not using seat belts in a high best use state. *Journal of Safety Research, 27*, 209–215.

Santelli, J. S., Brener, N. D., Lowry, R., Bhatt, A., & Zabin, L. S. (1998). Multiple sexual partners among U.S. adolescents and young adults. *Family Planning Perspectives, 30*, 271–275.

Santelli, J. S., Kaiser, J., Hirsch, L., Radosh, A., Simkin, L., & Middlestadt, S. (2004). Initiation of sexual intercourse among middle school adolescents: The influence of psychosocial factors. *Journal of Adolescent Health, 34*, 200–208.

Sayette, M., Kirchner, T., Moreland, R., Levine, J., & Travis, T. (2004). Effects of alcohol on risk-seeking behavior: A group-level analysis. *Psychology of Addictive Behaviors, 18*, 190–193.

Schweizer, T., Jolicoeur, P., Vogel-Sprott, M., & Dixon, M. (2004). Fast, but error-prone, responses during acute alcohol intoxication: Effects of stimulus-response mapping complexity. *Alcoholism: Clinical and Experimental Research, 28*, 643–649.

Siegel, D., Aten, M., Rogimann, K., & Enaharo, M. (1998). Early effects of a school based human immunodeficiency virus infection and sexual risk prevention intervention. *Archives of Pediatrics and Adolescent Medicine, 152*, 961–970.

Spear, L. P. (2004). Adolescence and the trajectory of alcohol use: Introduction to part IV. *Annals of the New York Academy of Sciences, 1021*, 202–205.

Stanford, M., Greve, K., Boudreaux, J., Mathias, C., & Brumbelow, J. (1996). Impulsiveness and risk taking behavior: Comparison of high-school and college students using the Barratt Impulsiveness Scale. *Personality and Individual Differences, 21*, 1073–1075.

Steele, C., & Josephs, R. (1990). Alcohol myopia: Its prized and dangerous effects. *American Psychologist, 45*, 921–933.

Steele, C., & Southwick, L. (1985). Alcohol and social behavior: 1. The psychology of drunken excess. *Journal of Personality and Social Psychology, 48*, 18–34.

Stein, K., Roeser, R., & Markus, H. (1998). Self-schemas and possible selves and predictors and outcomes of risky behaviors in adolescents. *Nursing Research, 47*, 96–106.

Steinberg, L. (2004). Risk taking in adolescences: What changes and why? *Annals of the New York Academy of Science, 1021*, 51–58.

Talashek, M., Norr, K., & Dancy, B. (2003). Building teen power for sexual health. *Journal of Transcultural Nursing, 14*, 207–216.

Testa, M. (2002). The impact of men's alcohol consumption on perpetration of sexual aggression. *Clinical Psychology Review, 22*, 1239–1263.

Testa, M., Livingston, J. A., & Collins, R. L. (2000). The role of women's alcohol consumption in evaluation of vulnerability to sexual aggression. *Experimental and Clinical Psychopharmacology, 8*, 185–191.

Testa, M., & Parks, K. A. (1996). The role of women's alcohol consumption in sexual victimization in sexual victimization. *Aggression and Violent Behavior: A Review Journal, 1*, 217–234.

Tjaden, P., & Thoennes, N. (1998). Prevalence, incidence and consequences of violence against women: National Institute of Justice Centers for Disease Control and Prevention: Research in Brief. Washington, DC: National Institute of Justice.

Tyler, K. A., Hoyt, D. R., & Whitbeck, L. B. (1998). Coercive sexual strategies. *Violence and Victims, 13*, 47–61.

Ulleberg, P. (2002). Personality and subtypes of young drivers. Relationship to risk-taking preferences, accident involvement, and response to a traffic safety campaign. *Transportation Research, Part F, 4*, 279–297.

Utter, D. (2001). *Passenger vehicle driver cell phone use: Results from the fall 2000 National Occupant Protection Use Survey* (U.S. Department of Transportation, National Highway Traffic Safety Administration DOT HS 809 293). Retrieved October 25, 2004, from http://www-nrd.nhtsa.dot.gov/pdf/nrd-30/NCSA/RNotes/2001/809-293.pdf

Weinhardt, L., Forsyth, A., Carey, M., Jawoski, B., & Durant, L. (1998). Reliability and validity of self-report behaviors for HIV-related sexual behavior: Progress since 1990 and recommendations for research and practice. *Archive of Sexual Behavior, 27*, 155–180.

Weinstein, N. (1984). Why it won't happen to me: Perceptions of risk factors and susceptibility. *Health Psychology, 3*, 431–457.

Wilson, G. T., & Lawson, D. M. (1978). Effects of alcohol on sexual arousal in women. *Journal of Abnormal Psychology, 85*, 489–497.

Wilson, G. T., & Niaura, R. (1984). Alcohol and the disinhibition of sexual responsiveness. *Journal of Studies on Alcohol, 46*, 219–224.

Wilson, G., Niaura, R., & Adler, J. (1985). Alcohol, selective attention, and sexual arousal in men. *Journal of Studies on Alcohol, 46*, 107–115.

Wilson, J., Fang, M., Wiggins, S., & Cooper, P. (2003). Collision and violation involvement of drivers who use cellular telephones. *Traffic Injury Prevention, 4*, 45–52.

Wingood, G. M., & DiClemente, R. J. (1998). The influence of psychosocial factors, alcohol, drug use on African American women's high-risk sexual behavior. *American Journal of Preventive Medicine, 15*, 54–59.

Yi, H., Williams, G., & Dufour, M. (2003). *Alcohol epidemiologic data system: Surveillance report #65—Trends in alcohol-related fatal traffic crashes, United States, 1977–2001.* Bethesda, MD: National Institute on Alcohol Abuse and Alcoholism, Division of Biometry and Epidemiology.

Zuckerman, M. (1991). *Psychobiology of personality.* Cambridge: Cambridge University Press.

PART IV

Alcohol Intervention Research

Chapter 11

Alcohol Brief Interventions

Deborah Finfgeld-Connett

ABSTRACT

A large proportion of Americans report binge or heavy drinking. The human and economic costs of alcohol misuse are extensive, with hundreds of thousands of lives lost or disrupted and billions of dollars spent due to impaired productivity, crime, and adverse health consequences. In an effort to reduce costs such as these, scientists and clinicians have developed brief interventions, characterized by their low intensity and short (5–60 minutes) duration, as well as by their intent to provide early intervention before drinkers develop alcohol abuse or dependence. The purpose of this review, therefore, is to analyze research studies related to brief intervention and critically analyze and critique their findings. In addition, both prospective randomized controlled trials and meta-analyses will be used to discuss the implications for clinical practice and make recommendations for future research.

Keywords: alcohol treatment, brief intervention, alcohol interventions

Alcohol abuse is a national and global epidemic. It is estimated that 47% of Americans age 12 and older use alcohol. Of those individuals, 21% (46 million) binge drink, and 6% (13 million) report heavy drinking (Substance Abuse and Mental Health Services Administration ([SAMHSA] 2001; see definitions in

Table 2.1, chapter 2). Consequences of alcohol abuse include premature death, impaired productivity, health-related adverse events such as injury from motor vehicle crashes, and crime. The cost of these and other alcohol-related adverse events are estimated to be $184.6 billion per year, and of this amount, $26.3 billion is spent on health care services (National Institute on Alcohol Abuse and Alcoholism [NIAAA], 2000). Because alcohol use spans a continuum that includes low-risk, at-risk, problem, and dependent drinking, scientists have developed and tested a variety of intervention strategies targeted to particular populations of drinkers. Alcohol dependence describes only a small portion of the drinking population and requires treatment from a specialist. For the 5% to 15% of the population who have problem or at-risk drinking (NIAAA, 2000; Saunders & Lee, 2000), strategies such as brief intervention have emerged as possible efficacious treatments.

Fleming, Barry, Manwell, Johnson, and London (1997) defined brief intervention as a clinically based strategy that includes assessment and direct feedback, contracting and goal setting, behavior modification techniques, and the use of written materials that serve as a self-help manual. Brief intervention is often conducted in general health care settings and is designed for use by health professionals who do not specialize in addictions treatment. It is most often used with people who are not alcohol dependent, and its goal is moderate drinking rather than abstinence (Fleming & Graham, 2001; Fleming & Manwell, 1999; NIAAA, 1999). As the evidence unfolds, brief intervention may be an appropriate nursing strategy in both inpatient and outpatient settings. It also serves as the foundation for reducing risky behaviors other than alcohol misuse, such as risky sexual behaviors associated with disease transmission or risky driving behaviors associated with injury.

Brief intervention typically consists of 5 to 60 minutes of counseling and education, with usually no more than four sessions. It addresses the specific problem behaviors such as at-risk or heavy drinking and is intended to provide early intervention before the onset of alcohol-related problems (Babor & Higgins-Biddle, 2000). The purpose of this review is to analyze and critique research studies related to alcohol brief intervention.

METHODS

In order to complete the review of relevant work, a literature search was completed with the following keywords: *alcohol, brief intervention, brief interventions, early interventions, prevention,* and *treatment.* The following electronic data bases were used for the search: Cumulative Index of Nursing and Allied Health Literature (CINAHL), Premedline, Medline, and PsycInfo. In addition, reference lists were scanned for relevant documents. The literature search was limited to peer-reviewed English-language publications. For purposes of this review, studies were organized according to the following categories: primary care, injury, women, miscellaneous large-scale studies, and meta-analyses.

BRIEF INTERVENTION: PHILOSOPHICAL/THERAPEUTIC UNDERPINNINGS AND HISTORY

Alcohol brief interventions are predicated on a harm reduction philosophy. This philosophy has been developed as a public health alternative to the moral/criminal and disease models associated with alcohol misuse and abuse. Abstinence is viewed as an ideal outcome, but other goals that focus on reducing harm are deemed appropriate (Marlatt, 1998). Alcohol abuse and misuse are thought to have multiple causes and range from mild to severe (Larimer et al., 1998). Hallmarks of harm reduction strategies include promoting personal changes in the "right direction" (Marlatt, 1998, p. 55), personal choice and responsibility (Larimer et al., 1998), and enhancement of self-efficacy (Bandura, 1997). Harm reduction services are nonstigmatizing, easily accessible, and meet clients "where they are" (Marlatt, 1998, p. 55).

An important component of harm reduction is screening to detect people with behavioral patterns that place them at risk before the consequences become pronounced (Babor & Higgins-Biddle, 2000). Harm reduction is a complementary philosophy to the principle of secondary prevention. Early recognition of hazardous drinking (pattern of drinking that poses a high risk of future damage to physical or mental health [Reinert & Allen, 2002]) and minimizing harm are basic principles of secondary prevention (Babor, Ritson, & Hodgson, 1986).

History

In the United States, many traditional alcohol abuse treatment programs originated from federal, state, and local efforts in the 1960s to upgrade care from punitive treatments such as the use of drunk tanks in jails to handle intoxication. By the 1980s, third-party payers were assuming a greater role in reimbursing for lengthy (~28 day) inpatient care. These programs were largely based on the Minnesota model and the philosophy espoused by Alcoholics Anonymous (AA). They were designed for people with alcohol abuse and dependence, and the goal of treatment was abstinence. Despite the widespread availability of these programs, a growing awareness developed that more flexible treatment options, such as brief intervention, might be appropriate for the large number of nondependent, problem, or heavy drinkers. These individuals were either at risk for adverse consequences of alcohol or had already experienced negative consequences of drinking but were not alcohol dependent (Barry, 1999). At the same time, international experts affiliated with the World Health Organization (WHO) began to explore methods to detect people with harmful alcohol consumption before health and social consequences became pronounced (WHO, 1980).

Alcohol brief interventions, therefore, evolved from several different initiatives. One of the earliest was an attempt to increase emergency care referrals for alcohol treatment services (Chafetz, 1961; Chafetz et al., 1962). These investigators found that medical patients given a single session of counseling and advice persisted longer in alcohol treatment programs. Other initiatives developed from international concern that global patterns of heavy drinking were escalating in many populations. International interest focused on the idea that controlled drinking might be a reasonable alternative to abstinence in certain populations of drinkers. Each of these initiatives is explored below.

WHO Collaborative Project

In 1982, the WHO Collaborative Project on Identification and Treatment of Persons with Harmful Alcohol Consumption was initiated to develop the scientific basis for screening and brief intervention in the primary care setting (Babor & Grant, 1992; Babor et al., 1986; WHO Brief Intervention Study Group, 1996). The second phase of the project was to test the effectiveness of screening and brief intervention in an international, (predominantly) primary care population ($N = 1,559$). Subjects who drank heavily (50–120 g of absolute alcohol daily for men and 32–80 g for women) were included in the study (see Table 2.1, chapter 2, for definitions of a standard drink). Dependent drinkers were excluded from the study.

Two interventions were tested: simple advice (screening, 5 minutes of advice about the importance of sensible drinking, and a pamphlet) and brief counseling (screening, simple advice, 15 additional minutes of counseling, and 3 optional sessions). Outcome measures from the randomized controlled trial (RCT) included alcohol consumption and alcohol-related health and social consequences. Male subjects exposed to either of two interventions reported significantly decreased daily alcohol consumption from baseline, whereas both control and experimental female subjects reduced their alcohol consumption regardless of condition (Babor & Grant, 1992; WHO Brief Intervention Study Group, 1996). At 10-year follow-up, results from the Sydney, Australia, arm ($n = 554$) indicated no differences in mean alcohol consumption (Wutzke, Conigrave, & Saunders, 2002).

Other Brief Intervention Protocols

During the same years of the WHO (1996) study, several other teams were also developing and testing brief intervention protocols. The investigators of the

Malmo Project in Sweden (Kristenson, Öhlin, Hultén-Nosslin, Trell, & Hood, 1983) studied men ($N = 473$) with elevated serum γ glutamyl transferase (GGT; GGT for inclusion needed to be from 83 to 200 units/liter). One group was offered consultations with a physician every third month, monthly GGT testing, and contacts with a nurse until GGT levels stabilized. The control group was informed by letter that they had impaired liver function, encouraged to restrict alcohol consumption, and invited for follow-up GGT testing 2, 4, and 6 years later. At 2- and 4-year follow-up, both groups experienced significantly decreased GGT values, and at 4, 5, and 6 years, significant differences were detected in absenteeism due to illness, hospital days, and mortality. Note that, in this study, treatment offered to the experimental group stretched the definition of brief intervention, and the control group received treatment more akin to brief treatment. Frequent contact with health care professionals over an extended period of time, therefore, seemed to result in better medical and social outcomes in the study population.

In a study from Great Britain, investigators for the Medical Research Council (MRC) trial (Wallace, Cutler, & Haines, 1988) recruited subjects from the offices of 47 general practitioners. Men who indicated that they drank 35 units (standard drinks) or more per week and women who consumed 21 units or more per week, or individuals who responded positively to two or more CAGE items, were invited to participate. An additional 25% of those who were not drinking excessively but indicated concern about their drinking were also invited to take part. Participants ($N = 909$) were randomized to control or treatment groups. The brief intervention consisted of counseling and distribution of a booklet and drinking diary. Optional follow-up sessions were offered to some participants at 4, 7, and 10 months. Proportionate reductions in drinking within treatment and control groups were 47.7% and 29.2%, respectively, with greater intervention effects among men than women. No significant differences were found in the number of sick days, morbidity, or health care use in the study population. The early studies, therefore, showed that brief intervention had a temporary effect lasting at least a year on the alcohol consumption of nondependent drinkers. These early findings sparked international interest in the strategy as a mechanism to reduce alcohol consumption in at-risk populations before they developed serious alcohol-related health effects.

Controlled Drinking

During this same time period of the WHO study, a growing interest in controlled drinking emerged as a treatment goal for problem drinkers. Lloyd and Salzberg (1975) suggested that controlled drinking was an appropriate goal for problem drinkers but that abstinence should be the goal for dependent drinkers. Miller and Hester's (1980) work showed that success rates for controlled drinking in the nondependent population were as high as 60% to 70%. Miller and his colleagues (Miller, 1975; Miller & Munoz, 1976; Miller, Pechacek, & Hamburg, 1981) developed and tested the behavioral self-control training (BSCT) approach to achieve controlled drinking. BSCT was an educational counseling approach that required 10 brief sessions with specific behavioral goal setting, self-monitoring, and training in self-control of alcohol consumption.

A brief intervention strategy was evolving from a variety of research teams. The intervention was time limited, driven by printed materials, and targeted to problem, harmful, or hazardous drinkers rather than dependent drinkers. Common elements of brief interventions included written materials, such as pamphlets or booklets, typically including didactic information and decision-making and goal-setting exercises (e.g., Heather, 1998; NIAAA, 1996). Follow-up sessions occurred in person or on the telephone and were focused on reinforcing information that was shared earlier and providing support (Fleming & Manwell, 1999).

BRIEF INTERVENTION APPROACHES AND COMMON ELEMENTS

Several approaches underpin brief interventions, including cognitive-behavioral therapy, strategic/interactional therapies, solution-focused therapy, humanistic and existential therapies, and interpersonal therapy (Barry, 1999). Brief interventions are predicated on behavioral self-control training in which clients are encouraged to develop an awareness of their personal drinking cues, effective self-change strategies, and progress toward drinking goals (Miller & Munoz, 1976). Brief interventions tend to (1) be problem- and solution-focused, (2) involve clearly delineated and measurable short-term goals, (3) be strongly influenced by individual counseling styles and active therapeutic relationships, and (4) hold the individual responsible for self-change (Barry, 1999).

FRAMES Model

In addition to the use of the aforementioned therapeutic approaches, Miller and Sanchez (1993) proposed six elements summarized by the acronym FRAMES (feedback, responsibility, advice, menu of strategies, empathy, and self-efficacy). Using this paradigm, emphasis is placed on personal responsibility and choice. Health care professionals provide clients with feedback on their risks for alcohol problems based on factors such as their current drinking patterns and medical consequences of their drinking. They emphasize the client's responsibility and choice for reducing drinking and give explicit advice to reduce or stop drinking. In addition, an essential element of brief intervention is to offer clients a variety of strategies (a menu) from which to choose. These may include setting a specific goal for alcohol consumption, developing skills to avoid drinking in high-risk situations, and pacing one's drinking (NIAAA, 1999). A warm, reflective, and understanding style (empathy) of delivering brief intervention is more effective than a more confrontational manner. This portion of the FRAMES model was empirically tested by Miller and Rollnick (1991), who found that when they used an empathetic as compared to confrontational counseling style, clients' drinking was reduced. Brief intervention often includes techniques such as eliciting and reinforcing self-motivating statements that are targeted to enhance self-efficacy. The NIAAA (1999) provides the following example of such as statement: "I am worried about my drinking and want to cut back." The professional usually focuses on strengths and encourages people to develop, implement, and commit to plans to stop drinking (NIAAA, 1999).

Other Elements

Graham and Fleming (1998) identified the following additional elements as important to the effectiveness of brief intervention: goal-setting, follow-up, and timing. The drinking goal is negotiated between the client and health care professional and may be presented in a written prescription or signed contract. Clients have their progress followed and have ongoing support to meet drinking goals. Follow-up may take the form of phone calls or repeat in-person visits. Findings from several studies suggest that timing is also important. At a time when individuals perceive that they have a problem such as an illness or injury, they may be more willing to make behavior changes than when they are in more problem-free situations (DiClemente et al., 1991; NIAAA, 1999; Prochaska & DiClemente, 1983). This idea has led to the concept of the "teachable moment," a window of opportunity for an intervention that encourages people to change a risky behavior such as heavy drinking (Waller, 1990).

Motivational Interviewing

The principles of motivational interviewing (MI) set the tone for brief interventions, although MI requires more time and training. MI employs five basic motivational strategies to mobilize the client's own change resources. In addition to expressing empathy and supporting self-efficacy, motivational techniques consist of developing discrepancy, avoiding argumentation, and rolling with resistance (Miller, 1999). Developing discrepancy involves helping individuals assess where they are and where they want to be. Avoiding argument means that the practitioner guards against covertly disagreeing with clients and helps them develop their own rationale for avoiding harmful drinking habits. Finally, the health care provider rolls with resistance by assisting clients to change their perceptions and develop their own solutions to problems (Miller, 1999).

BRIEF INTERVENTION RANDOMIZED CONTROLLED
TRIALS IN PRIMARY CARE

Space does not permit an extensive discussion of all primary care brief intervention studies. Four large-scale, multisite trials are offered as exemplars. Project TrEAT (Trial for Early Alcohol Treatment) represents the first large-scale brief intervention study conducted in primary care settings in the United States and was based on the materials, procedures, and measures of the MRC trial (Wallace et al., 1988). Problem drinkers ($N = 774$; men who drank more than 168 g of absolute alcohol per week and women who drank more than 132 g) were randomized to intervention and control groups. Dependent drinkers were excluded from the sample. Brief interventions consisted of two (10–15-minute) physician-conducted counseling sessions, a workbook, and two nurse-initiated follow-up phone calls (Fleming et al., 1997, 2002). At 1-year follow-up, the experimental group reduced alcohol consumption from 19.1 standard drinks per week at baseline to 11.5, whereas the control group decreased from 18.9 at baseline to 15.5. At 4-year follow-up, consumption differences between the groups were nonsignificant. Unlike the control group, however, health care utilization rates were significantly reduced in the experimental group (Fleming et al., 2002). Using 6- and 12-month follow-up data, a comprehensive cost–benefit analysis showed a total net benefit of $947 per study participant (Fleming et al., 2000).

The Lahti Project was part of a multicomponent study coordinated by the World Health Organization Regional Office for Europe. Subjects who were considered heavy drinkers (positive CAGE questionnaire and/or 280 g of absolute alcohol per week for men and 190 g per week for women) were secured from primary care clinics and occupational health centers in Finland. They were randomized to three groups: (1) 10 to 20 minutes of advice, self-help booklet, and six follow-up sessions; (2) 10 to 20 minutes of advice, self-help booklet, and two follow-up sessions; and (3) minimal advice (control). Baseline consumption was 237 (Group A), 269 (Group B), and 267 (control) g of alcohol per week for men (Aalto, Seppa, et al., 2001); and 216 (Group A), 180 (Group B), and 154 (control) g of alcohol per week for women (Aalto et al., 2000). Dependent drinkers were excluded from the sample. Of 414 randomized subjects, 280 (67.6%) participated in the 3-year follow-up assessment; men averaged 240 (Group A), 278 (Group B), and 320 (control) g of alcohol per week (Aalto, Seppa, et al., 2001), and women averaged 131 (Group A), 279 (Group B), and 146 (control) g of alcohol per week (Aalto et al., 2000). There were no statistically significant decreases in alcohol consumption among the three groups (Aalto et al., 2000; Aalto et al., 2001).

In a study conducted at three Kaiser Permanente health maintenance organization (HMO) facilities in the northwest United States, subjects ($N = 516$) were randomized to usual care (control) or brief intervention. Individuals scoring higher than 21 on the Alcohol Use Disorder Identification Test (AUDIT) were excluded for alcohol dependence. At baseline, mean drinking days per week were 3.3 and 3.5 for the intervention and control groups, respectively. Mean drinks per drinking day were 5 and 4.7, respectively. The brief intervention consisted of a 30-second message from the primary care physician, a 15-minute consultation with a health counselor, and printed material. At 12-month follow-up, 80% of the subjects were retained; subjects in the intervention group did not significantly reduce their drinking days per week as compared with controls (2.7 vs. 3.1) and had similar drinks per drinking day (Senft, Polen, Freeborn, & Hollis, 1997).

Project Health (Ockene, Adams, Hurley, Wheeler, & Hebert, 1999) was carried out in four primary care practices in northeastern United States with "high-risk" drinkers ($N = 530$; men who drank > 12 standard drinks per week or consumed ≥ 5 standard drinks on one occasion; women who consumed > 9 standard drinks per week or consumed ≥ 4 more standard drinks on one occasion). No subject was excluded for excessive or dependent drinking, but those subjects made up less than 2% of the total population. Subjects were randomized to one 5- to 10-minute counseling session or usual care. Client-centered brief interventions were carried out by nurses or physicians at regularly scheduled appointments. At 6 months, the experimental group had a statistically significant reduction in drinking from baseline (18.7 vs. 12.6 or −6.1 drinks per week) compared with controls (16.4 vs. 13.3 or −3.1 drinks per week).

Summary and Critique of Brief Intervention Studies in the Primary Care Setting

Several interesting trends occurred in the four studies reported above. When subjects were seen by their primary care providers several times prior to follow-up, reductions in drinking were greater. This trend may reflect a larger dosage effect (Ockene et al., 1999) or the fact that some individuals were more concerned about their health and, thus, sought out additional professional advice. It should be noted that regression toward the mean (Fleming & Graham, 2001) and self-resolution of mild to moderate alcohol problems are thought to be quite common (Sobell, Sobell, Toneatto, & Leo 1993) and may explain the negative results of several of the clinical trials.

Lack of significant findings may have resulted from small sample sizes. Alternatively, investigators may have underestimated the impact of minimal advice received by the control groups, or minimal advice could have served as an intervention itself (Aalto et al., 2000, 2001). In addition, the screening procedures may have served as an intervention with the same strength as the experimental interventions, thereby decreasing the likelihood of statistically significant differences among groups. Senft et al. (1997) suggested that their findings may have been influenced by the small sample size and a relatively short follow-up period. They also cautioned that even given positive results, the costs of screening and implementing a brief intervention protocol in primary care settings may be prohibitive (Freeborn, Polen, Hollis, & Senft, 2000). This concern may not be a valid one, however, because Fleming et al. (2002) found that the total cost per patient for the brief intervention was only $205, whereas a $43,000 reduction in future health care costs occurred for every $10,000 invested in early alcohol interventions in primary care.

Trials of brief intervention in the primary care population have shown variable results in drinking outcomes. Although the sample sizes were generally over 500, often the power analysis was not part of the published research report, which makes it difficult to determine if the sample sizes had adequate power to detect change and differences across groups.

Investigators have not determined the best target population for brief intervention in primary care and make no cogent arguments as to how they made decisions to include/exclude participants based on alcohol consumption. Is it the heavy episodic drinking population, heavy drinkers, or drinkers who merely exceed moderate drinking limits? Some investigators excluded alcohol-dependent subjects (Fleming et al., 1997), and others did not (Ockene et al., 1999), but none provided a rationale for this decision. Is brief intervention appropriate for dependent drinkers? The investigators did not make an argument one way or the other, and the lack of consensus on what constitutes an appropriate target population persists even in NIAAA documents. The NIAAA (1999) noted that variations of brief intervention have been found effective for helping non-alcohol-dependent patients reduce or stop drinking, for motivating alcohol-dependent patients to enter long-term alcohol treatment, and for treating some alcohol-dependent patients. They do not provide assistance to health care providers or scientists as to which dependent patients might be helped with brief intervention, nor do they explain what they mean by "variations" of brief intervention, nor which variation is more effective. To move the science forward, it is essential that scientists identify the specific population of drinkers most likely to respond to brief intervention, and begin to refine the intervention so that it contains effective content and a consistent dose.

Investigators in the WHO study in the primary care population (Babor & Grant, 1992, 1994; WHO, 1996) found gender differences in the response to brief intervention. Although men in the intervention group had a significantly lower weekly alcohol consumption than controls, both experimental and control female subjects decreased their weekly alcohol consumption. Although preliminary reports of these findings were widely available (Babor & Grant, 1992), future investigators (Aalto et al., 2000; Fleming et al., 1997; Okene et al., 1999) have not refined their protocols to deal with gender differences and continue to use the same variation of brief intervention regardless of gender. One might ask, is screening alone a successful strategy for women, whereas are men more responsive to a brief intervention plus screening? Until investigators begin to refine and test variations of the intervention based on findings from previous studies, and determine what comprises the intervention, the science will not progress.

There is little dialogue about outcome that leads to true harm reduction. Although Ockene et al. (1999) found a statistically significant reduction in drinking at 6 months, does a reduction of three drinks per week as compared with controls lead to long-term healthier outcomes for people? Fleming et al.'s (2002) finding that the intervention group had significantly reduced care utilization rates as compared with controls at 48 months after the intervention indicates harm reduction, but the other studies provided no such long-term follow-up. Studies in different populations, particularly with injured subjects, have some of the same methodological problems and are discussed below.

BRIEF INTERVENTION INJURY STUDIES

Alcohol use is associated with an increased number of injuries, including automobile crashes, falls, and fires (NIAAA, 2000). Despite the relationship between alcohol and injury, health care providers do not routinely screen injured individuals for drinking problems, nor are interventions generally offered when a problem is detected (D'Onofrio & Degutis, 2002). It is estimated that blood alcohol testing is standard practice in only 63.7% of U.S. level I and II trauma centers (Soderstrom, Dailey, & Kerns, 1994), and most trauma centers that do obtain a blood alcohol level do not use those data for assessment, screening, and intervention. Based on the apparent need for and promise of brief intervention, several RCTs have been conducted to examine the effectiveness in injured patients.

Four RCTs that examined the effectiveness of alcohol brief interventions in injury-related cases were located. In two instances, brief interventions were delivered in the emergency department (Longabaugh et al., 2001; Monti et al., 1999) and in two instances, during an inpatient hospitalization (Gentilello et al., 1999; Sommers, Dyehouse, & Howe, 2001). Interventions ranged from the simple advice and brief counseling interventions modeled on Babor and Grant's work (Sommers et al., 2001; WHO, 1996) to a 60-minute intervention followed by a booster session (Longabaugh et al., 2001).

Emergency Department Studies

Monti et al. (1999) studied older adolescents who were injured ($N = 94$; $M = 18.4$ years old) and seen in the ED. Subjects either had a positive blood alcohol concentration or reported drinking prior to the event that precipitated treatment; no discussion was made about an exclusion for alcohol dependence. The investigators delivered a brief motivational interview lasting 35 to 40 minutes during the ED visit. At 6 months, control and experimental subjects had no significant differences in alcohol consumption (drinks per episode and drinking days per month). Subjects in the experimental group, however, had a 32% reduction in self-reported drinking and driving and half the occurrence of alcohol-related injuries compared with the standard care cohort.

Longabaugh et al. (2001) studied the effects of a brief motivational intervention for injured drinkers seen in the ED for an injury that did not require hospitalization. For study inclusion, subjects had to be assessed as a hazardous or harmful drinker (positive breath test for alcohol, reported ingesting alcohol within 6 hours of injury, or a positive score for harmful or hazardous drinking on a screening instrument). Subjects were excluded if they had been previously diagnosed with alcohol dependence or abuse. Among similarly aged participants ($N = 539$, $M = 27$ years old), brief interventions alone and brief interventions followed by a booster session were not more effective than standard care in reducing consumption at 12-month follow-up. However, brief intervention plus booster proved to be significantly more effective than standard care in reducing intrapersonal and interpersonal consequences and improving social responsibility and impulse control. The findings that the intervention plus a booster session 7 to 10 days after the ED visit affected alcohol-related consequences 12 months after the intervention was a critical addition to the science being generated about brief intervention.

Inpatient Acute Care Studies

Gentilello et al. (1999) investigated the effectiveness of a brief intervention delivered to injured patients during hospitalization for an injury. Subjects were enrolled if they had problem or dependent drinking as assessed by a battery of laboratory and psychometric screening instruments. Injured patients received a 30-minute brief intervention by a clinical psychologist (Dunn, Donovan, & Gentilello, 1997) at or near discharge and a follow-up letter at 1 month; control patients received screening but no intervention. The intervention group decreased their weekly alcohol consumption by 21.8 standard drinks, whereas the control group decreased their intake by only 6.7 drinks per week. In addition, there was a 47% reduction in new injuries in the intervention group as compared with the control cohort. It should also be noted that among this sample of 762 individuals, the mean age was 36 (Gentilello et al., 1999), which is somewhat older than subjects in the Longabaugh et al. (2001) study. Age, therefore, may play a role in the effectiveness of brief interventions when injury has occurred. In addition, all interventions were delivered by a single, highly trained clinical psychologist, enabling the investigators to maintain a high level of consistency for the intervention throughout the study.

Sommers and colleagues (2001) investigated the effectiveness of two brief intervention strategies (simple advice and brief counseling) delivered to young adults (M = 29 years) during hospitalization for an alcohol-related vehicular crash. The interventions were based on the WHO (1996) brief intervention model. Subjects were enrolled based on the Fleming et al. (1997) inclusion criteria, and subjects who had a positive screen for dependence were excluded. Based on a sample of 186, no statistically significant decreases in drinking occurred across groups at 12-month follow-up. All groups significantly decreased their alcohol consumption from baseline (5.88 binges per month) to 12 months (2.02 binges per month). The authors concluded that either the injury itself or the screening alone served as an effective intervention.

Summary and Critique

Since Waller's (1990) discussion of a "teachable moment," a visit to a health care provider has been viewed theoretically as a window of opportunity to change risky patterns of behavior that may lead to injury. Investigators testing the effectiveness of brief intervention in the injury population have studied a variety of populations (adolescents vs. adults; dependent vs. problem drinkers) and settings (ED vs. hospital setting). In addition, the intervention has varied from the simple advice (screening and 5 minutes of advice) (Sommers et al., 2001) to a brief intervention lasting 40 to 60 minutes, with a booster session 7 to 10 days after the ED visit and lasting an undocumented time (Longabaugh et al., 2001). Finally, the intervention has been delivered by a variety of providers such as a single clinical psychologist (Gentilello et al., 1999), nurses (Sommers et al., 2001), health care providers with a variety of backgrounds (clinical psychology, social work, and educational preparation in other social/behavioral sciences; Longabaugh et al., 2001), and staff research assistants with unknown preparation (Monti et al., 1999).

Although variations in methods existed across these protocols, and although some investigators reported significant differences between intervention and control groups and some did not, all subjects decreased their drinking from baseline. For example, even though there were no differences among groups, both Longabaugh et al. (1999) and Sommers et al. (2001) reported significant decreases in drinking across all subjects regardless of group. Findings from all four studies seem to indicate that (1) the screening, even without an intervention, is an effective strategy to reduce drinking in the year after injury; and/or (2) the injury itself is a powerful deterrent to future drinking. Prospective work is needed to determine if screening alone can lead to a reduction in drinking after injury. Sommers (CDC, 2004) has a funded trial in progress to test the role of screening versus intervention in the ED population.

Results from the WHO (1996) primary care study suggested that women may respond to screening without intervention, whereas men may not. None of the investigators of the injury trials investigated whether or not this was true in their subjects. Finally, one issue that remains unresolved is whether or not dependent drinkers should be included in future RCTs of brief interventions for injured patients.

All of the four injury studies had rigorous designs with inclusion/exclusion criteria based on previous scientific work and randomization to group. All used interviewers blinded to group assignment for longitudinal data collection. In addition, all four studies employed well-developed strategies to maintain the integrity of the intervention across the life of the study and across all interviewers.

Four primary problems exist with current published studies of brief intervention in the injury population: a short follow-up period, lack of detailed descriptions of the sample with rationale for the sample size, the potential for a biased sample, and failure to use previous results of brief intervention trials to inform their data analyses procedures. As with the brief intervention studies in primary care, the follow-up time for outcome measures was relatively short (6–12 months depending on study) for the alcohol consumption outcome variables as well as alcohol-related adverse events. It is noteworthy, however, that Gentilello et al. (1999) performed a review of medical records to determine reinjury rates at 36 months. As long as brief intervention studies rely on a 12-month follow-up as compared with longer periods of time, overall rates of harm reduction and lasting effects of the intervention on health outcomes are difficult to ascertain.

As the science around brief intervention develops, investigators should use strategies for describing the sample as in most pharmaceutical trials. Investigators are inconsistent about reporting differential attrition rates and a priori power analyses. Gentilello et al. (1999) presents the flow of participants in the trial (p. 475), but the other investigators do not. In general, sample sizes are small (a low of 94 in Monti et al., 1999, and a high of 762 in Gentilello et al., 1999), and agreement to participate is also low (55% in Sommers et al., 2001, and 67% in Monti et al., 1999). With cell sizes at times in the 30 to 40 range in two of the reported studies, type II error (failure to detect a reliable difference due to insufficient power) is of concern. Small sample size is a reflection of the high cost of longitudinal trials; in an ideal world, no longitudinal trials would be initiated unless the project had adequate funding for an appropriate sample size and adequate time for follow-up.

Retention across the life of the study was variable, ranging from a low of approximately 55% at 12 months (Gentilello et al., 1999; Sommers et at., 2001), to a high of 89% at 6 months (Monti et al., 1999). Because of the difficulty in recruiting and retaining subjects in injury trials, the possibility exists that the findings from the trials are not generalizable.

Finally, the analyses procedure of all four brief intervention trials in injured subjects do not capitalize on findings from early brief intervention trials in the primary care population, particularly related to gender. Monti et al. (1999) and Sommers et al. (2001) had sample sizes that were too small to investigate gender differences in their outcome measures, and Longabaugh et al.'s (2001) total female sample was 120. Gentilello et al. (1999) reported that "we were unable to detect an intervention response in female trauma patients . . . however, the number of women in the study was relatively small, which may have biased gender-based analysis" (p. 479).

BRIEF INTERVENTION STUDIES
IN OTHER POPULATIONS

Several other trials of brief intervention provide additional information on its effectiveness and potential to alter management of heavy drinking. Gender-based conclusions of secondary analyses of Project TrEAT, the MRC trial, the Lahti Project, and the WHO Study Group are as follows, as well as supporting evidence from other trials: (1) Women may be more likely than men to respond to screening only as well as screening and brief intervention (Aalto et al., 2000; WHO, 1996); (2) at 48 months after intervention, women may be more likely than men to reduce their drinking, and women who become pregnant during the study period have the most dramatic decreases (Manwell et al., 2000). These findings are supported by those of Chang and colleagues (Chang, Goetz, Wilkins-Haug, & Berman, 2000; Chang, Wilkins-Haug, Berman, & Goetz, 1999), who showed that pregnant women ($N = 250$), in screening only and brief intervention groups, demonstrated a decline in antepartum alcohol consumption after initial assessment; and (3) women may be more likely than men to reduce excessive consumption following brief intervention (Sanchez-Craig, Leigh, Spivak, & Lei, 1989; Wallace et al., 1988).

Gender-based findings have been replicated in brief intervention studies with college students. Marlatt et al. (1998) found that women demonstrated significantly greater decrements in alcohol consumption than men. Using the same dataset, the investigators found that 508 high-risk (high risk was defined as experiencing negative consequences from drinking or having at least five drinks on one occasion in the past month) control as well as intervention subjects reduced total alcohol consumption but not the number of drinking days (Baer, Kivlahan, Blume, McKnight, & Marlatt, 2001). One important conclusion from brief intervention trials with women and college students seems to be that in these particular populations, both screening for alcohol use alone and screening and brief intervention together may be effective in reducing alcohol consumption in the short term (1–4 years following intervention).

REVIEW OF META-ANALYSES RELATED TO ALCOHOL BRIEF INTERVENTIONS

The first widely cited meta-analysis of brief intervention trials was published by Bien, Miller, and Tonigan (1993). The investigators reported on 32 controlled studies of brief intervention enrolling over 6,000 problem drinkers across multiple health care settings. They discussed the soundness of the study methods based on 12 criteria, such as randomization procedures, quality control of the intervention, and length of follow-up. The studies contained less severely impaired drinkers as compared with dependent drinkers, and the brief intervention consisted of 1 to 6 hours of assessment and counseling. Using all 32 RCTs, the investigators calculated a within and between effect size for the intervention on alcohol consumption. For the brief intervention versus control studies, mean effect size for the within-group computation (pretreatment and post-treatment means within the groups) was 0.70 and for the between-group computation (post-treatment means for the brief intervention and comparison groups), 0.38. Bien et al. (1993) noted that, although the between-group effect of brief intervention versus no intervention is reasonable and replicable across studies, it produced a relatively small effect size.

Results of a review by Kahan, Wilson, and Becker (1995) are not included in this review because of the lack of accepted meta-analyses techniques. However, a meta-analysis by Wilk, Jensen, and Havighurst (1997) presented a rigorous use of the technique. They located 99 references that were RCTs of brief intervention in adult drinkers and performed a meta-analysis on 12 that met inclusion criteria based on the Chalmers' scoring system (Chalmers et al., 1981). Trials were included with subjects who were heavy or problem drinkers (rather than dependent drinkers) and who had interventions lasting 10 to 60 minutes for up to three sessions. Outcome data were pooled, and a combined odds ratio was 1.91, with a 95% confidence interval (CI) of 1.61 to 2.27 in favor of brief alcohol intervention over no intervention. These findings were consistent across gender, intensity of intervention, type of clinical setting, and higher quality clinical trials. In addition, the researchers found that there was a likelihood of subjects' developing moderate drinking patterns after intervention if they were female versus male, had interventions with more than one session, and were treated in the inpatient rather than the outpatient medical setting.

Poikolainen's (1999) meta-analysis focused on studies ($N = 7$) published from 1987 to 1997. Subjects were generated from the general population and primary care settings and reflected the effects of brief interventions (5–20 minutes) versus lengthier treatments. Other selection criteria included random allocation of subjects to intervention and control groups, alcohol intake or GGT as the outcome variable, and 6- to 12-month follow-up time. Findings indicated a significant decrease in alcohol consumption among women exposed to lengthier treatments. The pooled effect estimate of change in alcohol consumption was

−51 g of alcohol per week (95%; CI = −74, −29). Due to the lack of homogeneity among studies, similar results could not be reported among men. In regard to very brief interventions, evidence of significant decreases in consumption were lacking for both genders.

Poikolainen (1999) suggested that differences among studies preclude any universal claims regarding the effectiveness of brief interventions in primary care populations. Treatment effectiveness could be greatly influenced by idiosyncratic differences in protocols and delivery methods, which are not customarily reflected in published reports. In future studies, it would be helpful if excessive drinking were based on standard criteria. Presently, criteria vary from study to study, making comparisons across investigations very difficult.

Moyer, Finney, Swearingen, and Vergun (2002) found 92 studies that reported outcomes of brief interventions and ultimately excluded 36 because they did not examine a treatment that was "brief" (no more than four sessions). However, they did include interventions that involved no contact with a health care provider but rather consisted solely of written self-help materials. Problem and heavy drinkers were included as well as subjects referred for more extensive treatment (most likely alcohol-dependent subjects). Effect sizes were calculated for multiple drinking-related variables such as alcohol consumption (both time-based and quantity-based), abstinence, biological markers of alcohol use, and a variety of "drinking problems." Positive mean effect sizes (indicating better outcome for brief intervention conditions as compared with control conditions) were 0.26 (95%; CI = 0.20–0.32) for alcohol consumption at 6 to 12 months after intervention and 0.20 (95%; CI = −0.008–0.41) for alcohol consumption at more than 12 months. The largest effect size (0.67) occurred at 3 months after the intervention.

Critique of Meta-Analyses

The meta-analyses included in this review were conducted using accepted meta-analysis techniques and offer important insights into the effectiveness of brief intervention. That said, the value of meta-analyses is limited by the studies that are available for analysis. Study selection criteria were clearly outlined, and in two cases (Bien et al., 1993; Wilk et al., 1997) overall methodological quality scores were calculated. In general, the meta-analyses included studies in which subjects were largely recruited via opportunistic methods, and their problems were not severe. Follow-up periods were generally short (≤ 12 months), and conclusions regarding long-term outcomes are difficult to infer.

BRIEF INTERVENTION TRIALS: STATE OF THE ART, UNANSWERED QUESTIONS, AND FUTURE DIRECTIONS

RCTs testing the effectiveness of brief intervention to reduce alcohol consumption and alcohol-related consequences have been occurring for more than 20 years. The clinical trials as well as meta-analyses indicate that some variations of brief intervention, when used in the problem and/or heavy drinking population, are effective in reducing short-term alcohol consumption and adverse alcohol-related consequences such as injury. The exact nature of the "best" brief intervention is unknown, but certain characteristics seem related to its effectiveness. The more contact the patient has with the provider, the stronger the effect of the intervention. Investigators who reported trials that showed significant decreases in alcohol consumption and alcohol-related adverse events used at least one follow-up session or booster dose of the intervention and often more than one additional session (Babor & Grant, 1994; Fleming et al., 1997; Gentilello et al., 1999; Longabaugh et al., 2001; WHO, 1996). The intervention can be provided by a generalist rather than an addictions specialist, but the generalist needs special training, and the intervention is best delivered in an inpatient setting (Wilk et al., 1997). Women may be more susceptible to screening and screening/intervention than men (WHO, 1996; Wilk et al., 1997).

Unanswered Questions

Many unanswered questions exist about the nature and effectiveness of brief intervention and how generalizable the research findings are to the real-world setting. From a research standpoint, there are many unanswered questions for investigators to consider. One critical issue that has not yet been explored is, who should deliver the intervention? To date, no investigators have studied effectiveness of the same intervention delivered by different practitioners such as physicians, social workers, nurses, or clinical psychologists. Is the intervention more effective if delivered by someone of the same gender or race as the patient? Should the intervention be delivered by the patient's own health care provider, or should the patient be referred to an unknown consultant for the intervention? It is critical that these subtle differences in the delivery of the intervention be tested.

What is the appropriate target population for brief intervention? Brief intervention was designed for the problem and heavy (non-alcohol-dependent) population, and most clinicians and scientists continue to view that population as most appropriate. However, the NIAAA (1999) acknowledges that, although it is most often used with patients who are not alcohol dependent, and its goal may be moderate drinking rather than abstinence, it can be used to assist alcohol-dependent patients with a goal of abstinence. It has also been used to motivate alcohol-dependent patients to enter specialized treatment (Chafetz et al., 1962) and has been studied as an alternative to long-term treatment in specialized alcohol treatment settings (Project MATCH Research Group, 1997). RCTs are needed to investigate the effectiveness of brief intervention in the alcohol-dependent population to clarify the target population and to enable health care providers to understand its role in both alcohol misuse and abuse.

What should the dose of the intervention be? Although the Babor and Higgins-Biddle (2000) and Fleming et al. (1997) definitions are commonly used for brief intervention, they leave open many questions about the nature of the intervention. Generally, written materials are used to guide the discussion, but no standardized written materials are currently available. The length of the intervention is generally 30 to 60 minutes, but there is variation in the amount of time providers spend with subjects. Although the more contact the provider has with the subject, the more effective the intervention is, no standard recommendations exist as to how long and how often the intervention should be. Much work, therefore, needs to be done on the refinement of past procedures. Several investigative teams have built on each others' work; for example, Fleming et al. (1997) used the materials from the MRC trial (Wallace et al., 1988), and Fleming et al. (1997) passed materials from the TrEAT trial on to Sommers et al. (2001) for their trial with injured subjects and the current ED study (CDC, 2004). None of these investigators, however, have used their knowledge and experience to publish these materials or provide them for general use.

What outcome measures should be used? Is it appropriate to use self-reported measures? Review of the clinical trials and meta-analyses indicates that a large variety of outcome measures for alcohol consumption and alcohol-related adverse events have been used by investigators. The most common measures for quantity and frequency are drinks per week, drinks per drinking day, and occurrences of heavy episodic drinking (binges or 4+/5+ drinking) per month (Bien et al., 1993; Fleming et al., 1997; WHO, 1996). Many investigators are using the three quantity and frequency questions from AUDIT (Saunders, Aasland, Babor, de la Fuenta, & Grant, 1993) that was created and tested during the WHO (1996) trial to gather alcohol consumption data (Fleming et al., 1997; Sommers et al., 2001). Variables used to measure alcohol-related adverse events (also called alcohol-related negative consequences) have included sick days, mortality, and GGT (Kristenson et al., 1983), postintervention injury rates (Gentilello et al., 1999), cost of health care following intervention (Fleming et al., 1997), and traffic citations and crashes (Fleming et al., 1997; Sommers et al., 2001). Most brief intervention studies use both alcohol consumption and alcohol-related adverse events as baseline and outcome measures in a brief intervention trial.

One research issue that is supported by a large body of scientific work is the validity of self-reported alcohol consumption. In the early clinical trials implemented prior to 1995, investigators used strategies such as collecting data from collateral informants (WHO, 1996) or using biological measures to assess the criterion-related validity of self-reported alcohol consumption (Sillanaukee, 1997). However, neither strategy has shown to be more accurate than self-report alone. Collaterals consistently reported lower amounts of alcohol use than subjects reported (Fleming et al., 1997) or the same amounts as the subjects (Baer et al., 2001; Ockene et al., 1999). There is no single or combined biological measure with sensitivity and specificity higher than 80% (Sommers, Savage, Wray, & Dyehouse, 2003) that could be used as a "gold standard" comparison with self-reported alcohol consumption except for measures of ethanol in body fluids, which would have to be obtained immediately after a drinking session.

Fleming et al. (1997, p. 42) addressed this issue: "Project TrEAT did not assess biological markers such as blood alcohol level (BAL), GGT, and carbohydrate deficient transferring (CDT) due to the low sensitivity of these tests. . . . " Articles across decades of science have supported the validity of self-reported alcohol use, and a detailed review of these articles is beyond the scope of this chapter. In several classic articles, leading scientists have provided methodological advice to investigators on how to enhance the validity of self-reported alcohol consumption (Babor, Brown, & Del Boca, 1990; Maisto, McKay, & Connors, 1990; Midanik, 1988; Sobell & Sobell, 1990). As Midanik (1988, p. 1027) noted: "Whether an individual gives accurate information about his or her alcohol use is based on many factors: the interview situation, the respondent him/herself, how the specific information is elicited, and the context of the interview." It is up to the investigator to make the arguments that the methods provided the milieu within which self-reported measures most closely reflected actual patterns of drinking. Investigators may use biological measures to corroborate self-report, or may interview collaterals, or may use interview methods that have been shown in past studies to improve the accuracy of self-reported alcohol consumption. No single method of corroboration is appropriate for all investigations.

What is the appropriate length of follow up to determine if harm reduction has occurred or the desired outcome has occurred? Brief intervention trials present challenges to investigators. They are expensive to implement. Subject retention across many years of a longitudinal study is difficult. For these reasons, most brief intervention trials have used a 12-month follow-up; this tradition provides little information on the long-term effects of the intervention. Given the number of investigators who have reported on 12-month outcomes and the number of meta-analyses that have been published, it is time for funding agencies to focus their awards on those large scale trials that have the capability to recruit and retain subjects across at least 3- to 5-years of follow-up. Because the effect of the brief intervention decays over time (Moyer et al., 2002), booster sessions have the potential to enhance the effectiveness of the intervention during the 3 to 5 year follow-up. Until more is known about how to strengthen the long-term effects of the intervention, scientists will be hard pressed to make the argument that brief intervention can lead to long term behavioral change in problem and heavy drinkers.

CONCLUSION

Investigators are urged to focus on delineating the most effective and least costly form of brief intervention. Important factors include who is best prepared to deliver brief intervention, who has the greatest potential to benefit, and what constitutes the most effective treatment strategy. Researchers need to determine what outcome measures reflect behavior change and what is the most appropriate length of follow-up. Nurses have an important stake in how these questions are answered because they are in key positions to deliver brief intervention.

Based on current findings, and the potentially high cost of routinely offering alcohol brief interventions, it is difficult to give unwaveringly support to their wide-spread adoption. Moreover, given the complexities of carrying out well-designed alcohol brief intervention research (Sibthorpe et al., 2002), remaining questions may be difficult to answer. What appears appropriate for the time being is for all health care providers to implement routine screening for risky and problem drinking. At the same time, they also need to become better informed about safe drinking guidelines so that when a teachable moment presents itself, accurate information can be provided in an efficient and low-cost manner.

REFERENCES

Aalto, M., Saksanen, R., Laine, P., Forsstrom, R., Raikaa, M., Kiviluoto, M., et al. (2000). Brief intervention for female heavy drinkers in routine general practice: A 3-year randomized, controlled study. *Alcoholism: Clinical and Experimental Research, 24,* 1680–1686.

Aalto, M., Seppa, K., Mattila, P., Mustonen, H., Ruuth, K., Hyvarinen, H., et al. (2001). Brief intervention for male heavy drinkers in routine general practice: A three-year randomized controlled study. *Alcohol and Alcoholism, 36,* 224–230.

Babor, T., Brown, J., & Del Boca, F. (1990). Validity of self-reports in applied research on addictive behaviors: Fact or fiction. *Behavioral Assessment, 12,* 5–31.

Babor, T., & Grant, M. (1992). Project on identification and management of alcohol-related problems. Report on phase II: A randomized clinical trial of brief interventions in primary health care. Geneva: World Health Organization.

———. (1994). Comments on the WHO report "Brief Intervention for Alcohol Problems": A summary and some international comments. *Addiction, 89,* 657–678.

Babor, T., & Higgins-Biddle, J. C. (2000). Alcohol screening and brief intervention: Dissemination strategies for medical practice and public health. *Addiction, 95,* 677–686.

Babor, T., Ritson, E. B., & Hodgson, R. J. (1986). Alcohol-related problems in the primary health care setting: A review of early intervention strategies. *British Journal of Addiction, 81,* 23–46.

Baer, J. S., Kivlahan, D. R., Blume, A. W., McKnight, P., & Marlatt, G.A. (2001). Brief intervention for heavy drinking college students: 4 year follow-up and natural history. *American Journal of Public Health, 91,* 1310–1306.

Bandura, A. (1997). *Self-efficacy: The exercise of control.* New York: W. H. Freeman.

Barry, K. L. (1999). Brief interventions and brief therapies for substance abuse. Treatment Improvement Protocol (TIP) Series 34 (DHHS Publication No. (SMA) 99-3353). Rockville, MD: Substance Abuse and Mental Health Services Administration Center for Substance Abuse Treatment.

Bien, T. H., Miller, W. R., & Tonigan, J. S. (1993). Brief interventions for alcohol problems: A review. *Addiction, 88,* 315–336.

Centers for Disease Control and Prevention. (2004). Acute health care, rehabilitation and disability prevention research, National Center for Injury Prevention and Control. Retrieved September 15, 2004, from http://www.cdc.gov/ncipc/profiles/acutecare/default.htm

Chafetz, M. E. (1961). A procedure for establishing therapeutic contact with the alcoholic. *Quarterly Journal of Studies on Alcohol, 22,* 325–328.

Chafetz, M. E., Blane, H. T., Abram, H. S., Golner, J., Lacy, E., McCourt, W. F., et al. (1962). Establishing treatment relations with alcoholics. *Journal of Nervous and Mental Diseases, 134,* 395–409.

Chalmers, T. C., Smith, H., Blackburn, B., Silverman, B., Schroeder, B., Reitman, B., et al. (1981). A method for assessing the quality of a randomized control trial. *Controlled Clinical Trials, 2,* 31–49.

Chang, G., Goetz, M. A., Wilkins-Haug, L., & Berman, S. (2000). A brief intervention for prenatal alcohol use. *Journal of Substance Abuse Treatment, 18,* 365–369.

Chang, G., Wilkins-Haug, L., Berman, S., & Goetz, M. A. (1999). Brief intervention for alcohol use in pregnancy: A randomized trial. *Addiction, 94,* 1499–1508.

DiClemente, C. C., Fairhurst, S. K., Velasquez, M. M., Prochaska, J. O., Velicer, W. F., & Rossi, J. S. (1991). The process of smoking cessation: An analysis of precontemplation, contemplation, and preparation stages of change. *Journal of Consulting and Clinical Psychology, 59,* 295–304.

D'Onofrio, G., & Degutis, L. C. (2002). Preventive care in the emergency department: Screening and brief intervention for alcohol problems in the emergency department—a systematic review. *Academic Emergency Medicine, 9,* 627–638.

Dunn, C., Donovan, D., & Gentilello, L. (1997). Practical guidelines for performing alcohol interventions in trauma centers. *Journal of Trauma, 42,* 299–304.

Fleming, M. F., Barry, K. L., Manwell, L. B., Johnson, K., & London, R. (1997). Brief physician advice for problem alcohol drinkers: A randomized controlled trial in community-based primary care practices. *Journal of the American Medical Association, 277,* 1039–1045.

Fleming, M. F., & Graham, A. W. (2001). Screening and brief interventions for alcohol use disorders in managed care settings. *Recent Developments in Alcoholism, 15,* 393–416.

Fleming, M. F., & Manwell, L. B. (1999). Brief intervention in primary care settings. *Alcohol Research and Health, 23,* 128–137.

Fleming, M. F., Mundt, M. P., French, M. T., Manwell, L. B., Stauffacher, E. A., & Barry, K. L. (2000). Benefit-cost analysis of brief physician advice with problem drinkers in primary care settings. *Medical Care, 38,* 7–18.

————. (2002). Brief physician advice for problem drinkers: Long-term efficacy and benefit-cost analysis. *Alcoholism: Clinical and Experimental Research, 26,* 36–43.

Freeborn, D. K., Polen, M. R., Hollis, J. F., & Senft, R. A. (2000). Screening and brief intervention for hazardous drinking in an HMO: Effects on medical care utilization. *Journal of Behavioral Health Services & Research, 27,* 446–453.

Gentilello, L. M., Rivara, F. P., Donovan, D. M., Jurkovich, G. J., Daranciang, E., Dunn, C. W., Villaveces, A., Copass, M., & Ries, R. R. (1999). Alcohol interventions in a trauma center as a means of reducing the risk of injury recurrence. *Annals of Surgery, 230,* 473–483.

Graham, A. W., & Fleming, M. F. (1998). Brief interventions. In A. W. Graham, T. K. Schultz, & B. B. Wilford (Eds.), *Principles of addiction medicine* (2nd ed., pp. 615–630). Chevy Chase, MD: American Society of Addiction Medicine.

Heather, N. (1998). *So you want to cut down your drinking?* Edinburgh, Scotland: Health Education Board.

Kahan, M., Wilson, L., & Becker, L. (1995). Effectiveness of physician-based interventions with problem drinkers: A review. *Canadian Medical Association Journal, 152,* 851–859.

Kristenson, H., Öhlin, H., Hultén-Nosslin, M. B., Trell, E., & Hood, B. (1983). Identification and intervention of heavy drinking in middle-aged men: Results and follow-up of 24–60 months of long-term study with randomized controls. *Alcoholism: Clinical and Experimental Research, 7,* 203–209.

Larimer, M. E., Marlatt, G. A., Baer, J. S., Quigley, L. A., Blume, A. W., & Hawkins, E. H. (1998). Harm reduction for alcohol problems: Expanding access to and acceptability of prevention and treatment services. In G. A. Marlatt (Ed.), *Harm reduction: Pragmatic strategies for managing high-risk behaviors* (pp. 69–121). New York: Guilford.

Lloyd, R. W., & Salzberg, H. C. (1975). Controlled social drinking: An alternative to abstinence as a treatment goal for some alcohol abusers. *Psychological Bulletin, 82,* 815–842.

Longabaugh, R., Woolard, R. F., Nirenberg, T. D., Minugh, A. P., Becker, B., Clifford, P. R., et al. (2001). Evaluating the effects of a brief motivational intervention for injured drinkers in the emergency department. *Journal of Studies on Alcohol, 62,* 806–816.

Maisto, S., McKay, J., & Connors, G. (1990). Self-report issues in substance abuse: State of the art and future directions. *Behavioral Assessment, 12,* 117–134.

Manwell, L. B., Fleming, M. F., Mundt, M. P., Stauffacher, E. A., & Barry, K. L. (2000). Treatment of problem alcohol use in women of childbearing age: Results of a brief intervention trial. *Alcoholism: Clinical and Experimental Research, 24,* 1517–1524.

Marlatt, G. A. (1998). Basic principles and strategies of harm reduction. In G. A. Marlatt (Ed.), *Harm reduction: Pragmatic strategies for managing high-risk behaviors* (pp. 49–69). New York: Guilford.

Marlatt, G. A., Baer, J. S., Kivlahan, D. R., Dimeff, L. A., Larimer, M. E., Quigley, L. A., et al. (1998). Screening and brief intervention for high-risk college student drinkers: Results from a 2-year follow-up assessment. *Journal of Consulting and Clinical Psychology, 66,* 604–615.

Midanik, L. (1988). Validity of self-reported alcohol use: A literature review and assessment. *British Journal of Addiction, 83,* 1019–1029.

Miller, W. R. (1975). A behavioral intervention program for chronic pubic drunkenness offenders. *Archives of General Psychiatry, 32,* 915–918.

————. (1999). *Enhancing motivation for change in substance abuse treatment: Treatment Improvement Protocol (TIP) Series 35* (DHHS Publication No. (SMA) 99-3354). Rockville, MD: Substance Abuse and Mental Health Services Administration, Center for Substance Abuse Treatment. Retrieved October 30, 2004, from http://www.ncbi.nlm.nih.gov/books/bv.fcgi?rid=hstat5.chapter.61302

Miller, W. R., & Hester, R. K. (1980). Treating the problem drinker: Modern approaches. In W. R. Miller (Ed.), *The addictive behaviours: Treatment of alcoholism, drug abuse, smoking, and obesity* (pp. 11–141). Oxford: Pergamon.

Miller W. R., & Munoz, R. F. (1976). *How to control your drinking.* Englewood Cliffs, NJ: Prentice-Hall.

Miller, W. R., Pechacek, R., & Hamburg, S. (1981). Group behavior therapy for problem drinking. *International Journal of the Addictions, 16,* 827–837.

Miller, W. R., & Rollnick, S. (1991). *Motivational interviewing: Preparing people to change addictive behavior.* New York: Guilford.

Miller, W. R., & Sanchez, V. C. (1993). Motivating young adults for treatment and lifestyle change. In G. Howard (Ed.), *Issues in alcohol use and misuse in young adults* (pp. 55–82). South Bend, IN: University of Notre Dame Press.

Monti, P. M., Colby, S. M., Barnett, N. P., Spirito, A., Rohsenow, D. J., Myers, M., et al. (1999). Brief intervention for harm reduction with alcohol-positive older adolescents in a hospital emergency department. *Journal of Consulting and Clinical Psychology, 67,* 989–994.

Moyer, A., Finney, J. W., Swearingen, C. E., & Vergun, P. (2002). Brief interventions for alcohol problems: A meta-analytic review of controlled investigations in treatment-seeking and non-treatment-seeking populations. *Addiction, 97,* 279–292.

National Institute on Alcohol Abuse and Alcoholism (NIAAA). (1996). *How to cut down on your drinking.* Retrieved October 30, 2004, from http://www.niaaa.nih.gov/publications/handout.htm

————. (1999, April). Brief intervention for alcohol problems. *Alcohol Alert, 43,* 1–4. Retrieved October 30, 2004, from http://www.niaaa.nih.gov/publications/aa43.htm

————. (2000). *Tenth special report to the U.S. Congress on alcohol and health* (NIH Pub. No. 00-1583). Rockville, MD: Author. Retrieved October 30, 2004, from http://www.niaaa.nih.gov/publications/10report/intro.pdf

Ockene, J. K., Adams, A., Hurley, T. G., Wheeler, E. V., & Hebert, J. R. (1999). Brief physician- and nurse practitioner–delivered counseling for high-risk drinkers. *Archives of Internal Medicine, 159,* 2198–2205.

Poikolainen, K. (1999). Effectiveness of brief interventions to reduce alcohol intake in primary health care populations: A meta-analysis. *Preventive Medicine, 28,* 503–509.

Prochaska, J. O., & DiClemente, C. C. (1983). Stages and processes of self-change of smoking: Toward an integrative model of change. *Journal of Consulting and Clinical Psychology, 51,* 390–395.

Project MATCH Research Group. (1997). Matching alcoholism treatments to client heterogeneity: Project MATCH posttreatment drinking outcomes. *Journal of Studies on Alcohol, 58,* 7–29.

Reinert, D. F., & Allen, J. P. (2002). The alcohol use disorders identification test (AUDIT): A review of recent research. *Alcoholism: Clinical and Experimental Research, 26,* 272–279.

Sanchez-Craig, M., Leigh, G., Spivak, K., & Lei, H. (1989). Superior outcome of females over males after brief treatment for the reduction of heavy drinking. *British Journal of Addiction*, 84, 395–404.

Saunders, J. B., Aasland, O. G., Babor, T. F., de la Fuenta, J. R., & Grant, M. (1993). Development of the Alcohol Use Disorders Identification Test (AUDIT): WHO collaborative project on early detection of persons with harmful alcohol consumption. *Addiction*, 88, 791–804.

Saunders, J. B., & Lee, N. K. (2000). Hazardous alcohol use: Its delineation as a subthreshold disorder, and approaches to its diagnosis and management. *Comprehensive Psychiatry*, 2, 95–103.

Senft, R. A., Polen, M. R., Freeborn, D. K., & Hollis, J. F. (1997). Brief intervention in a primary care setting for hazardous drinkers. *American Journal of Preventive Medicine*, 13, 464–470.

Sibthorpe, B. M., Bailie, R. S., Brady, M. A., Ball, S. A., Sumner-Dodd, P., & Hall, W. D. (2002). The demise of a planned randomised controlled trial in an urban Aboriginal medical service. *Medical Journal of Australia*, 176, 273–276.

Sobell, L., & Sobell, M. (1990). Self-report issues in alcohol abuse: State of the art and future directions. *Behavioral Assessment*, 12, 77–90.

Sobell, L. C., Sobell, M. B., Toneatto, T., & Leo, G. I. (1993). What triggers the resolution of alcohol problems without treatment? *Alcoholism: Clinical and Experimental Research*, 17, 217–224.

Soderstrom, C. A., Dailey, J. T., & Kerns, T. J. (1994). Alcohol and other drugs: An assessment of testing and clinical practices in U.S. trauma centers. *Journal of Trauma*, 36, 68–73.

Sommers, M. S., Dyehouse, J. M., & Howe, S. R. (2001). Binge drinking, sensible drinking, and abstinence after alcohol-related vehicular crashes: The role of intervention versus screening. *45th Annual Proceedings of the Association for the Advancement of Automotive Medicine*, 45, 317–328.

Sommers, M. S., Savage, C., Wray, J., & Dyehouse, J. M. (2003). Laboratory measures of alcohol (ethanol) consumption: Strategies to assess drinking patterns with biochemical measures. *Biological Research for Nursing*, 4, 203–217.

Substance Abuse and Mental Health Services Administration (SAMHSA). (2004). *Results from the 2002 National Survey on Drug Use and Health: National findings*. Retrieved October 1, 2004, from http://www.oas.samhsa.gov/NHSDA/2k2NSDUH/Results/2k2 results.htm#chap3

Wallace, P., Cutler, S., & Haines, A. (1988). Randomised controlled trial of general practitioner intervention in patients with excessive alcohol consumption. *British Medical Journal*, 297, 663–668.

Waller, J. A. (1990). Management issues for trauma patients with alcohol. *Journal of Trauma*, 30, 1548–1553.

Wilk, A. I., Jensen, N. M., & Havighurst, T. C. (1997). Meta-analysis of randomized control trials addressing brief intervention in heavy alcohol drinkers. *Journal of General Internal Medicine*, 12, 274–283.

World Health Organization. (1980). *Problems related to alcohol consumption: Report of a WHO Expert Committee* (Tech. report series 650). Geneva: Author.

World Health Organization (WHO) Brief Intervention Study Group. (1996). A cross-national trial of brief interventions with heavy drinkers. *American Journal of Public Health*, 86, 948–955.

Wutzke, S., Conigrave, K., & Saunders, J. (2002). The long-term effectiveness of brief interventions for unsafe alcohol consumption: A 10-year follow-up. *Addiction*, 97, 665–675.

Index

5% drinking. *see* Drinking, heavy and episodic
12-step programs, 165. *see also* Alcoholics Anonymous (AA)

AARP (American Association of Retired Persons), 262
"Abbreviated food frequency questionnaire," 74
Abstaining populations, 4, 6, 29, 54, 73, 79–80, 90–91, 102, 114–117, 202, 267, 367–368, 380
  Brief intervention (BI) outcome, desired, 367–368, 380
  definitions, and, 6, 29, 73, 79–80, 90–91, 91, 267
  disease, and, 90–91
  pregnancy, and, 102, 114–117
  research analysis, college students, and, 202
  "sick-quitter problem," 73, 79–80, 91
ACSVS (American Cancer Society Volunteer Study), 80, 84, 87, 91
Adolescent Alcohol Prevention Trial Information, 146
Adolescent Resident Task Force, 165
Adolescent Transitions Program (ATP), 157, 161
Adolescents, 41, 135–170, 188–189, 328–346. *see also* Children; College students; Interventions
  behaviors, 41, 137–168, 328–346
  drug use, and, 135–139, 188–189
  interventions
    community-based, 139, 162–168
    Emergency Departments, and, 373–374
    family-based, 139, 155–162
    school-based, 138–155, 160–161
  peers
    interventions, effectiveness, 152–154, 160–161
    publications regarding, 141–151, 163, 165
    risk factors, and, 139
  phases of (age-based), 136
  risk perception, risky behaviors and, 334
Adolescents Training and Learning to Avoid Steroids (ATLAS), 145
Adulthood, 214–240, 246–269, 337–338. *see also* Women
  developmental changes, 221–231, 237
  middle-aged adults, 214–221
  older adults
    alcohol abuse and dependence
      disease and death, and, 251–252
      drug use, and, 260–262
      early- *vs.* late-onset, 249–251, 267
      gender differences, alcohol and aging, and, 252–253
      genetics, and, 251–252
      intervention, treatment, and, 262–266
      physiologic effects, and, 253–259
      psychological effects, and, 259–260
    consumption, and, 246–269
    work settings, employment and, 231–236
  young adults, 214–215, 337–338
AEQ. *see* Alcohol Expectancy Questionnaire (AEQ)
African American populations, 52, 83–87, 119–120, 136, 152–155,

African American populations (continued)
162, 190–192, 200–202, 216–
217, 299, 337, 344
adolescents, and, 136, 162
college students, and, 190–192, 202
drinking, risky and, 344
drinking norms, women, and, 299
FAS (Fetal alcohol syndrome), and,
119–120
interventions, school-based, and,
152–155
moderate drinking, effects of, 83,
84–87
Age differences, 46–54, 69, 108, 221,
230–231, 294–295, 301, 310,
337–338
alcohol sequelae, effects of, 246
college students, consumption and,
187, 192–194
consumption, and, 221, 230–231, 294–
295, 310
driving, risky, 337–338
moderate drinking, defined, 69
pregnancy, alcohol consumption during, 108
therapy, consumption patterns, and,
301
Agency for Health Care Research and
Policy (AHRQ), 66–68, 84–86
AHRQ. see Agency for Health Care Research and Policy (AHRQ)
Alcohol, abuse/dependence, and, 5–16,
118, 245–269, 290–292, 302–
303, 335, 363–365, 371–373,
383. see also Alcoholism;
Death; Disease; Drinking,
heavy and episodic; Drinking,
problem; Genetics
assessment of, 5, 256, 262–264, 268,
269, 302–303, 373, 383
Brief Intervention (BI), and, 365,
371–373
Child Sexual Abuse (CSA), and,
290–292
definitions, 30

disease and death, caused by, 6–10,
251–252
early- vs. late-onset, 249, 267
mental disorder, DSM and, 335
multi-generational nature of, 118
prevalence of, 363–364
Alcohol biometrics. see laboratory tests,
consumption
Alcohol consumption. see Consumption,
of alcohol
Alcohol dependence syndrome. see
Alcoholism
Alcohol Expectancy Questionnaire
(AEQ), 236, 342
Alcohol Misuse Prevention Study
(AMPS), 148–149, 153
Alcohol myopia behavior model, 342,
345–346. see also Behaviors,
risky; Expectancy behavior
model; Problem behavior
model; Risk perception behavior model
Alcohol-Related Birth Defects (ARBD).
see under FAS (Fetal Alcohol
Syndrome)
Alcohol-Related Neurodevelopmental Defects (ARND). see under FAS
(Fetal Alcohol Syndrome)
Alcohol treatment. see Treatment, alcohol
Alcohol Use Disorders Identification Test
(AUDIT), 34, 54–55, 111,
115–116, 198–199, 224, 370–
371, 381
adults, and, 224
Brief Intervention (BI), and, 370–371,
381
college students, and, 198–199
history of, 54–55
pregnant women, consumption and,
111, 115–116
Alcoholics Anonymous (AA), 230, 231,
236, 239, 250–251, 260, 266,
267, 303–304, 365. see also Alcohol, abuse/dependence, and;
Alcoholism; Drinking, heavy
and episodic

Brief Intervention (BI), and, 365
early- vs. late-onset, long-term sobriety
    and, 250–251, 267
Social Support Network Inventory
    (SSNI), and, 236
study populations, and, 239
treatment effectiveness, 266, 303–304
Alcoholism. see also Alcohol, abuse/de-
    pendence, and; Alcoholics
    Anonymous (AA)
adulthood, and, 214
college students, consumption and
    motivations, 192–194
defined, 31
drinking, harmful, 31
drinking, hazardous, 31
next generation (women), effect on,
    237
representation, consumption studies, 54
syndrome, alcohol dependence, 30
AMA (American Medical Association),
    88, 249, 262
American Association of Retired Persons
    (AARP), 262
American Cancer Society Volunteer
    Study (ACSVS), 80, 84, 87,
    91
American Indian/Alaska Native popula-
    tions, 119–120, 216–217. see
    also Native American
    populations
American Medical Association (AMA),
    88, 249, 262
American Nurses Association (ANA),
    10–11, 262
American Nurses Foundation, 15–16
American Psychological Association
    (APA), 306
American Society of Addiction Medi-
    cine, 31
AMERSA (Association for Medical Edu-
    cation & Research in Sub-
    stance Abuse), 16–17
AMPS (Alcohol Misuse Prevention
    Study), 148–149, 153

ANA (American Nurses Association),
    10–11, 262
AOD (alcohol and other drugs) treat-
    ment. see under drugs
APA. see American Psychological Associ-
    ation (APA)
ARBD (alcohol-related birth defects). see
    under FAS (Fetal Alcohol
    Syndrome)
ARND (alcohol-related neurodevelop-
    mental defects). see under FAS
    (Fetal Alcohol Syndrome)
Asian populations, 136, 189, 190–192,
    200–201
adolescents, and, 136
alcohol-flush reaction, and, 189
college students, and, 190–192
drug use, consequences of, 200–201
Assessing Alcohol Problems: A Guide for
    Clinicians and Researchers
    (NIAAA), 199
Association for Medical Education & Re-
    search in Substance Abuse
    (AMERSA), 16–17
At-risk drinking. see Drinking, risky
AUDIT. see Alcohol Use Disorders Iden-
    tification Test (AUDIT)
Australian Twin Study, 247

BACs (Blood Alcohol Concentrations),
    36–37, 44–50, 115–116, 261,
    382. see also Biological mark-
    ers; Laboratory tests, consump-
    tion of alcohol
alcohol types, and, 36–37
aspirin, 261
Brief Intervention (BI), and, 382
Mental Developmental Index (MDI),
    and, 115–116
testing, and, 44–50
Behavioral Risk Factor Surveillance Sys-
    tem (CDC), 262, 330, 341
Behavioral Risk Factors Surveillance Sur-
    vey (BRFSS), 105–109
Behavioral Self-Control Training
    (BSCT), 368

Behaviors, risky, 36–37, 327–353, 364, 369, 375, 383. *see also* Alcohol Myopia Behavior Model; disease; Expectancy behavior model; Problem behavior model; Protective factors; Risk perception behavior model; Sensation-seeking model
Brief Intervention (BI), and, 364
definition of, 330
drinking/driving, risky
  alcohol, types and, 36–37
  Emergency Department (ED) interventions, and, 350–351
  theoretical models, and, 340–341
driving, risky, 331, 336–341
factors, risk and protective, 349–350
preventable death, teenagers and, 328–329
sexual behavior, risky, 331, 341–349, 351
  interventions, and, 351
  prevalence of, 343–344
  types of, 343
"teachable moment," and, 369, 375, 383
theoretical models (diagram), 333
Bias, 88–89, 105, 107, 286–287, 308–309
Binge drinking. *see* Drinking, heavy and episodic
Biological markers, 45–53, 112–115. *see also* BACs (Blood Alcohol Concentrations); Laboratory tests, consumption of alcohol
Bisexual populations. *see* GLBT populations
Blood alcohol concentrations (BAC). *see* BACs (Blood Alcohol Concentrations)
BRFSS (Behavioral Risk Factors Surveillance Survey, 105–109
Brief Intervention (BI), 8, 28, 114–115, 164, 167, 202, 264, 363–383. *see also* Consequences, of alcohol consumption; Drinking, problem; Interventions; Motivational Interviewing (MI); Prevention; World Health Organization (WHO)
adolescents, and, 164, 167
college students, and, 202
controlled drinking, as goal of, 367–368, 380
definition of, 364
effectiveness, optimizing, 380–382
elements of, 368–369
harm reduction, and, 365, 373, 382
history of, 365–368
intimate partner violence (IPV), and, 8
older adults, and, 264
outcome, desired, 367–368, 380–381
as prevention, 365
Screening and Brief Intervention (SBI), 28
studies of, 366–367, 370–371, 373–375, 377
study analysis, 371–373, 375–377, 378–383
"teachable moment," and, 369, 375, 383
theoretical approaches, 368–369
Brief Situational Confidence Questionnaire, 116
British Regional Health Study, 73
BSCT (Behavioral Self-Control Training), 368

CAD (coronary artery disease). *see* Disease
CAGE (screening test), 109–112, 197–199, 219, 302, 367, 370, 377. *see also* CUGE (screening test)
Brief Intervention (BI), and, 367, 370, 377
college students, and, 197–199
GLBT populations, and, 302
incidence & prevalence studies, 219
pregnancy, risky drinking, and, 110–112
women, and, 109–110
Canadian Study of Health and Aging, 251

Cancer Prevention Study, 87
Cardiovascular disease, 68–92. see also
        Disease
    moderate drinking, and
        conclusions, 87
        definitions, 68–70
        historical background, 70
        literature critique, 84–92
        literature review, 70–84
        population variances, and, 69, 80–89
CARF (Commission on the Accredita-
        tion of Rehabilitation Facili-
        ties), 306
CAS (College Alcohol Study), 184–203
CDC. see Centers for Disease Control
        and Prevention (CDC)
Center for Science in the Public Interest,
        39
Center for Substance Abuse Treatment
        (CSAT), 16–17
Centers for Disease Control and Preven-
        tion (CDC), 12–16, 104, 106–
        107, 262, 328–329, 337–338,
        341
    alcohol abuse, screening for, 262
    driving, risky, 337–338, 341
    National Center on Birth Defects and
        Developmental Disabilities
        (NCBDDD), and, 104
    nursing research, and, 12–16
    preventable death, teenagers and,
        328–329
Children. see also Adolescents; Interven-
        tions; Prevention
    interventions, family-based, 157
    interventions, school-based, 147–148,
        153
    prevention strategies, school-based, 152
Cochrane Review of Primary Prevention
        for Alcohol Misuse in Young
        People, 155
Cognition, 4, 187–194, 236, 257–258,
        285, 334, 342, 345–346, 347.
        see also Expectancy behavior
        model; Motivations

anticipated experiences, of consump-
        tion, 236
    behaviors, and, 334, 342, 345–346, 347
    college students, and, 187–194
    effects, of consumption, 257–258
    memory disabilities, and alcohol, 4
    sexual orientation, definition, 285
Collaborative Study on the Genetics of
        Alcoholism (CSGA), 237–238
College Alcohol Study (CAS), 184–203
College students, 39, 179–204, 377. see
        also Adolescents
    Brief Intervention (BI), and, 377
    consumption, and, 39, 179–204
        assessing, 39
        cognition, and, 187–194
        consequences of, 183, 199–201
        domain-based analysis, 189–196
        housing, and, 194–196
        identity formation, and, 190–192
        peer affiliations, and, 194–195
        prevalence of, 183–184
        studies, history of, 183–187
    defined, 181
    motivations, and, 192–194
Commission on the Accreditation of Re-
        habilitation Facilities (CARF),
        306
Consequences, of alcohol consumption,
        36–37, 181–182, 187–188,
        199–201, 216–220, 336–337,
        365. see also Brief Intervention
        (BI); Interventions; Preven-
        tion; Protective factors; Sexual
        abuse/assault
    adulthood, and, 216–220
    alcohol, types and, 36–37
    Brief Intervention (BI), and, 365
    college students, and, 194, 199–201
    driving, risky, and, 336–337
    drug use, and, 200–201
    sexual assault, and, 200
Consumption, of alcohol, 1–383. see also
        Measurement, alcohol use and;
        Pregnancy, alcohol consump-

Consumption, of alcohol (continued)
  tion during; Self-reported mea-
    surements, alcohol use
  drinking categories, 29–33 (see also un-
    der individual drinking categories)
  prevalence of, 4
  recommendations for (U.S.), 35
  terminologies, 29–33, 30, 38–40, 181
CORE Survey, 184–203
Costs, of alcohol abuse, 4, 364, 372
Cox proportional hazards model, 80,
    91–92
CSAT (Center for Substance Abuse
    Treatment), 16–17
CSGA (Collaborative Study on the Ge-
    netics of Alcoholism),
    237–238
CUGE (screening test), 198. see also
    CAGE (screening test)
Cultural Enhancement Program, 162

DARE (Drug Abuse Resistance Educa-
    tion) program, 153
Death. see also Alcohol, abuse/depen-
    dence, and; Disease
  alcohol, caused by, 3, 4, 80, 180
  risky behavior, teenagers and, 328–329
Dependence syndrome, alcohol. see Alco-
    hol, abuse/dependence, and;
    Alcoholism
DHHS. see U.S. Department of Health
    and Human Services (HHS)
Diagnostic and Statistical Manual of Men-
    tal Disorders (DSM-III &
    DSM-IV), 196, 198, 218–219,
    223–226, 260, 284, 335
  alcohol dependence, mental health
    and, 335
  consumption, and, 196, 198, 218–219,
    223–226
  depression criteria, and alcohol/depres-
    sion relationship, 260
Disease, 3, 4, 54, 246, 251–252, 258, 267.
    see also Alcohol, abuse/depen-
    dence, and; Behaviors, risky;
    Cardiovascular disease; Death;

Drinking, risky; FAS (Fetal Al-
    cohol Syndrome); Health pro-
    motion; Intrauterine growth
    restriction (IUGR)
  alcohol use, and, 3, 4, 54
  Alzheimer's, ERT and, 258
  vulnerability to, 246, 251–252, 267
Disinhibition/impulsivity, 339–341
Drink, standard
  concept of, 34–35
  definition of, 29, 68–69
  self-reported data, and, 43
Drinkers, former. see Abstaining popula-
    tions; "Sick quitters"
Drinking, at-risk. see Drinking, heavy and
    episodic; Drinking, problem
Drinking, controlled, 367–368
Drinking, dependent. see Alcoholism;
    Drinking, heavy and episodic
Drinking, harmful. see Drinking, problem
Drinking, hazardous. see Alcoholism;
    Drinking, heavy and episodic;
    Drinking, problem
Drinking, heavy and episodic, 4, 31–32,
    38–41, 102, 107–108, 181–
    196, 289–301, 366. see also Al-
    cohol, abuse/dependence, and;
    Brief Intervention (BI); Con-
    sumption, of alcohol; Drink-
    ing, problem; Drinking, risky;
    Laboratory tests, consumption
  5-HTTLPR, behavior differences, and,
    189
  ALDH (aldehyde dehydrogenase), 189
  college students, and, 184, 187, 188
  GLBT population, and, 289–301
  pregnancy, alcohol consumption dur-
    ing, 102, 107–108
  terminology, 31–32, 38–40, 181
Drinking, high-risk. see Drinking, risky
Drinking, low-level. see drinking, low-
    volume
Drinking, low-risk. see drinking, low-
    volume
Drinking, low-volume, 4, 32, 254–257,
    255

defined, 32
older adults, and, 254–257
prevalence of, 4
"sick quitters" data, vs other data, 255
Drinking, moderate, 33, 54, 65–97, 69–
70, 254–257, 378, 380
Brief Intervention (BI), and, 378, 380
cardiovascular disease, and, 65–97
defined, 33, 69–70
older adults, and, 254–257
representation, consumption studies, 54
Drinking, non-binge, 181
Drinking, problem, 4, 31–33, 54, 365–
380, 369, 375, 383. see also Alcohol, abuse/dependence, and;
Brief Intervention (BI); Drinking, heavy and episodic
Brief Intervention (BI), 365–380
prevalence of, 4
"teachable moment," and, 369, 375,
383
terminology, 31–33
Drinking, risky, 33, 181, 331, 335–336,
339–351. see also Behaviors,
risky; Disease; Protective
factors
defined, 33, 181, 331
disinhibition/impulsivity, and, 335–336
driving, risky, and, 339–341, 350–351
factors, risk and protective, 349–350
incidence, 335
sexual behavior, and, 341–347
Drinking limits, recommended, 33, 35
Drug Abuse Resistance Education
(DARE) program, 153
Drug Prevention in Higher Education Program, 185
Drugs, 12–16, 135–136, 138–139, 163,
165, 188–189, 200–201, 260–
262, 297–298, 300
adolescents, environments and,
138–139
AOD (alcohol and other drugs)
adolescent interventions, and, 163,
165

intimate partner violence (IPV),
and, 297–298
treatment, and, 165, 300
Monitoring the Future (MTF) project,
135–136, 188–189
nursing research, and, 12–16
OTC, use with alcohol and, 260–262
Substance Abuse and Mental Health
Services Administration
(SAMHSA), 136
use with alcohol, consequences and,
200–201
DSM-III/DSM-IV. see Diagnostic and Statistical Manual of Mental Disorders (DSM-III & DSM-IV)

EAP. see Employee Assistance Program
(EAP)
ED. see Emergency Department (ED)
Emergency Department (ED), 164, 167,
350–351, 366, 373–377, 381
Brief Intervention (BI), 164, 167, 366
injury studies, 373–374
risky drinking/driving, interventions,
and, 350–351
study analysis, 375–377, 381
Employee Assistance Program (EAP),
233, 235
Enzymatic method, 45–46
Epidemiologic Catchment Area Study,
230
ER. see Emergency Department (ED)
Estrogen replacement therapy (ERT),
258–259
Ethanol consumption. see consumption,
of alcohol
Ethnic differences. see also racial
differences
college students, consumption and, 188
Expectancy behavior model, 342–348. see
also Alcohol myopia behavior
model; Behaviors, risky; Problem behavior model; Risk perception behavior model

Faculty Development Program (FDP),
11–18

FAE (Fetal Alcohol Effects). *see* FAS (Fetal Alcohol Syndrome)
FAEE (Fatty Acid Ethyl Esters), 112–113. *see also* Biological markers
Families, 155–162, 190, 192–194, 216–220, 236, 237–238, 246, 265–266, 289–290, 292, 297–298, 301–302
    adolescents, interventions and, 155–162
    consumption, and, 192–194, 216–220, 236
    dependence, generational, 237–238
    drinking history, college students transitional development and, 190
    genetics, generational, 237–239
    GLBT populations, 289–290, 292, 297–298, 301–302
    older adults, and, 246, 265–266
FAS (Fetal Alcohol Syndrome), 8, 101–134. *see also* Disease
    alcohol consumption, and, 119–123
    ARBD (alcohol-related birth defects), 103–104, 120
    ARNDs (alcohol-related neurodevelopmental defects), 115
    awareness, history of, 103–104
    criteria for, 102
    FAE (fetal alcohol effects), 8, 103–104, 120, 122
    PAE (Prenatal Alcohol Effects), 103–104
    screening for, 109–114
    studies of, 117–118
    susceptibility, and, 123
FDP (Faculty Development Program), 11–18
Framingham Osteoporosis Study (FOS), Hannan Group, 77, 79–81, 259
"French paradox," 70. *see also* Disease; Health promotion
Fund for the Improvement of Postsecondary Education (FIPSE), 185

Gay populations. *see* GLBT populations
Gender differences, 5, 39, 46–54, 69, 73–80, 87, 109–110, 113–114, 136, 184, 187–188, 190–194, 200–201, 216–217, 221, 236–238, 251–253, 256–261, 266, 268, 286, 288–289, 296, 334, 337, 338, 344, 348, 372–373, 376–380
    adulthood, and, 54, 216–217, 221, 236–238
    among heterosexual *vs.* homosexual populations, 288–289
    behaviors, risky, and, 334, 337, 338, 344, 348
    Biological markers, and, 113–114
    Brief Intervention (BI), responses, 372–373, 376–380
    drug use, consequences, and, 200–201
    effects of, drinking, 39, 73–80, 87, 256–260
    GLBT community, and, 286, 288, 296
    laboratory tests, and, 46–54, 109–110
    older adults, 251–253, 256–261, 266, 268
    terminology, 5, 69
Genetics, 20, 189, 190, 237–238, 250–252, 267, 334–335
    5-HTTLPR, drinking behavior differences, and, 189
    college students, and, 190
    dependence, generational patterns of, 237–238
    older adults, 250–252, 267
    Problem behavior model definition, 334–335
    studies, and, 20
GGT (test). *see under* Laboratory tests, consumption
GLBT populations, 190–192, 283–313
    assessment and treatment, 302–308
    college students, identity formation, and, 190–192
    consumption (of alcohol), and, 287–302
        aging, and, 294–295
        drinking expectancies, and, 298–299
        peer contexts and social norms, and, 299–300
        psychological adjustment, and, 292–294, 300–301

relationships, and, 297–298
self-definition, and, 288
social roles, and, 294–296
distinctions, self-definitions, and, 286,
    308
identity (sexual), 286, 288, 292, 295
Global Status Report on Alcohol
    (WHO), 4

Hanes Survey, 248
Hannan Group (Framingham Osteoporo-
    sis Study (FOS)), 77, 79–81,
    259
Hazelden Foundation, 262
Health Care Professionals Follow-up
    Study (HCPFS), 74–78
Health promotion, 65–97, 73, 93. see also
    Disease
Healthy People 2010, 102
Healthy School and Drugs, 144
Heath Resources and Services Administra-
    tion, 16–17
Heavy, episodic drinking. see Drinking,
    heavy and episodic
HHS (U.S. Department of Health and
    Human Services), 11, 68, 102
High unconventionality behavior model.
    see Problem behavior model
Hispanic populations, 52, 83–87, 152–
    155, 190–192
    college students, identity formation,
        and, 190–192
    interventions, school-based, 152–155
    laboratory tests, and, 52
    moderate drinking, effects of, 83–87
Homosexual populations. see GLBT
    populations
Honolulu Heart Study, 82–83
Housing, college, 181–182, 187, 194–196,
    199–202

Imperial Cancer Research Fund's Cancer
    Studies Unit, 71
Institute of Medicine, 104
International Council of Nurses (ICN),
    17–18
International Council on Alcohol and
    Addiction (ICAA), 17–18

International Guide for Monitoring Alco-
    hol Consumption and Rela-
    tional Harm, 169
International Nurses Society on Addic-
    tions, 18
Interventions, 8–9, 114–117, 138–168,
    237–238, 246, 262, 328, 332,
    336, 350–351, 373–374. see
    also Adolescents; Brief Inter-
    vention (BI); Children; Conse-
    quences; Prevention;
    Protective factors
adolescents, and, 155–162, 328
behaviors, risky, 332, 336, 350–351,
    373–374
    drinking, perceived benefits and, 336
    drinking/driving, risky, 350–351
    Emergency Departments, and,
        373–374
    sexual, interventions, and, 351
community-based, 139, 162–168
drug and alcohol mixing, older adults
    and, 262
family-based, 139, 155–162, 246
    effectiveness of, 160–162
    older adults, hindrances to, 246
    publications regarding, 157–160
    and school-based interventions, in-
        corporation into, 160–161
genetic predispositions, counteracting,
    238
injury hospitalization, screening and, 8
older adults, myths and, 246
peers, and, 152–154
pregnancy, and, 114–117
school-based, 138–155, 160–161
    effectiveness of, 152–155
    and family-based interventions, in-
        corporating, 160–161
    publications regarding, 141–151
sobriety, support systems and, 237
Intimate partner violence (IPV), 7–8,
    297–298. see also Sexual abuse/
    assault
Intrauterine growth restriction (IUGR),
    118, 119, 122. see also Disease

Japanese populations, 82–83, 84–87
Joint Commission on Accreditation of Healthcare Organizations (JCAHO), 306

Keep a Clear Mind intervention, 161

Laboratory tests, consumption of alcohol, 45–54, 112–114, 366–367, 380–382. *see also* BACs (Blood Alcohol Concentrations); consumption, of alcohol
analysis, 53
aspects of, 45
biology of, 45–54
Blood, saliva, urine alcohol tests, 48–50
Brief Intervention (BI), and, 380–382
combining, 53
GGT (test), 45, 47, 51–52, 53, 366–367
long-range period, 51–52
MCV (mean corpuscular volume), 45, 47, 51–52
population specificity, and, 53
pregnant women, applicability to, 112–114
short- and medium-range period, 50–51
testing data, 47
WBAA (whole blood associated acetaldehyde), 47
Lahti Project, The (WHO), 370, 372–373, 377
Latino populations. *see* Hispanic populations
Lesbian populations. *see* GLBT populations
Life Skills Training, 141–143, 153
Low-level drinking. *see* Drinking, low-volume

MacAndrew Scale of the Minnesota Multiphasic Personality Inventory (MMPI), 197

MACDP. *see* Metropolitan Atlanta Congenital Defects Program (MACDP)
Malmo Project, 366–367
MAST (Michigan Alcoholism Screening Test), 109–110, 110–112, 120, 197, 226
adults, developmental stage, consumption and, 226
college students, and, 197
FAS (fetal alcohol syndrome), and, 120
pregnancy, risky drinking, and, 110–112
women, and, 109–110
Maternal Health Practices and Child Development Project, 121–122
MCV (mean corpuscular volume). *see under* Laboratory tests, consumption
MDI (Mental Developmental Index). *see* Mental Developmental Index (MDI)
Measurement, alcohol use and, 27–64, 111–112. *see also* Alcohol Use Disorders Identification Test (AUDIT); Quantity/frequency measurements, alcohol use; Self-reported measurements, alcohol use
definitions, 29–33
diary methods, 38
drunkenness, perception of, 40–41
graduated frequency measures, 37, 40
laboratory tests, 45–54
short-term recall methods, 37–38
Timeline Followback (TLFB) method, 38, 42, 111–112
variability measures, and, 40–42
Medical Research Council (MRC), 367, 370, 377
"Medicinal purposes," 66. *see also* Cardiovascular disease; Disease
Mental Developmental Index (MDI), 115–116
Metropolitan Area Child Study, 161

Metropolitan Atlanta Congenital Defects Program (MACDP), 108
Michigan Alcoholism Screening Test. *see* MAST (Michigan Alcoholism Screening Test); SMAST (Shortened Michigan Alcoholism Screening Test)
Midwest Nursing Research Society (MNRS), 18
Midwestern Prevention Project, 159, 160–161
Million Dollar Machine (MDM), 147
Minnesota Heart Health program, 163
Minnesota model, 365
Minnesota Multiphasic Personality Inventory (MMPI), 197
Minorities. *see* racial differences
MMPI (MacAndrew Scale of the Minnesota Multiphasic Personality Inventory), 197
Moderate drinking. *see* Drinking, moderate
Monitoring the Future (MTF) study, 135–136, 184–203, 228, 335
Motivational Interviewing (MI), 115–116, 369. *see also* Brief Intervention (BI)
Motivations, 192–194, 236. *see also* Cognition
MRC (Medical Research Council), 367, 370, 377
MTF. *see* Monitoring the Future (MTF) study
Multi-site Women's Health Study (MWHC), 300

N. Hanes Survey, 248
National Advisory Council on Alcohol Abuse and Alcoholism, 203
National Center for Injury Prevention and Control (NCIPC), 328–329
National Center on Addiction and Substance Abuse (NCASA), 248, 261

National Center on Birth Defects and Developmental Disabilities (NCBDDD), and, 104
National Committee on Quality Assurance (NCQA), 306
National Comorbidity Study, 307
National Health and Nutrition Examination Survey, 307
National Health and Retirement Survey, 216
National Health and Social Life Survey (NHSLS), 286–287
National Health Interview Follow-up Study, 83
National Health Interview Survey, 231, 232
National Highway Traffic Safety Administration (NHTSA), 337
National Household Survey on Drug Abuse (NHSDA), 105–109, 307
National Injury Center (CDC), 12–16
National Institute
  Brief Intervention (BI), population target
  study analysis, 372
National Institute of Nursing Research, 5
National Institute on Alcohol Abuse and Alcoholism (NIAAA), 4, 5, 11–16, 29–33, 35, 107, 155–156, 180, 199, 214, 246, 253, 264, 267, 328–329, 338, 364, 368–369, 380
  adolescents, 107, 328–329
  adulthood, consumption and, 214
  alcohol, abuse/dependence, and, 4, 364
  alcohol-related studies, funding of, 5
  behaviors, risky, and, 338
  Brief Intervention (BI), 368–369, 380
  college students, and, 180, 199
  drinking limits, recommended, 35
  interventions, family-based, 155–156
  nursing curricula, and, 11, 15–16
  nursing research, and, 11–15
  older adults, and, 246, 253, 264
  terminology, and, 29–33, 35, 267

National Institute on Drug Abuse (NIDA), 11–16, 107
National Institutes of Health (NIH), 11, 44, 104, 269
National Lesbian Health Care Survey (NLHCS), 295, 300
National Longitudinal Alcohol Epidemiologic Survey, 260, 294
National Longitudinal Survey of Youth, 233, 343
National Nurses Society on Addictions, 18
National Organization on Fetal Alcohol Syndrome (NOFAS), 104
National Pregnancy and Health Survey (NPHS), 107
National Safety Council (NSC), 337
National Study of Health and Life Experiences of Women (NSHLEW), 294
National Survey on Drug Use and Health (NSDUH), 105–109, 307
National Task Force on Fetal Alcohol Syndrome and Fetal Alcohol Effects (FAS), 104
National Violence Against Women (NVAW), 343
Native American populations, 119–120, 120, 153, 154, 162, 190–192, 216–217, 221
  adulthood, alcohol consumption and, 216–217, 221
  children and adolescents, interventions and, 153, 154, 162
  college students, identity formation, and, 190–192
  FAS (Fetal alcohol syndrome), and, 119–120
  FAS (fetal alcohol syndrome), and, 120
NCASA (National Center on Addiction and Substance Abuse), 248, 261
NCBDDD (National Center on Birth Defects and Developmental Disabilities), 104

NCIPC (National Center for Injury Prevention and Control), 328–329
NCQA (National Committee on Quality Assurance), 306
New Mexico Elder Health Survey, 83–84
NHS (Nurses Health Study), 74–78
NHSDA (National Household Survey on Drug Abuse), 105–109
NHSLS (National Health and Social Life Survey), 286–287
NIAAA. see National Institute on Alcohol Abuse and Alcoholism (NIAAA)
NIDA (National Institute on Drug Abuse), 11–16, 107
NIH (National Institutes of Health), 11, 44, 104, 269
NLHCS (National Lesbian Health Care Survey), 295, 300
NOFAS (National Organization on Fetal Alcohol Syndrome), 104
NPHS (National Pregnancy and Health Survey), 107
NSC (National Safety Council), 337
NSDUH (National Survey on Drug Use and Health), 105–109, 307
NSHLEW (National Study of Health and Life Experiences of Women), 294
Nurses Health Study (NHS), 74–78
Nurses in Substance Abuse, 18
Nursing Interest Group (ICAA), 17–18

Office of Substance Abuse Prevention (OSAP), 11–12
Older populations. see under Adulthood
"One-stop shop" of services, 116. see also Interventions
Orientation, sexual. see GLBT populations
OTC drugs. see drugs

PDI (Psychomotor Developmental Index), 115
Physicians' Health Study (PHS), 74–77, 84, 88–89

Positive Youth Development Program, 143

PRAMS (Pregnancy Risk Assessment Monitoring), 105–109

Pregnancy, alcohol consumption during, 101–134. *see also* women
  Brief Intervention (BI), 114–115, 377
  effects of, during stages of, 122
  epidemiology, 105–109
  FAE (Fetal Alcohol Effects)
    moderate use, and, 122
    nursing, and, 8
    relationship between, 8
  FAS (Fetal Alcohol Syndrome)
    alcohol consumption, and, 119–123
    criteria for, 102
    nursing, and, 8
    studies of, 117–118
    susceptibility to, 123
  moderation of, and effects, 122–123
  Motivational Intervention (MI), 115–116
  nursing, and, 8
  "one-stop shop" of services, 116
  studies, history of, 9–

Pregnancy Risk Assessment Monitoring (PRAMS), 105–109

Prevention. *see also* Brief Intervention (BI); interventions; Protective factors
  drug and alcohol mixing, older adults and, 262
  harm reduction philosophy, and, 365
  National Advisory Council on Alcohol Abuse and Alcoholism college students, and, 203
  older adults, alcohol abuse and dependence, and, 251
  programs, effectiveness of, 203–204
  programs, ideas for
    anxiety sensitivity, and, 190
    cognitive expectancies, and, 193–194
    More!!
  secondary, defined, 365

www.collegedrinkingprevention.com, 203

Pride Institute, 303, 306

Problem behavior model, 334–335, 340–341, 346. *see also* Alcohol myopia behavior model; Behaviors, risky; Expectancy behavior model; Risk perception behavior model

Problem drinking. *see* Drinking, problem

Project ALERT, 145, 153

Project GOAL, 264

Project Health, 370–371

Project MAINSTREAM (**M**ulti-**A**gency **IN**itiative on Substance Abuse **TR**aining and **E**ducation for **Am**erica), 16–17

Project Naja, 162

Project Northlands
  conceptual framework of, 162
  effectiveness of, 167–168
  publications regarding, 146, 158, 166–167

Project PALS, 162

Project TrEAT (Trial for Early Alcohol Treatment), 370, 377, 381–382

Protective factors. *see also* Behaviors, risky; Interventions; Prevention; Risk factors
  ALDH (aldehyde dehydrogenase), 189
  children, school-based interventions, and, 152
  college students, negative consequences and, 194
  GLBT community, and, 289–302, 301, 310–311
  pregnancy, FAS and, 123

Psychomotor Developmental Index (PDI), 115

Public Affairs Committee of the Teratology Society on Fetal Alcohol Syndrome (FAS), 117

Quantity/frequency measurements, alcohol consumption, 28, 36–38, 41–42

Quantity/frequency measurements, alcohol consumption (continued)
adulthood, work settings, and, 233
Alcohol Use Disorders Identification Test (AUDIT), and, 55, LFM!
Brief Intervention (BI), outcomes, 381
CAGE (screening test), use with college students, and, 198
consumption, determination of, 36–40
GLBT populations, and, 302
interventions, school-based effectiveness of, 152–155
moderate drinking, heart disease and, 71, 73, 76, 83
older adults, alcohol use and, 248, 268
pregnancy, alcohol use during, 108, 110–111
and routine screening, absence of, 7
utility of, older adults and, 268
variability measures, and, 40–42
variations in definitions of, and research problems, 118–119

Racial differences. see also African American populations; Hispanic populations; Japanese populations; Native American populations
5-HTTLPR
drinking behavior differences, and, 189
adulthood, consumption and, 216–217, 238
college students, consumption and, 187, 190–192
drug use
consequences, of alcohol consumption, and, 200–201
FAS (Fetal alcohol syndrome), and, 119–120
GLBT populations
identity (sexual)
development of, 292
psychological distress, and, 292–294, 310
therapy, consumption patterns, and, 301

moderate drinking
definition of, 69
effects of, 81–82
older adults, 266, 268
pregnancy, alcohol consumption during, 108, 109, 119–120
representation, consumption studies, 54
Recommended drinking limits
defined, 33
Residence halls. see housing
Residential Student Assistance Program (RSAP), 165, 167–168
Resisting Pressure to Drink and Drive, 147
Risk factors, for alcohol abuse/dependence. see also Protective factors
adolescents, and, 152–169
college students, and, 194–195
GLBT community, and, 289–302, 309–311
Risk perception behavior model. see also Alcohol myopia behavior model; Behaviors, risky; Expectancy behavior model; Problem behavior model
definition, 334
drinking/driving, risky and, 340–341
model diagram, 333
Risky behaviors. see Behaviors, risky
Risky single-occasion drinking. see Drinking, heavy and episodic
Robert Wood Johnson Foundation, 185
RSAP (Residential Student Assistance Program), 165, 167–168

SAMHSA. see Substance Abuse and Mental Health Services Administration (SAMHSA)
SBI. see under Brief Intervention (BI)
School interventions, 139–155, 160–161. see also Adolescents; Children
Self-reported measurements, alcohol use
adults, developmental stage, consumption and, 226
blood alcohol concentrations (BAC) correlations, and, 44

Brief Intervention (BI), outcome of, 381–382
consumption measurement, 42–45
effectiveness, elements of, 42–43
moderate drinking and disease, 74, 76, 89–90
older adults and, 247–248
pregnancy, alcohol consumption during, 105–109, 119
research, opportunities for, 44–45, 381–382
seasonal variation in, 44
sexual behavior, risky and, 344
standard variables, lack of, 44
untruthful, causes of, 43
validity of, 42–45
variations in definitions of, and research problems, 118–119, 381–382
Sensation-seeking model, 332–341. *see also* Behaviors, risky
Sexual abuse/assault. *see also* consequences, of alcohol consumption; interventions; intimate partner violence (IPV); prevention
child sexual abuse (csa), consumption and, 290–292
college students, consequences and, 200
consumption, effects on, 236
intimacy, consumption and, 237, 238
Sexual orientation. *see* GLBT populations
SFP (Strengthening Families Program), 159, 162
Shifting Gears, 162–163
Shortened Michigan Alcoholism Screening Test (SMAST), 224
"Sick quitters," 73, 91. *see also* abstaining populations
within abstaining population, 73, 79–80, 91
data integrity, and -probably in above entry?!!-, 255
definition of, 6, 91, 267

SMAST (Shortened Michigan Alcoholism Screening Test), 224
Social factors
adolescents and children, consumption and, GET!!!
college students, consumption and, GET!!!
GLBT populations
GLB populations within college students, studies and, 187
homosexuality, removal from DSM, 284
identity (sexual)
definition, 285–286
intimate partner violence (IPV), and, 297–298
orientation (sexual)
definition, 285–286
and gender identity, distinctions between, 286
prevalence of, in U.S., 286–287
research analysis, college students, and, 202
societal stigma (model) and, 289–302
older adults, consumption and, 249–250
problem behavior model definition, 334–5
Social Support Network Inventory (SSNI), 236
Speas Memorial Trust, 15–16
Standard drink. *see* drink, standard
STARS (Start Taking Alcohol Risks Seriously), 150–151, 160, 161
Strengthening Families Program (SFP), 159, 162
Student Assistance Service Corp, 165
Substance Abuse and Mental Health Services Administration (SAMHSA), 106, 329
adolescents, and, 136
GLBT population, and, 304, 306
prevalence, alcohol abuse and dependence, 363–364

Substance Abuse and Mental Health Services Administration (SAMHSA) *(continued)*
 Project MAINSTREAM (Multi-Agency INitiative on Substance Abuse TRaining and Education for America)
 substance abuse, health professional education and, 16–17
 terminology, defining, 31–33
Substance Abuse Subtle Screening Inventory 2, 197
Substance use. *see* drugs
Syndrome, alcohol dependence. *see* Alcoholism

T-ACE (screening test), 110–112, 114–115, 117
"Teachable moment," 369, 375, 383. *see also* Brief Intervention (BI); Interventions
Teenagers. *see* Adolescents
The Exciting and Entertaining Northland Students (TEENS), 158
Timeline Followback (TLFB) method, 38, 42, 111–112
Toward No Drug Abuse (TND), 149
Transgender populations. *see* GLBT populations
TrEAT. *see* Project TrEAT (Trial for Early Alcohol Treatment)
Treatment, alcohol, 43, 250–251, 263–267, 303–305
TWEAK (screening test), 110–111, 197–199

University Life Transitions Project Telephone Diary Study, 188

U.S. Department of Health and Human Services (HHS), 11, 68, 102
U.S. Preventive Services Task Force, 262–264

Veterans Administration, 230, 268
Violence, 4. *see also* Intimate Partner Violence (IPV); Sexual abuse/assault

WHO. *see* World Health Organization (WHO)
WHO Collaborative Project on Identification and Treatment of Person with Harmful Alcohol Consumption, 366, 375
Women, 43, 54, 101–134, 236–239, 258–259, 343, 347. *see also* GLBT populations; pregnancy, alcohol consumption during
 estrogen replacement therapy (ERT), 258–259
 families, and, 236–239
 pregnant women, 43, 101–134
 sexual behavior, risky, 347
 sexual violence, prevalence of, 343
 studies, and, 54
Women's Health Initiative, 307
Women's Health Study, 77
World Health Organization (WHO), 4, 54, 370. *see also* Brief Intervention (BI)

Youth Risk Behavior Surveillance System, 307, 329–330
Youth Risk Behavior Survey (YRBS), 343–344

Contents of Previous 10 Volumes

VOLUME XXII: Eliminating Health Disparities Among Racial and Ethnic Minorities in the United States

Joyce Fitzpatrick, Series Editor; Antonio M. Villarruel and Cornelia P. Porter, Volume Editors

1. Introduction: Eliminating Health Disparities Among Racial and Ethnic Minorities in the United States   ANTONIA M. VILLARRUEL
2. Race and Racism in Nursing Research: Past, Present, and Future   CORNELIA P. PORTER AND EVELYN BARBEE
3. Structural and Racial Barriers to Health Care   LINDA BURNES BOLTON, JOYCE NEWMAN GIGER, AND C. ALICIA GEORGES
4. Language Barriers and Access to Care   SEONAE YEO
5. Health Disparities Among Men from Racial and Ethnic Minority Populations   CONSTANCE DALLAS AND LINDA BURTON
6. Immigration and Health   DEANNE K. HILFINGER MESSIAS AND MERCEDES RUBIO
7. Health Disparities Among Asian Americans and Pacific Islanders   M. CHRISTINA ESPERAT, JILLIAN INOUYE, ELIZABETH W. GONZALEZ, DONNA C. OWEN, AND DU FENG
8. African American and Asian American Elders: An Ethnogeriatric Perspective   MELEN R. MCBRIDE AND IRENE D. LEWIS
9. Cancer in U.S. Ethnic and Racial Minority Populations   SANDRA MILLON UNDERWOOD, BARBARA POWE, MARY CANALES, CATHY D. MEADE, AND EUN-OK IM
10. Mental Health and Disabilities: What We Know About Racial and Ethnic Minority Children   MARY LOU DE LEON SIANTZ AND BETTE RUSK KELTNER
11. Utilization of Complementary and Alternative Medicine Among Racial and Ethnic Minority Populations: Implications for Reducing Health Disparities   ROXANNE STRUTHERS AND LEE ANNE NICHOLS

12.   Community Partnerships: The Cornerstone of Community Health Research   CARMEN J. PORTILLO AND CATHERINE WATERS

VOLUME XXI: Research on Child Health and Pediatric Issues

Joyce Fitzpatrick, Series Editor; Margaret Shandor Miles and Diane Holditch-Davis, Volume Editors

1.   Enhancing Nursing Research With Children and Families Using a Developmental Science Perspective   MARGARET SHANDOR MILES AND DIANE HOLDITCH-DAVIS
2.   Care of Preterm Infants: Programs of Research and Their Relationship to Developmental Science   DIANE HOLDITCH-DAVIS AND BETH PERRY BLACK
3.   Developmental Transition From Gavage to Oral Feeding in the Preterm Infant   SUZANNE M. THOYRE
4.   Physical Symptoms in Children and Adolescents   HYEKYUN RHEE
5.   Symptom Experiences of Children and Adolescents With Cancer   SHARRON L. DOCHERTY
6.   Growing Up With Chronic Illness: Psychosocial Adjustment of Children and Adolescents With Cystic Fibrosis   BECKY CHRISTIAN
7.   Children's Psychological Responses to Hospitalization   JUDITH A. VESSEY
8.   Children Living With Chronic Illness: An Examination of Their Stressors, Coping Responses, and Health Outcomes   JANET L. STEWART
9.   Parents of Children With Chronic Health Problems: Programs of Nursing Research and Their Relationship to Developmental Science   MARGARET SHANDOR MILES
10.   The Sibling Experience of Living With Childhood Chronic Illness and Disability   MARCIA VAN RIPER
11.   Maternal Mental Health and Parenting in Poverty   LINDA S. BEEBER AND MARGARET SHANDOR MILES
12.   A Review of the Second Decade of the *Annual Review of Nursing Research* Series   JOYCE J. FITZPATRICK AND JOANNE S. STEVENSON

VOLUME XX: Research on Geriatrics

Joyce Fitzpatrick, Series Editor; Patricia Archbold and Barbara Stewart, Volume Editors

1.   Maintaining and Improving Physical Function in Elders   JILL A. BENNETT
2.   Pressure Ulcer Prevention and Management   COURTNEY H. LYDER

3. Pain in Older Adults   LOIS L. MILLER AND KAREN AMANN TALERICO
4. Interventions for Persons with Irreversible Dementia   SANDY C.
       BURGENER AND PRUDENCE TWIGG
5. Transitional Care of Older Adults   MARY D. NAYLOR
6. Interventions for Family Members Caring for an Elder with
       Dementia   GAYLE J. ACTON AND MARY A. WINTER
7. End of Life Care for Older Adults in ICU's   JUDITH GEDNEY BAGGS
8. Nursing Homes and Assisted Living Facilities as Places for
       Dying   JULIANNA C. CARTWRIGHT
9. Home Health Services Research   ELIZABETH A. MADIGAN, SUSAN
       TULLAI-MCGUINNESS, AND DONNA FELBER NEFF
10. Telehealth Interventions to Improve Clinical Nursing of
       Elders   JOSETTE F. JONES AND PATRICIA FLATLEY BRENNAN
11. Genetics and Gerontological Nursing: A Need to Stimulate
       Research   LORRAINE FRAZIER AND SHARON K. OSTWALD
12. Hearing Impairment   MARGARET I. WALLHAGEN
13. Elder Mistreatment   TERRY FULMER

VOLUME XIX: Research on Women's Health

   **Joyce Fitzpatrick, Series Editor; Diana Taylor and Nancy Fugate-
   Woods, Volume Editors**
1. What We Know and How We Know It: Contributions from Nursing to
       Women's Health Research and Scholarship   DIANA TAYLOR AND
       NANCY WOODS
2. Conceptual Models for Women's Health Research: Reclaiming
       Menopause As an Exemplar of Nursing's Contributions to Feminist
       Scholarship   LINDA C. ANDRIST AND KATHLEEN I. MACPHERSON
3. Women As Mothers and Grandmothers   ANGELA BARRON MCBRIDE
       AND CHERYL PROHASKA SHORE
4. Women and Employment: A Decade Review   MARCIA GRUIS KILLIEN
5. Interventions for Women As Family Caregivers   MARGARET J. BULL
6. Lesbian Health and Health Care   LINDA A. BERNHARD
7. Immigrant Women and Their Health   KAREN J. AROIAN
8. Women and Stress   CHERYL A. CAHILL
9. Sleep and Fatigue   KATHRYN A. LEE
10. Intimate Partner Violence Against Women   JANICE HUMPHREYS,
       BARBARA PARKER, AND JACQUELYN C. CAMPBELL
11. Health Decisions and Decision Support for Women   MARILYN L.
       ROTHERT AND ANNETTE M. O'CONNOR
12. Female Troubles: An Analysis of Menstrual Cycle Research in the
       NINR Portfolio As a Model for Science Development in Women's
       Health   NANCY KING REAME

VOLUME XVIII: Research on Chronic Illness

Joyce Fitzpatrick, Series Editor; Jean Goeppinger, Volume Editor
1. Two Decades of Insider Research: What We Know and Don't Know About Chronic Illness Experience   SALLY E. THORNE AND BARBARA L. PATERSON
2. Children with Epilepsy: Quality of Life and Psychosocial Needs   JOAN K. AUSTIN AND DAVID W. DUNN
3. Adherence in Chronic Disease   JACQUELINE DUNBAR-JACOBS, JUDITH A. ERLEN, ELIZABETH A. SCHLENK, CHRISTOPHER M. RYAN, SUSAN M. SEREIKA, AND WILLA M. DOSWELL
4. Heart Failure Management: Optimal Health Care Delivery Programs   DEBRA K. MOSER
5. Cancer Care: Impact of Interventions on Caregiver Outcomes   JEANNIE V. PASACRETA AND RUTH McCORKLE
6. Interventions for Children with Diabetes and Their Families   MARGARET GREY
7. Management of Urinary Incontinence in Adult Ambulatory Care Populations   JEAN F. WYMAN
8. Family Interventions to Prevent Substance Abuse: Children and Adolescents   CAROL J. LOVELAND-CHERRY
9. School-Based Interventions for Primary Prevention of Cardiovascular Disease: Evidence of Effects for Minority Populations   JANET C. MEININGER
10. Breakthroughs in Scientific Research: The Discipline of Nursing, 1960–1999   SUE K. DONALDSON

VOLUME XVII

Joyce Fitzpatrick, Editor
1. Music Therapy   MARIAH SNYDER AND LINDA CHLAN
2. Sleep Promotion in Adults   JUDITH A. FLOYD
3. Guided Imagery Interventions for Symptom Management   LUCILLE SANZERO ELLER
4. Patient-Centered Communication   SARAH JO BROWN
5. Acute Pain   MARION GOOD
6. The Chronobiology, Chronopharmacology, and Chronotherapeutics of Pain   SUSAN E. AUVIL-NOVAK
7. Chronic Low Back Pain: Early Interventions   JULIA FAUCETT
8. Wandering in Dementia   DONNA L. ALGASE
9. Cognitive Interventions Among Older Adults   GRAHAM J. McDOUGALL, JR.

10. Primary Health Care   BEVERLY J. MCELMURRY AND GWEN BRUMBAUGH
       KEENEY
11. Uncertainty in Chronic Illness   MERLE H. MISHEL
12. Nursing Research in Italy   RENZO ZANOTTI

VOLUME XVI

Joyce Fitzpatrick, Editor
1. Childhood Nutrition   CHRISTINE M. KENNEDY
2. Health Care for the School-Age Child   KATHLEEN ANN LONG AND
       DAVID WILLIAMS
3. Childhood Diabetes: Behavioral Research   PATRICIA BRANDT
4. Prevention of Mental Health Problems in Adolescence   SUSAN KOOLS
5. The Development of Sexual Risk Taking in Adolescence   ROSEMARY
       A. JADACK AND MARY L. KELLER
6. Motivation for Physical Activity Among Children and
       Adolescents   NOLA J. PENDER
7. Health Promotion in Old Age   SUSAN M. HEIDRICH
8. Health Promotion for Family Caregivers of Chronically Ill
       Elders   BARBARA A. GIVEN AND CHARLES W. GIVEN
9. Prenatal and Parenting Programs for Adolescent Mothers   PAULETTE J.
       PERRONE HOYER
10. Chronic Obstructive Pulmonary Disease: Strategies to Improve
       Functional Status   JANET L. LARSON AND NANCY KLINE LEIDY
11. Schizophrenia   JEANNE C. FOX AND CATHERINE F. KANE

VOLUME XV

Joyce Fitzpatrick and Jane Norbeck, Editors
1. Parenting the Prematurely Born Child   DIANE HOLDITCH-DAVIS AND
       MARGARET SHANDOR MILES
2. Interventions for Cognitive Impairment and Neurobehavioral
       Disturbances of Older Adults   DIANE CRONIN-STUBBS
3. Uncertainty in Acute Illness   MERLE H. MISHEL
4. Violence in the Workplace   JEANNE BEAUCHAMP HEWITT AND PAMELA
       F. LEVIN
5. Interventions to Reduce the Impact of Chronic Disease: Community-
       Based Arthritis Patient Education   JEAN GOEPPINGER AND KATE
       LORIG
6. Parent–Adolescent Communication in Nondistressed Families   SUSAN
       K. RIESCH

7. Adherence to Therapy in Tuberculosis   FELISSA L. COHEN
8. Health Promotion and Disease Prevention in the Worksite   SALLY LECHLITNER LUSK
9. Nursing at War: Catalyst for Change   QUINCEALEA BRUNK
10. Long-Term Vascular Access Devices   JANET S. FULTON
11. Nursing Research in Taiwan   SHYANG-YUN PAMELA KOONG SHIAO AND YU-MEI YU CHAO

VOLUME XIV

Joyce Fitzpatrick and Jane Norbeck, Editors
1. Blood Pressure   SUE A. THOMAS AND FREDA DEKEYSER
2. Psychoneuroimmunological Studies in HIV Disease   NANCY L. MCCAIN AND JANICE M. ZELLER
3. Delirium Intervention Research in Acute Care Settings   DIANE CRONIN-STUBBS
4. Smoking Cessation Interventions in Chronic Illness   MARY ELLEN WEWERS AND KAREN L. AHIJEVYCH
5. Quality of Life and Caregiving in Technological Home Care   CAROL E. SMITH
6. Organizational Redesign: Effect on Institutional and Consumer Outcomes   GAIL L. INGERSOLL
7. Organizational Culture   BARBARA A. MARK
8. Oncology Nursing Education   M. LINDA WORKMAN
9. Moral Competency   VIRGINIA R. CASSIDY
10. Nursing Research in Israel   HAVA GOLANDER AND TAMAR KRULIK
11. The Evolution of Nursing Research in Brazil   ISABEL AMÉLIA COSTA MENDES AND MARIA AUXILIADORA TREVIZAN

VOLUME XIII

Joyce Fitzpatrick and Joanne Stevenson, Editors
1. Quality of Life and the Spectrum of HIV Infection   WILLIAM L. HOLZEMER AND HOLLY SKODOL WILSON
2. Physical Health of Homeless Adults   ADA M. LINDSEY
3. Child Sexual Abuse: Initial Effects   SUSAN J. KELLEY
4. The Neurobehavioral Effects of Childhood Lead Exposure   HEIDI VONKOSS KROWCHUK
5. Case Management   GERRI S. LAMB
6. Technology and Home Care   CAROL E. SMITH

7. Nursing Minimum Data Set   POLLY RYAN AND CONNIE DELANEY
8. Pediatric Hospice Nursing   IDA M. MARTINSON
9. Faculty Practice: Interest, Issues, and Impact   PATRICIA HINTON WALKER
10. The Professionalization of Nurse Practitioners   BONNIE BULLOUGH
11. Feminism and Nursing   PEGGY L. CHINN
12. Health Risk Behaviors for Hispanic Women   SARA TORRES AND ANTONIA M. VILLARRUEL

Dictionary of Nursing Theory and Research, *3rd Edition*

Bethel Ann Powers, PhD, RN
Thomas R. Knapp, EdD

"The exceptional readability and convenient size of this dictionary make it a wonderful companion for any nurse seeking to demystify the phenomena of nursing theory and research."

—**Nursing Research,** praise for previous edition

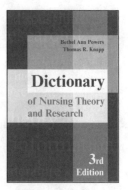

"An excellent collection of information essential to all nurses, not only those involved in research but also practicing nurses interested in innovation and change. Students at all academic levels will find it particularly useful. The definitions of terms are clear and accurate and the range of topics is comprehensive, with frequent cross-referencing and citations given from relevant literature..."

—**Nursing Times,** praise for previous edition

The new edition of this concise reference includes updated terminology and the addition of many new terms with examples and references that reflect current nursing practice. With the inclusion of research, theory, statistical, and epidemiological definitions and cross-reference notes at the end of each entry, this compilation is a handy and up-to-date dictionary for students, clinicians, and researchers.

Partial Contents:

- Preface to the Third Edition
- Explanatory Notes
- Alphabetical Listing of Research and Theory Terms
- References
- About the Authors

August 2005   224pp   0-8261-1774-0   softcover

11 West 42nd Street, New York, NY 10036-8002 • Fax: 212-941-7842
Order Toll-Free: 877-687-7476 • Order On-line: www.springerpub.com

Subscribe to the Annual Review of Nursing Research Series and save 10%

When you become a subscriber to the Annual Review of Nursing Research Series, you will automatically receive new books in the series upon publication at 10% off the list price. If you do not choose to keep the book, simply return it for a full refund.

Why not start your subscription and receive these new titles—

Annual Review of Nursing Research, Volume 24
Focus on Patient Safety
0-8261-4136-6 Publishing in 2006

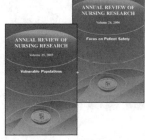

Annual Review of Nursing Research, Volume 25
Vulnerable Populations
0-8261-4137-4 Publishing in 2007

In addidtion, when you subscribe, keep the new book in the series and receive a 10% discount on any other Springer title purchased that year.

Please sign up below

✂

❑ *YES, I would like to subscribe to* the Annual Review of Nursing Research Series

Charge to: ❑ VISA ❑ MasterCard ❑ American Express

Card # _____ Expires _____

Signature _____

Ship to:

Name _____

Title _____

Institution _____

Address _____

City/State/Zip _____

Telephone _____

E-mail _____

Springer Publishing Company
11 West 42nd Street
New York, NY 10036
www.SpringerPub.com

Four Easy Ways to Order

☎ **Toll free phone: 1-877-687-7476**

📠 **Fax: 212-941-7842**

✉ **Mail: Detach order form and mail**

🖱 **E-mail: www.springerpub.com**